# Liver Transplantation and Hepatobiliary Surgery

*500 Practice Questions*

# Liver Transplantation and Hepatobiliary Surgery

*500 Practice Questions*

Valeria Ripa, MD

Fady M. Kaldas, MD

Copyright © 2025 Valeria Ripa, MD and Fady M. Kaldas, MD
All rights reserved.

No part of this publication may be reproduced, stored in a retrieval system, or transmitted in any form or by any means - electronic, mechanical, photocopying, recording, or otherwise - without prior written permission from the authors, except for brief quotations used in reviews, articles, or scholarly works.
This publication is intended for educational and informational purposes only. It is designed as a study and review guide for medical professionals and trainees. While every effort has been made to ensure the accuracy of content, the authors and publisher make no guarantees and disclaim liability for any outcomes resulting from the use of this material. Any resemblance to actual individuals, cases, or institutions is purely coincidental unless otherwise stated.

Authors:

**Valeria Ripa, MD,**
Abdominal Transplant and Hepatobiliary Surgery Fellow,
Division of Liver and Pancreas Transplantation,
David Geffen School of Medicine at UCLA

**Fady M. Kaldas, MD, FACS,**
Professor of Surgery,
Kelly Lee Tarantello Chair in Liver Transplantation,
Director, Transplant and Hepatobiliary Surgery Fellowship,
Co-Director, Heart-Liver Disease Program,
Division of Liver and Pancreas Transplantation,
David Geffen School of Medicine at UCLA

ISBN: 979-8-9987815-2-0
e-ISBN: 979-8-9987815-1-3
First Edition
Published independently by Valeria Ripa, MD and Fady M. Kaldas, MD

# Table of Contents

*Introduction* ............................................................................................ 1
*Abbreviations* ......................................................................................... 2
1. Basic Concepts of Surgical Anatomy and Pathophysiology ............ 4
2. Organ Donation and Allocation ...................................................... 13
3. Indications for Liver Transplantation ............................................. 23
4. Indications for Liver Transplantation in the Pediatric Population ... 61
5. Special Consideration in Patient Evaluation ................................. 89
6. Organ Donation and Technical Aspects of Liver Transplantation 121
7. Split and Living Donor Transplantation ........................................ 139
8. Complex Operative Scenarios ....................................................... 157
9. Medical Care of Transplant Recipents .......................................... 171
10. Transplant Pathology and Immunology ..................................... 201
11. Immunosuppression ................................................................... 215
12. Machine Perfusion ...................................................................... 235
13. Liver Transplant Survival and Results ........................................ 249
*References* ........................................................................................ 253

Liver Transplantation and Hepatobiliary Surgery: 500 Practice Questions

# Introduction

This book is designed to serve as a comprehensive resource for medical professionals seeking to deepen their understanding of clinical questions related to liver transplantation and hepatobiliary surgery. It is meticulously designed to facilitate both knowledge assessment and the acquisition of new information in this specialized field. Each clinical question is accompanied by a concise explanation that elucidates the underlying concepts and rationale, supported by references from reputable sources. The structured format of this book aims to enhance the learning experience, providing clinicians, surgeons, and students with a valuable tool for self-assessment and review.

Valeria Ripa, MD and Fady M. Kaldas, MD

# Abbreviations

AFP - alpha-fetoprotein
ALP - alkaline phosphatase
ALT - alanine aminotransferase
APC – antigen presenting cell
ARDS - acute respiratory distress syndrome
AST - aspartate aminotransferase
ATP - adenosine triphosphate
BID- "bis in die", twice a day
BMI - body mass index
BUN - blood urea nitrogen
CMV - cytomegalovirus
CNS - central nervous system
CRRT - continuous renal replacement therapy
CSF - cerebrospinal fluid
CT - computed tomography
CUSA - cavitron ultrasonic surgical aspirator
DBD - donation after brain death
DCD - donation after circulatory death
EBV - Epstein-Barr virus
ERCP - endoscopic retrograde cholangiopancreatography
ESRD - end-stage renal disease
FFP - fresh frozen plasma
GABA - gamma-aminobutyric acid
GFR - glomerular filtration rate
GGT - gamma-glutamyl transferase
GSC - Glasgow coma scale
HCC - hepatocellular carcinoma
HIDA - hepatobiliary iminodiacetic acid
HLA - human leukocyte antigen
ICU - intensive care unit
Ig - immunoglobulin
INR - international normalized ratio
IV - intravenous
IVC - inferior vena cava
LDH - lactate dehydrogenase
LDL - low-density lipoprotein

LFT - liver function tests
MAP - mean arterial pressure
MASH - metabolic dysfunction-associated steatohepatitis
MELD - model for end-stage liver disease
MHC - major histocompatibility complex
MRCP - magnetic resonance cholangiopancreatography
MRI - magnetic resonance imaging
NADH - nicotinamide adenine dinucleotide (reduced form)
OCS - organ care system
OPO - organ procurement organization
OPTN - Organ Procurement and Transplantation Network
PCR - polymerase chain reaction
PEEP - positive end-expiratory pressure
PELD - Pediatric end-stage liver disease
PET - positron emission tomography
PRBC - packed red blood cells
SCS – standard cold storage
TGF-β - transforming growth factor-beta
TIPS - transjugular intrahepatic portosystemic shunt
TPN - total parenteral nutrition
UNOS - United Network for Organ Sharing
γ-GTP - gamma-glutamyl transpeptidase

Valeria Ripa, MD and Fady M. Kaldas, MD

# 1. Basic Concepts of Surgical Anatomy and Pathophysiology

1. Which statement is false?
a) Thomas Starzl performed the first human liver transplant in 1963
b) The introduction of cyclosporine for liver transplantation occurred in 1979
c) Development of the University of Wisconsin (UW) solution occurred in 1987
d) The Food and Drug Administration approved tacrolimus for use in liver transplantation in 1993
e) The development of the MELD score in the United States for organ allocation took place in 1990
**Answer: e**
MELD score was introduced in 2002.[1–5]

2. In 1897, James Cantlie proposed a functional rather than surface division of the liver into two lobes ("Cantlie's line"), which correlates with:
a) The plane from the gallbladder fossa to the middle hepatic vein
b) The falciform ligament
c) The plane from the gallbladder fossa to the right hepatic vein
d) The plane from the portal vein bifurcation to the middle hepatic vein
e) The plane from the portal vein bifurcation to the right hepatic vein
**Answer: a**
Cantlie's line is a virtual plane that divides the gallbladder fossa and the suprahepatic vena cava; its path overlaps with the course of the middle hepatic vein.[6]

3. Considering the anatomy and function of Glisson's capsule, which of the following statements best describes the structural characteristics and its roles?
a) It is a thick layer of submucosal tissue that provides a rigid barrier around the liver
b) It is a thin, elastic layer of visceral fascia that encases the liver, playing a critical role in fluid exchange and accommodating daily size fluctuations in response to metabolic activities
c) It is a thick elastic layer of connective tissue primarily serving protective and nutritional functions for the liver
d) It is a fibrous layer that predominantly contains macrophages, inhibiting cell migration within the hepatobiliary system
e) It is a membranous elastic tissue enriched with abundant elastic fibers, essentially constituting the parietal peritoneum covering the liver

**Answer: b**
Glisson's capsule is a thin layer of interstitial tissue and visceral fascia that surrounds the liver, plays a crucial role in fluid exchange and cell migration, and serves to protect and enclose the liver parenchyma.[7]

4. During a surgical resection for a biliary malignancy in a 55-year-old female patient, which anatomical feature of the common hepatic duct is critical for safely identifying and accessing the biliary confluence during hilar dissection?
a) Muscular sheath around the duct for bile flow control
b) Peritoneal covering of the duct for structural rigidity
c) Connective tissue encasing the duct, forming the hilar plate, guiding dissection
d) Fatty layer surrounding the duct, granting surgical protection
e) Venous plexus over the duct, marking the confluence
**Answer: c**
The common hepatic duct is enveloped in connective tissue that forms the hilar plate within the hepatoduodenal ligament. This structure aids surgeons in identifying and dissecting the biliary confluence, providing access to the right and left hepatic ducts during procedures for biliary malignancies.[8]

5. A 38-year-old male is being evaluated for a living liver donation to his 2-year-old daughter. An MRI of the liver was performed to assess the liver anatomy and to plan for a left lateral segmentectomy. What is the most common biliary variation?
a) Segment II and III ducts merge near the umbilical fissure, forming the left lateral segment duct, which joins a segment IV duct to form the left hepatic duct
b) Segment II and III ducts merge near the umbilical fissure, then unite with two segment IV ducts to form the left hepatic duct
c) A single segment III duct receives drainage from segment IV and merges with the segment II duct close to the hepatic hilum
d) Segment II and III ducts merge lateral to the umbilical fissure, forming a short channel that joins a segment IV duct to form the left hepatic duct
e) Segment II duct joins segment IV duct near the umbilical fissure, then merges with segment III duct to form the left hepatic duct
**Answer: a**
This is the most common anatomical variant, seen in 55% of cases.[9]

6. A 52-year-old female patient presents for a left hepatic lobe resection due to HCC. Although the surgical procedure was completed without complications, her postoperative course is notable for persistently elevated white blood cell count, ALP, and bilirubin levels. Further evaluation with an MRCP reveals dilated hepatic ducts in the right posterior liver lobe (segments VII and VIII), which appear to converge and

become obstructed at the site of liver transection. This surgical complication is attributed to:
a) Bile duct transection low in the hilar plate, causing partial obstruction of the right-sided liver drainage
b) Missed identification of the posterior branch of the right hepatic duct originating from the left hepatic duct, leading to disrupted bile flow
c) Iatrogenic injury to the right hepatic artery, causing ischemic cholangiopathy
d) Insufficient drainage from the left hepatic lobe post-resection, resulting in biliary obstruction
e) Postoperative bile leak from the resection site, affecting biliary drainage
**Answer: b**
A significant surgical variant in biliary anatomy involves the posterior branch of the right hepatic duct originating directly from the left hepatic duct, approximately 1 cm beyond the hilar plate, crossing Cantlie's line to drain segments VII and VIII. This anatomical variant must be carefully considered during liver resections. In this case, the complication arose from missed identification of the posterior branch of the right hepatic duct originating from the left hepatic duct, leading to disrupted bile flow.[10]

7. A 21-year-old female with a previous history of bipolar disorder presents to the hospital in acute liver failure and hepatic encephalopathy after ingesting half a bottle of acetaminophen in a suicide attempt, following a breakup with her boyfriend one day prior. Her laboratory results show AST level of 3298 U/L, ALT level of 4650 U/L, a bilirubin of 3.5 mg/dL, and an INR of 5.8. According to her parents, the patient began college one year ago and reports occasional alcohol use and smoking. This clinical picture is most consistent with:
a) Fulminant hepatic failure (FHF)
b) Acute liver decompensation
c) Acute-on-chronic liver disease
d) Acute viral hepatitis
e) Acute decompensation of Wilson's disease
**Answer: a**
FHF is defined as the onset of hepatic encephalopathy within 8 weeks of the first symptoms of liver disease, with the absence of preexisting liver disease. Specific laboratory criteria demonstrating severe hepatic dysfunction allow these patients to receive the highest priority for organ allocation, given that their life expectancy without a liver transplant is less than 7 days.[11]

8. All of the following are commonly associated with acute liver failure (ALF), except:
a) Hepatic encephalopathy
b) Coagulopathy

c) Renal failure
d) Jaundice
e) Portal hypertensive bleeding
**Answer: e**
ALF is a clinical syndrome resulting from the rapid loss of hepatocyte function. Hepatic encephalopathy is, by definition, present to some degree in all patients with ALF. Cerebral edema is a cardinal feature and can lead to uncal herniation, resulting in brainstem compression and death. In contrast, portal hypertensive bleeding and severe fluid retention are distinctly uncommon in the context of ALF.[11]

9. What is the most common cause of acute liver failure (ALF) in the United States?
a) Drugs/toxins
b) Infections
c) Unknown (indeterminate acute liver failure)
d) Metabolic and genetic disorders (e.g., Wilson's disease, pregnancy-associated acute liver failure)
e) Autoimmune disorders
f) Vascular causes (e.g., shock, acute liver ischemia, hepatic vein occlusion)
**Answer: a**
The most common causes of ALF in the United States are drugs and toxins, particularly acetaminophen, which accounts for approximately 46% of cases. Other causes include ALF of indeterminate origin (14%), viral infections such as hepatitis A and B (11%), autoimmune disorders (5%), ischemic events (4%), Wilson's disease (2%), and a variety of other metabolic, structural, and undetermined causes (14%).[12]

10. Which of the following statements about liver stellate cells is not correct?
a) Stellate cells constitute approximately 5% to 8 % of the healthy liver mass
b) Stellate cells store vitamin E
c) Stellate cells store vitamin A
d) Stellate cells synthesize extracellular matrix components
e) Stellate cells support the homeostasis of hepatocytes and endothelial cells
**Answer: b**
Hepatic stellate cells represent a highly versatile cell type that plays a significant role in liver development and differentiation, regeneration, response to xenobiotics, immunoregulation, control of hepatic blood flow, and inflammatory responses. They do serve as a storage site for vitamin A, but not for vitamin E.[13]

11. A 23-year-old male from Russia presents to the hospital while visiting the United States, exhibiting signs of acute liver failure (ALF). His laboratory results indicate AST level of 10,987 U/L, ALT level of 12,518 U/L, a bilirubin level of 11.2 mg/dL, and

an INR of 5.1. Further investigation is consistent with acute hepatitis A-induced liver damage. The prognosis of ALF primarily depends on which of the following factors?
a) Clearance of the hepatitis A virus
b) The balance between liver cell death and liver repair and regeneration
c) The speed of liver regeneration and remodeling
d) The duration of ongoing hepatic necrosis
e) The age of the patient and comorbidities

Answer: b

Survival in cases of acute liver failure critically depends on the ability to achieve rapid and robust recovery of liver cell function before life-threatening complications, such as cerebral edema and sepsis, arise. The adequacy of liver repair and regeneration following acute liver injury is as important as the extent of the injury in determining the overall outcome; both components significantly influence prognosis.[14]

12. Which of the following statements regarding the role of oval cells in liver regeneration following massive liver injury is most accurate?
a) Oval cells are primarily responsible for the immediate response to acute liver injury by directly supporting hepatocyte function
b) Oval cells are derived from immature liver sinusoidal cell within the liver parenchyma
c) The proliferation of oval cells is a critical compensatory mechanism when normal regenerative pathways are insufficient
d) Oval cells are mostly involved in the regeneration of non-parenchymal liver cells, such as Kupffer cells and endothelial cells
e) Oval cells have been shown to promote bile duct regeneration but do not contribute to hepatocyte replacement

Answer: c

A population of small portal zone cells in the Canal of Hering with a high nuclear-to-cytoplasmic ratio known as oval cells. The proliferation of oval cells serves as a critical compensatory mechanism in the context of massive liver injury, where the conventional regenerative pathways are overwhelmed, enabling the differentiation of these progenitor cells into hepatocytes to facilitate liver regeneration.[15]

13. Cirrhosis is defined as the histological development of regenerative nodules surrounded by fibrous bands in response to chronic liver injury, ultimately leading to portal hypertension and end-stage liver disease. The initial signs of advanced cirrhosis often manifest as abnormalities in laboratory test results, except for which of the following?
a) Thrombocytopenia
b) Neutropenia

c) Prolonged prothrombin time
d) Hyperbilirubinemia
e) Hypoalbuminemia
**Answer: b**
The first signs of advanced cirrhosis frequently include laboratory test abnormalities such as thrombocytopenia, prolonged prothrombin time, hyperbilirubinemia, and hypoalbuminemia; however, neutropenia is not typically one of the initial manifestations.[11]

14. Which of the following is the most common cause of liver cirrhosis in the United States?
a) Chronic hepatitis B virus infection
b) Chronic hepatitis C virus infection
c) Alcoholic liver disease
d) Nonalcoholic fatty liver disease (NAFLD)
e) Autoimmune hepatitis
**Answer: c**
Alcoholic liver disease is the most common cause of liver cirrhosis in the United States, followed by NAFLD and chronic viral hepatitis.[16]

15. All of the following are complications of end-stage liver disease, except:
a) Cerebral edema
b) Portal hypertension
c) Ascites
d) Hepatic encephalopathy
e) Synthetic dysfunction
f) Impaired metabolic capacity
**Answer: a**
While hepatic encephalopathy is a complication often associated with chronic liver failure; cerebral edema is commonly observed in acute liver failure. Cirrhosis leads to altered extracellular matrix deposition, causing vascular distortion that compromises hepatocyte function and leads to complications such as portal hypertension, ascites, synthetic dysfunction, and impaired metabolic capacity.[11]

16. What is the primary role of toll-like receptor 4 (TLR4) in liver fibrosis?
a) TLR4 on Kupffer cells enhances inflammation, indirectly supporting fibrosis progression
b) TLR4 on stellate cells promotes fibrosis by suppressing a regulator TGF-β1
c) TLR4 on stellate cells limits fibrosis by up-regulating anti-fibrogenic proteins
d) TLR4 on hepatocytes amplifies inflammatory signals that contribute to fibrosis

e) TLR4 polymorphisms accelerate fibrosis in hepatitis C virus infection by altering signaling

**Answer: b**

TLR4 on stellate cells promotes liver fibrosis by down-regulating bone morphogenic protein and activin membrane-bound inhibitor, a suppressor of TGF-β1, the key fibrogenic cytokine. While option a suggests TLR4 on Kupffer cells indirectly supports fibrosis through inflammation, this is less direct and less critical than the stellate cell pathway, which actively drives fibrosis.[17]

17. Which of the following statements regarding the pathogenesis of liver fibrosis and its clinical implications is most accurate?
a) Liver fibrosis develops uniformly in all individuals with chronic liver diseases, regardless of the duration or etiology of the injury, ultimately leading to cirrhosis in every ca
b) Fibrosis of the liver is mediated by different molecular signals and cellular processes based on the causes of liver insult
c) In most forms of chronic liver injury, including hepatitis C and autoimmune hepatitis, fibrosis is characterized by early lobular injury and initially displays lobular fibrosis, especially around the sinusoids
d) The progression of liver fibrosis is determined by the intensity, duration, and location of the hepatic injury, suggesting an individual-specific threshold that must be surpassed for significant fibrosis to occur
e) Removal of the source of chronic liver injury has consistently been shown to have no effect on the existing fibrotic tissue, making the reversal of liver fibrosis unachievable

**Answer: d**

The progression of liver fibrosis is determined by the intensity, duration, and location of the hepatic injury, suggesting an individual-specific threshold that must be surpassed for significant fibrosis to occur. This recognition underscores the varied clinical outcomes in patients with chronic liver diseases and points to the potential for fibrosis reversal upon removal of the injurious stimulus. In most forms of chronic liver injury, including hepatitis C and autoimmune hepatitis, fibrosis is initially most prominent in the portal region, which is the location most affected by these diseases. In contrast, alcoholic and nonalcoholic steatohepatitis—both characterized by early lobular injury—initially display lobular fibrosis, especially around the sinusoids.[17]

18. What is the principal collagen in liver fibrosis?
a) Type I collagen
b) Type II collagen
c) Type III collagen

d) Type IV collagen
e) Type V collagen
**Answer: a**
Type I collagen is the main collagen in liver fibrosis, creating the interstitial scar matrix that persists when not broken down. Matrix metalloproteinase-1 primarily degrades this collagen, however, sources of this enzyme are not as clearly established.[17]

19. Which of the following statements is correct regarding hepatocyte apoptotic cell death?
a) Cytosolic transaminases AST and ALT cannot be released into the serum by this mode of cell death
b) It leads to secondary necrosis when apoptotic bodies are not efficiently cleared
c) It does not produce an inflammatory effect
d) It occurs without forming apoptotic bodies, causing direct tissue damage
e) Apoptotic cells are rapidly engulfed by Kupffer cells and cleared from the liver
**Answer: b**
A common misconception is that apoptosis does not release cytosolic enzymes like AST and ALT into the serum; however, studies have shown that hepatocyte apoptosis can lead to elevated serum transaminases. Another misconception is that apoptosis is non-inflammatory. In the liver, if apoptotic bodies are not promptly cleared, they undergo secondary necrosis, releasing intracellular contents that provoke inflammation. Unlike other epithelial cells, hepatocytes cannot shed apoptotic bodies into a lumen, making the liver more susceptible to secondary necrosis during extensive apoptotic injury.[18]

20. During liver injury, the behavior of stellate cells is regulated by paracrine interactions with damaged hepatocytes and endothelial cells, as well as activated platelets, Kupffer cells, infiltrating leukocytes, and other stellate cells and hepatic myofibroblasts. These interactions are mediated by growth factors, regulatory peptides and lipids, cytokines, extracellular matrix components, and toxic metabolites. Which of the following molecules does not utilize receptor tyrosine kinase ligands?
a) Insulin-like growth factor (IGF)
b) Epidermal growth factor (EGF)
c) Endothelin-1
d) Platelet-derived growth factor (PDGF)
e) TGF-β
**Answer: c**
Endothelin-1 is a G-protein–coupled receptor (GPCR) ligand.[19]

21. A 64-year-old female is undergoing a right lateral hepatectomy for HCC. The right lobe is mobilized, and hilar structures are identified. To optimize surgical outcomes and minimize blood loss during this procedure, which surgical technique should be employed?
a) Intermittent right portal triad clamping with 15-minute clamp and 5-minute unclamp cycles
b) Continuous right portal triad clamping throughout the procedure
c) Selective clamping of the hepatic artery while maintaining portal vein flow
d) Using electrocautery at a high setting to divide liver parenchyma rapidly
e) Use of a vascular stapler for rapid transection of the liver parenchyma
**Answer: a**
Intermittent hilar clamping is the recommended technique to minimize hepatic blood loss and improve surgical outcomes during liver resection.[20]

## 2. Organ Donation and Allocation

22. An equitable liver allocation scheme must adequately balance the principles of justice, utility, autonomy, benevolence, and nonmalfeasance. Which of the following ethical principle primarily supports the allocation of organs to individuals who exhibit the greatest likelihood of survival?
a) Justice
b) Utility
c) Autonomy
d) Benevolence
e) Nonmalfeasance
**Answer: b**
A utilitarian approach prioritizes the allocation of organs to those with the best chance of survival, reflecting the ethical principle of utility.[21]

23. In the context of liver transplantation, which of the following best illustrates the principle of patient autonomy?
a) A patient may choose to participate in a tolerance program and minimize immunosuppression despite a history of rejection
b) Patient autonomy allows individuals to participate in selecting organ offers and determining their position on the transplant list
c) Patient autonomy permits an individual to become a living liver donor for their adult child who requires a second transplant due to alcohol relapse
d) A patient may refuse an organ offer based on personal values and preferences
e) Patient autonomy allows patients to request the use of normothermic machine perfusion for their transplant
**Answer: d**
An example of patient autonomy is when a patient chooses to refuse a liver organ from a hepatitis-positive donor.[21]

24. In the context of liver transplantation, which scenario best illustrates the principle of benevolence as it relates to the actions of a patient or donor in the organ allocation process?
a) A living liver donor prioritizes their own health concerns over the potential impact on recipients by choosing not to disclose a minor medical history to the transplant team

b) A patient in need of a liver transplant advocates for equitable access to organs for all candidates, regardless of socioeconomic status or medical history, demonstrating compassion for others in similar situations
c) A transplant recipient refuses to share information about their positive outcome with other patients, focusing solely on their personal recovery without regard for the broader community
d) A family member of a liver donor insists on certain conditions for the donation that may limit the available options for recipients, prioritizing their own values over the needs of patients in need
e) A transplant center limits organ offers to only those candidates deemed most likely to succeed, disregarding the needs and circumstances of other patients awaiting transplantation

**Answer: b**

The principle of benevolence emphasizes the importance of acting in a manner that promotes the well-being of others and aligns with ethical responsibilities to do what is morally right.[21]

25. A 35-year-old woman with acute liver failure presents to the emergency department. She is not a U.S. citizen and does not have health insurance. Despite this, her clinical condition qualifies her for urgent liver transplantation. The transplant team must decide whether to list her for a donor organ, knowing that resources are limited and multiple patients are already on the waiting list. The team decides to proceed with listing her based on established medical criteria and fairness in resource distribution. Which of the following ethical principle is most directly applied in this decision?
a) Justice
b) Utility
c) Autonomy
d) Benevolence
e) Nonmalfeasance

**Answer: a**

The principle of justice refers to fairness in the distribution of healthcare resources. In transplantation, this means allocating organs based on medical need and established criteria, without discrimination based on socioeconomic status, citizenship, or other unrelated factors.[21]

26. The MELD score was originally designed to estimate the three-month mortality risk for patients with cirrhosis who are undergoing transjugular portosystemic shunt placement. The UNOS has since modified the scoring system, establishing lower and upper limits of 6 and 40, respectively. Within donor service areas, livers are allocated

to candidates based on their MELD scores. In cases where multiple candidates possess identical scores, the liver allocation is determined by which of the following factors?
a) Length of waiting time
b) Current hospitalization in the ICU
c) Status 1A
d) Younger age of the candidate
e) Presence of cancer exception points

**Answer: a**

Waiting list mortality increases directly in proportion to the listing MELD score; the longer a patient is waiting, the higher the risk of dying. MELD allocation does not apply to status 1A or 1B candidates.[22]

27. The PELD score has been proposed as an objective tool for prioritizing children who are awaiting liver transplantation. This scoring system is applicable to all children younger than:
a) 10 years of age
b) 12 years of age
c) 14 years of age
d) 16 years of age
e) 18 years of age

**Answer: b**

The PELD score is utilized for children aged 12 years and under. Livers from donors aged 18 years or younger are prioritized for allocation to pediatric candidates. In situations where the MELD and PELD scores are equivalent, the organ will be assigned to the child, despite the higher mortality risk typically associated with the MELD score.[23]

28. Which of the following is not a component of the PELD score?
a) Age
b) Bilirubin
c) Albumin
d) Creatinine
e) INR
f) History of growth failure

**Answer: d**

The PELD score is a model that uses five objective parameters to accurately predict death or transfer to the ICU in children awaiting liver transplantation.[23]

29. A 17-year-old female patient with bipolar disorder has been admitted with fulminant hepatic failure secondary to an acetaminophen overdose. She is currently intubated, and her INR is 5.6. Considering the current liver allocation system in the United States, how will the liver be allocated to her?
a) The livers from all deceased donors are offered for status 1A candidates listed at transplant hospitals within a radius of 500 nautical miles from the donor hospital
b) The liver will be prioritized for her as a pediatric candidate, but only if there are no local candidates with a MELD score of 35 or higher
c) The liver will be allocated nationally to her as a status 1 adult candidate, ahead of all pediatric candidates in the region
d) The liver will be allocated to her as a status 1B candidate
e) The liver will be allocated directly to her as a pediatric candidate without consideration of MELD/PELD scores

**Answer: a**

As a status 1A candidate, this patient will receive offers for liver transplants from all diseased donors located within a 500 nautical mile radius from the hospital where she is listed. Furthermore, if any of the livers are not used within their own region, they will subsequently be offered at a national level to status 1 candidates.[24]

30. In patients with cirrhosis, which of the following statements best describes the implications of incorporating serum sodium into the MELD score, implemented in January 2016?
a) The MELD-sodium score has shown benefit only in patients with massive refractory ascites
b) The addition of serum sodium to the MELD score was primarily intended to assess renal function in patients awaiting liver transplantation
c) The MELD-sodium score did not improve mortality prediction in patients with cirrhosis
d) A low serum sodium level significantly enhances the predictive accuracy of the MELD score for 3- and 6-month mortality in cirrhotic patients
e) The MELD-sodium score improved long-term predictive power for 5-year survival in cirrhotic patients

**Answer: d**

A serum sodium level below 126 mEq/L significantly enhances the predictive power of the MELD score for 3- and 6-month mortality in cirrhotic patients.[24]

31. In the context of organ allocation for deceased liver donors who are not donating upon cardiorespiratory death and are under age 70, which of the following statements accurately describes the prioritization protocol for waitlist candidates?

a) Candidates with a PELD score of 30 or higher are prioritized over MELD score of 33-37
b) The initial offers for liver donations are first made to candidates within a 150 nautical mile radius, followed by offers to candidates with scores of 37 or higher, regardless of distance
c) After status 1A/1B candidates, waitlist candidates with MELD or PELD scores of 37 or higher are prioritized for offers, initially within 150 nautical miles, then expanding in a sequential manner
d) Offers are sequentially distributed first to candidates within a 500 nautical mile radius and then to those with MELD scores of 37 or higher
e) Candidates with PELD scores between 15 and 28 have the highest priority in the allocation process following status 1A/1B candidates

**Answer: c**

After status 1A/1B candidates, waitlist candidates with MELD or PELD scores of 37 or higher are prioritized for offers, initially within 150 nautical miles, then expanding in a sequential manner. The liver offers will then be extended to candidates within a 250 nautical mile radius, and finally to those within 500 nautical miles. The prioritization for MELD/PELD scores will continue in descending ranges, specifically from 33 to 36, then from 29 to 32, and finally from 15 to 28.[24]

32. A 64-year-old male patient with alcohol-induced liver cirrhosis has been diagnosed with HCC, measuring 4.2 cm in size, four months ago. His current MELD score is 25. Which of the following statements is true regarding his eligibility for liver transplantation and the associated MELD exception points?
a) The patient can receive 2 additional MELD points immediately upon listing
b) Since his HCC is diagnosed within 6 months, he will automatically qualify for the HCC MELD exception points
c) He must wait an additional two months to complete the six-month observation period before he can request MELD exception points, provided he remains within the Milan criteria at that time
d) The patient's MELD score will automatically increase every three months regardless of any updates in tumor size
e) The patient is not qualified for MELD exception points based on his tumor size

**Answer: c**

Under the organ allocation policy, the patient with HCC must undergo a 6-month observation period during which his tumor characteristics and overall health can be adequately assessed. After this period, if he still meets the Milan criteria for transplantation and maintains his current MELD score, he will qualify for additional MELD exception points. The maximum points granted for HCC MELD exceptions are capped at a fixed score (MMaT).[24]

33. The MELD allocation system does not apply to Status 1A candidates. Which of the following conditions is not classified under Status 1A?
a) Fulminant hepatic failure
b) Primary nonfunction of a transplanted liver
c) Wilson's disease with acute liver decompensation
d) Cystic fibrosis with acute liver decompensation
e) Hepatic artery thrombosis following liver transplantation

**Answer: d**
Cystic fibrosis with acute liver decompensation does not automatically qualify as a Status 1A condition. While cystic fibrosis can lead to liver disease, acute liver decompensation in this context does not fall under the immediate life-threatening conditions that define Status 1A candidates.[24]

34. In which year was the Uniform Brain Death Act passed, establishing the legal recognition of brain death in the United States?
a) 1954
b) 1968
c) 1978
d) 1984
e) 2007

**Answer: c**
The Uniform Brain Death Act was enacted in 1978, providing a standardized legal framework for the determination of brain death across the United States.
In 1954, the first successful human kidney transplant was performed between identical twins.
In 1968, the Uniform Anatomical Gift Act was passed, which laid the legal groundwork necessary for organ donation.
In 1984, the National Organ Transplant Act was enacted, instituting comprehensive guidelines for organ transplantation and creating the OPTN to enhance organ allocation.
In 2007, the Medicare Conditions of Participation for organ transplant programs became effective, ensuring quality standards for transplant centers.[25]

35. The OPTN and Intestinal Organ Transplantation Committee has established regulations regarding requests for MELD exceptions and extensions for non-HCC adult patients. Which of the following conditions is not currently qualified for standardized MELD exception requests?
a) Cholangiocarcinoma
b) Primary hyperoxaluria

c) Portopulmonary hypertension
d) Hepatopulmonary syndrome
e) Alpha-1 antitrypsin deficiency
**Answer: e**
Alpha-1 antitrypsin deficiency is typically not included in the standardized MELD exception criteria. While patients with this condition may experience liver dysfunction, they generally do not have the same urgent need for transplantation as patients with the other listed conditions.[24]

36. A 42-year-old male patient presents with nonresectable hilar cholangiocarcinoma. Importantly, there is no evidence of extrahepatic or intrahepatic metastases, and he has preserved liver synthetic function. The patient is interested in whether he can be listed for liver transplantation with MELD exception points. Which of the following statements is true regarding the patient's eligibility for MELD exception points?
a) Given the aggressive nature of the tumor, the patient can be listed for liver transplant with a MELD score of 35
b) The patient is eligible for MELD exception points as long as he provides evidence of the diagnosis through imaging and biopsy, and there is no evidence of metastatic disease
c) The presence of hilar cholangiocarcinoma disqualifies the patient from receiving MELD exception points
d) As a patient with an unresectable malignancy, he can be listed for liver transplant, but he must demonstrate significant liver dysfunction to qualify for MELD exception points
e) The patient must undergo palliative chemotherapy prior to being considered for MELD exception points, based on guidelines set by UNOS
**Answer: b**
In the context of hilar cholangiocarcinoma, if the diagnosis is confirmed through appropriate imaging techniques, biopsy, or tumor markers, and there is no evidence of metastatic disease, the patient is indeed eligible for MELD exception points.[24]

37. In the context of liver transplantation criteria, which of the following statements correctly describes the Status 1B category for pediatric patients?
a) Status 1B is reserved for extremely sick, chronically ill pediatric patients with cirrhosis who are younger than 12 years of age
b) Status 1B is reserved for extremely sick, chronically ill pediatric patients with cirrhosis who are younger than 18 years of age
c) Pediatric patients classified as Status 1B typically have a MELD score that automatically qualifies them for prioritized transplantation

d) Patients categorized under Status 1B represent the majority of the pediatric liver transplant waitlist
e) Status 1B patients are eligible for liver transplantation only after they turn 12 years of age

**Answer: b**

Status 1B is specifically designated for pediatric patients under the age of 18 who are experiencing severe illness due to chronic liver disease and cirrhosis.[24]

38. A 22-year-old male sustained a traumatic brain injury in a severe motor vehicle accident. After comprehensive medical evaluation, he was diagnosed with a severe, irreversible brain injury with minimal residual neurological function. He began treatment for bacteremia three days ago. Given this diagnosis, which statement best reflects his eligibility for organ donation?
a) He is eligible for organ donation, as a persistent vegetative state is equivalent to brain death
b) His severe, irreversible brain injury alone qualifies him for organ donation
c) If medical futility is confirmed and the family or legal representative consents to withdrawal of life support, he may be eligible for organ donation under controlled DCD protocols
d) His recent bacteremia renders him ineligible for organ donation
e) Organ donation discussions with the family or legal representative should be deferred until he is declared brain dead

**Answer: c**

Patients with severe, irreversible brain injuries often rely on intensive cardiopulmonary support to sustain life. Despite appearing permanently unconscious, they do not meet brain death criteria due to the presence of residual neurological function. When medical futility is established and the family or legal representative agrees to withdraw life support, the patient may qualify for organ donation under controlled DCD protocols. A cornerstone of DCD protocols is that the decision to withdraw life support precedes any consideration of organ donation, ensuring ethical clarity in the process.[26]

39. During a liver recovery procedure from an organ DCD donor, the procuring surgeon was informed that life support had been withdrawn in the operating room. Outside the operating room, the anesthesiologist asked the surgeon whether it would be appropriate to administer opioids to the patient, noting an elevated heart rate, to ensure comfort. What is the appropriate course of action?
a) The surgeon should state that administering opioids is contraindicated due to the patient's imminent cardiac death

b) The surgeon should agree that opioids are permissible to relieve discomfort and provide dosage recommendations
c) Opioids should not be administered unless the patient exhibits clear signs of acute pain or distress
d) The surgeon should clarify that they are not permitted to participate in patient management decisions
e) The surgeon should advise waiting for a formal declaration of death before administering any medications, including heparin

**Answer: d**

In controlled DCD, it is essential that members of the transplant team, including the procuring surgeon, refrain from participating in the patient's care management during the withdrawal of life support. This includes abstaining from decisions regarding the administration of non-procurement-specific medications, such as opioids or sedatives. Involvement of the transplant team in such decisions could create a perceived conflict of interest, potentially suggesting an intent to hasten death to optimize organ quality for transplantation.[27]

40. A 36-year-old male was involved in a severe car accident that resulted in significant neurological injuries. After thorough evaluation in the ICU, his clinical status raised concerns regarding brain death. Which of the following findings would not be consistent with a diagnosis of brain death?
a) Absence of pupillary response to light and lack of oculovestibular reflex (cold calorics)
b) Presence of spinal reflexes
c) Absent gag reflex and cough reflex during airway manipulation
d) A positive apnea test showing spontaneous respiratory effort with elevated arterial carbon dioxide levels
e) Unresponsive coma with no evidence of purposeful motor response or any brainstem reflexes

**Answer: d**

The positive apnea test involves disconnecting the patient from the ventilator while closely monitoring for spontaneous respirations. Prior to the test, the patient is pre-oxygenated and ventilator settings are adjusted to achieve a target $PaCO_2$ between 35 and 45 mmHg. During the test, supplemental oxygen is delivered via a catheter to ensure adequate oxygenation. The test is considered positive if there are no spontaneous breaths and the arterial blood gas indicates a rise in $PaCO_2$ to $\geq$ 60 mmHg after eight to ten minutes. Special considerations are made for patients with chronic $CO_2$ retention, where the $CO_2$ target may be adjusted based on their baseline levels.[28]

41. A 28-year-old female patient with decompensated cirrhosis is currently on the liver transplant waiting list. Her MELD score was recently updated to the new MELD 3.0 system. Which of the following factors related to her MELD 3.0 score is least likely to influence her transplant prioritization compared to traditional MELD-Na scoring?
a) Serum sodium levels adjusted for sex-based variations
b) Serum albumin levels reflecting her nutritional status and liver function
c) INR, indicating coagulopathy and liver synthetic function
d) Recent history of liver-related complications, including hepatic encephalopathy
e) Serum bilirubin levels correlated with the severity of liver injury and cholestasis
**Answer: d**
The MELD 3.0 score has been developed to replace the MELD-Na score for prioritizing liver transplants in cirrhotic patients in the United States. This new scoring system incorporates factors such as patient sex and serum albumin levels, along with modified weights for serum sodium, bilirubin, INR, and creatinine. It aims to modestly decrease waitlist mortality and enhance access for female candidates.[29]

# 3. Indications for Liver Transplantation

42. Consider the following patients being evaluated for liver transplantation. Based on the criteria for candidacy, which of the following individuals is likely to be an appropriate candidate for liver transplant therapy?
a) A 66-year-old female with recently diagnosed HCC of the left liver lobe and no underlying liver disease
b) A 57-year-old male with liver cirrhosis, a MELD score of 38, and a recently diagnosed lymphoma
c) A 45-year-old male with alcoholic induced liver cirrhosis, who has been sober for three months but is non-compliant with his medication regimen for bipolar disorder and diabetes
d) A 45-year-old male with alcoholic induced liver cirrhosis who is currently homeless
e) A 48-year-old male with MASH cirrhosis, a MELD score of 33, and a history of coronary artery disease post-cardiac stent placement four weeks ago
**Answer: e**
The 66-year-old female with recently diagnosed HCC confined to the left liver lobe may be a candidate for a left lobectomy, which can effectively address her malignancy without necessitating liver transplantation.
The 57-year-old male with liver cirrhosis and a MELD score of 38 who has a recently diagnosed lymphoma is not an appropriate candidate for transplantation due to the presence of active malignancy, which typically contraindicates liver transplantation until the cancer is adequately cured or in remission.
The 45-year-old male with alcoholic liver disease, while having achieved sobriety for three months, demonstrates non-compliance with his medication for bipolar disorder and diabetes.
The 45-year-old male with alcoholic liver disease is currently homeless, which presents a substantial barrier to transplant eligibility. Secure housing is generally a prerequisite for transplantation to ensure proper post-operative care and follow-up; however, if this patient secures stable housing, he may be considered a candidate.
The 48-year-old male with MASH cirrhosis and a recent history of coronary artery disease managed with a cardiac stent can still be eligible for liver transplantation. Typically, a waiting period of four to six weeks post-stent placement is acceptable.[30]

43. Which of the following patients is most suitable for liver transplantation, considering specific absolute contraindications?
a) A 17-year-old female with acetaminophen-induced acute liver failure and elevated intracranial pressure resulting in brainstem herniation

b) A 68-year-old male with acute hepatic necrosis secondary to septic shock and concurrent Candida auris infection isolated from urine and blood specimens
c) A 53-year-old male with liver failure due to a myeloproliferative disorder causing hepatic vein thrombosis, as well as extensive thrombosis of the portal, splenic, and mesenteric veins
d) A 43-year-old female with MASH, a BMI of 56, and a MELD score of 35
e) A 27-year-old male with liver disease secondary to TPN dependence due to short gut syndrome following a motor vehicle accident, currently residing in a long-term care facility

**Answer: d**

The 43-year-old female with MASH, a BMI of 56, and a MELD score of 35 is the most suitable candidate for liver transplantation among the options provided. Although her elevated BMI increases the risk of surgical complications, patients with MASH can achieve significant clinical improvement post-transplant, particularly if they commit to lifestyle modifications and weight management after the procedure.

The 17-year-old female has a severe complication of elevated intracranial pressure leading to brainstem herniation, indicating irreversible cerebral injury, which contraindicates transplantation.

The 68-year-old male's active Candida auris infection poses a significant risk of poor outcomes in the immunosuppressed post-transplant state.

The 53-year-old male's extensive thrombosis of the portal, splenic, and mesenteric veins renders liver transplantation technically unfeasible.

The 27-year-old male likely requires a multivisceral transplant due to short gut syndrome, but his long-term care facility residence and complex medical needs may result in suboptimal post-transplant outcomes.[30]

44. A 57-year-old Hispanic male with MASH and a MELD score of 34 is being evaluated for liver transplantation. His echocardiogram reveals normal structural findings, but a nuclear stress test indicates abnormal myocardial perfusion with reduced blood flow in certain areas during stress compared to baseline. What is the next step in his evaluation?
a) Schedule cardiac catheterization
b) Repeat the stress test in one week
c) Plan for simultaneous coronary artery bypass grafting and liver transplantation
d) Exclude the patient from transplantation based on the stress test findings
e) Proceed with listing for liver transplantation

**Answer: a**

The nuclear stress test indicated abnormal myocardial perfusion patterns during stress, suggesting that further evaluation of the cardiac status is warranted. Scheduling a cardiac catheterization is the appropriate next step in this patient's evaluation for liver transplantation, as it will allow for direct assessment of coronary artery patency.[31]

45. A 62-year-old male undergoes liver transplantation due to decompensated cirrhosis secondary to chronic hepatitis B virus (HBV) infection. During the surgical procedure, the anesthesiologist administered 1,000 IU of hepatitis B immunoglobulin (HBIG) during the anhepatic phase. Which of the following factors is most likely to contribute to the early recurrence of HBV in this patient?
a) Insufficient dosing of HBIG in the perioperative period
b) Emergence of mutations in the HBV polymerase enzyme
c) Insufficient innate antibodies production
d) Emergence of mutations in the HBV surface protein
e) The drug should be administered 12 to 24 hours before the anhepatic phase to decrease HBV DNA

**Answer: a**
Early recurrence of HBV following liver transplantation is predominantly associated with insufficient dosing of HBIG during the perioperative period. The current recommended dose of HBIG for prophylaxis after liver transplantation in patients with HBV infection is typically 10,000 IU administered IV once during the anhepatic phase. Inadequate HBIG prophylaxis is particularly concerning for patients with high pre-transplant levels of HBV replication.[32]

46. A 52-year-old Asian female with chronic hepatitis B virus (HBV) is under evaluation for liver transplantation. Due to the organ shortage, the transplant team is considering a marginal graft from an anti-HBc-positive donor. Which statement accurately reflects the risks and management of her transplantation?
a) HBV recurrence risk is higher with anti-HBc-positive grafts despite prophylaxis
b) Anti-HBc-positive grafts reduce long term graft but not patient survival in HBsAg-positive recipients
c) Anti-HBc-positive grafts reduce both graft and patient survival in HBsAg-positive recipients
d) HBV recurrence risk is not increased with anti-HBc-positive grafts using prophylaxis
e) HBV recurrence risk is approximately 40% with anti-HBc-positive grafts despite prophylaxis

**Answer: d**
In HBsAg-positive recipients, the risk of HBV recurrence with anti-HBc-positive grafts, when managed with post-transplant prophylaxis, is comparable to that with anti-HBc-negative grafts. These grafts are suitable for patients with HBV-related liver

disease requiring lifelong prophylaxis. Recent studies suggest that anti-HBc-positive grafts do not negatively impact graft or patient survival in this population.[32]

47. A 40-year-old male is being evaluated as a potential living donor. His hepatitis B virus (HBV) testing results show the following: HBsAg is negative, anti-HBc is positive, and anti-HBs is positive. Given this infectivity status, which of the following statements regarding the donor's suitability and potential risk to the recipient is correct?
a) The donor is at high risk of transmitting HBV to the recipient due to the presence of anti-HBc
b) The donor is considered non-infectious because he has cleared the virus and has protective antibodies against HBV
c) The donor should not be considered for donation, as his positive anti-HBc indicates an active HBV infection
d) The recipient will require aggressive antiviral prophylaxis post-transplant with this donor
e) The recipient can accept the donor liver only if he is positive for both anti-HBc and anti-HBs

**Answer: b**
Despite the absence of HBsAg and the presence of anti-HBs in a potential living donor, the risk of HBV transmission to the recipient remains. This is primarily due to the presence of anti-HBc, which indicates previous exposure to HBV. Furthermore, even after years of serological and virological suppression, the viral genome can persist latent in the liver as covalently closed circular DNA. Under certain conditions, such as immunosuppression or alterations in the immune response, this latent HBV can reactivate, leading to viral replication and potential infection in the recipient. Therefore, thorough assessment and vigilant monitoring of both the donor and recipient are essential in managing the risks associated with HBV during liver transplantation.[33]

48. A 53-year-old male with chronic hepatitis B virus (HBV) infection and liver cirrhosis undergoes liver transplantation. Considering his viral infection and post-transplant hepatitis B management protocols, how long will he likely need to remain on antiviral medication?
a) Six months, to allow full immune system recovery post-transplant
b) Lifelong antiviral therapy
c) One year, as this is the most common period for HBV recurrence
d) No antiviral therapy after transplantation
e) He can discontinue antiviral medication after 3 months if his HBV DNA levels remain undetectable

**Answer: b**
Patients with HBV-related cirrhosis who undergo liver transplantation require lifelong antiviral medication. The persistence of covalently closed circular DNA in the liver, combined with post-transplant immunosuppression, poses a lifelong risk of HBV reactivation.[33]

49. A 52-year-old female underwent liver transplantation for chronic hepatitis B virus (HBV) infection. During the procedure, the anesthesiologist administered 10,000 IU of hepatitis B immunoglobulin (HBIG) in the anhepatic phase. Her postoperative course was uncomplicated, and she continued HBIG and entecavir therapy. Four months later, she developed elevated LFT and a significant increase in HBV DNA levels. What is the most likely cause of these findings?
a) Emergence of HBV escape mutants due to mutations in the pre-S/S genome
b) Entecavir resistance from mutations in the HBV polymerase gene
c) Reinfection with wild-type HBV from the donor liver
d) Inadequate HBIG dosing
e) Coinfection with hepatitis D virus
**Answer: a**
In compliant patients on antiviral therapy post-liver transplantation, HBV recurrence is most commonly caused by escape mutants arising from mutations in the pre-S/S region of the HBV genome. These mutations enable the virus to evade immune control and HBIG. Entecavir resistance is unlikely within this timeframe, and reinfection with wild-type HBV from the donor liver or inadequate HBIG dosing is rare with a standard 10,000 IU dose and adherence to protocols. Hepatitis D coinfection is not supported by the clinical presentation.[32]

50. A 60-year-old male with chronic hepatitis B virus (HBV) infection and significant liver fibrosis is being evaluated for liver transplantation. His pretransplant viral load is recorded at $1.4 \times 10^6$ copies/mL. He receives appropriate antiviral prophylaxis post-transplantation with both hepatitis B immunoglobulin (HBIG) and entecavir. What is the most significant risk factor that increases the recurrence of HBV infection following transplantation?
a) Fulminant hepatic B infection
b) Negative hepatitis B e antigen (HBeAg) status at listing
c) The presence of co-infection with hepatitis D virus (HDV)
d) The pretransplant HBV viral load exceeding $10^4$-$10^5$ copies/mL
e) The timing of the initiation of antiviral therapy post-transplant
**Answer: d**
The primary risk factor for HBV recurrence after liver transplantation is the pretransplant HBV viral load. Higher viral loads (greater than $10^4$-$10^5$ copies/mL)

significantly increase the likelihood of recurrence, regardless of the prophylaxis employed. Additionally, infection with lamivudine-resistant HBV variants (YMDD mutants) increases the risk for recurrence, regardless of viral load.[34]

51. A 53-year-old Asian male recently underwent liver transplantation for acute-on-chronic liver failure secondary to chronic hepatitis B virus (HBV) and hepatitis D virus (HDV) coinfection. Which statement accurately describes the risk of HBV reinfection in this patient?
a) HBV reinfection risk is higher due to HDV's stimulatory effect on HBV replication
b) HBV reinfection risk is higher due to post-transplant immunosuppressive therapy
c) HBV reinfection risk is lower due to HDV's inhibitory effect on HBV replication
d) HBV reinfection risk is unaffected, as both viruses remain dormant immediately post-transplant
e) HBV reinfection risk is higher immediately post-transplant but decreases after 6 months

**Answer: c**
Regardless of HBV prophylaxis, patients with chronic HBV and HDV coinfection have a lower risk of HBsAg reappearance post-transplantation compared to those with HBV alone, resulting in improved survival rates. This reduced risk in HDV-coinfected patients is attributed to the inhibitory effect of HDV on HBV replication, with 70% to 90% of these patients being HBeAg-negative and having low serum HBV DNA levels.[35]

52. Hepatitis C virus (HCV) exhibits several unique characteristics that significantly influence its natural history. Which of the following statements about HCV is most accurate?
a) HCV has a double-stranded DNA genome that integrates into the host's DNA, facilitating persistent infection
b) HCV's inability to proofread during replication leads to a high mutation rate, allowing for significant genomic heterogeneity
c) HCV replicates primarily in the nucleus of hepatocytes, contributing to high levels of viral variation compared to other viruses
d) The high replication rate of hepatitis C virus (HCV), up to $10^{12}$ virions per day, can be observed in patients coinfected with hepatitis D virus
e) HCV consistently produces stable genomic variants that enhance the immune response against the virus

**Answer: b**
HCV is a single-stranded RNA virus that lacks the proofreading capability. This means that errors made during RNA replication are not corrected, resulting in a high mutation rate. It replicates entirely within the hepatocyte cytoplasm; there is no

nuclear replication or viral genomic integration into host DNA. With an estimated replication of up to 10^12 virions per day, the sheer volume of replication allows for the emergence of a diverse array of viral variants. While most of these mutations may not lead to viable virus strains, the presence of these variants enhances the virus's ability to escape immune detection and response.[36]

53. A 58-year-old female with hepatitis C virus (HCV)-related cirrhosis is listed for liver transplantation with a MELD score of 14. She recently completed direct-acting antiviral (DAA) therapy and achieved a sustained virological response (SVR). What is the most likely implication for her liver transplant eligibility?
a) Significant MELD score reduction, potentially allowing delisting from the transplant list
b) No significant change in liver function or transplant eligibility
c) Significant MELD score reduction and decreased HCC risk
d) Need for additional antiviral therapy due to viral mutation, while remaining transplant-eligible
e) Increased risk of liver decompensation immediately post-treatment
**Answer: a**
Successful HCV eradication with DAA therapy can significantly improve liver function in patients with cirrhosis, particularly those with MELD scores below 20. For this patient, with a MELD score of 14, achieving SVR may lead to a substantial reduction in her MELD score, potentially justifying delisting from the transplant waiting list. Studies indicate that patients with MELD scores above 18 are less likely to achieve sufficient improvement for delisting. Current guidelines recommend DAA therapy for patients with decompensated cirrhosis and lower MELD scores pre-transplant, as they are more likely to experience significant recovery.[37]

54. A 62-year-old male with a history of hepatitis C virus (HCV) infection achieved a sustained virological response (SVR) after completing direct-acting antiviral (DAA) therapy. His LFT have shown significant improvement. Which statement best reflects the ongoing management recommendations for HCC surveillance in this patient?
a) SVR after DAA therapy eliminates the need for HCC monitoring
b) Continuous HCC surveillance is required, as SVR reduces but does not eliminate the risk
c) HCC monitoring can be discontinued if MELD score improves and SVR persists
d) HCC surveillance is only needed if symptoms or abnormal LFT develop
e) HCC surveillance is needed for the first 5 years after achieving SVR, as HCC risk is highest initially
**Answer: b**

Achieving SVR with DAA therapy reduces but does not eliminate the risk of de novo HCC in patients with a history of HCV, particularly those with cirrhosis. Continuous surveillance for HCC is recommended, as eradication of HCV does not fully mitigate the oncogenic potential in the liver. However, SVR can lower mortality rates for patients on the transplant waiting list by improving overall liver function.[37]

55. A 37-year-old female with alcohol-related cirrhosis is listed for liver transplantation with a MELD score of 26. A donor offer becomes available from a 24-year-old DCD male who is hepatitis C virus (HCV)-positive, currently hospitalized following a drug overdose and anoxia. Which statement best reflects the transplant considerations and potential outcomes if she accepts this donor offer?
a) This donor graft is discouraged due to a higher risk of post-transplant liver failure compared to HCV-negative grafts
b) Recipients of DCD HCV-positive grafts have significantly worse outcomes
c) A donor liver biopsy is required to assess fibrosis, as it predicts poorer outcomes compared to HCV-negative grafts
d) Transplantation with this donor may yield similar graft and patient outcomes as HCV-negative donors if liver fibrosis is minimal
e) The donor's HCV status requires the recipient to start antiviral therapy before transplantation to reduce transmission risk
**Answer: d**
Recent studies indicate that patient and graft survival rates are similar between HCV-positive and HCV-negative DCD liver transplantation despite minimal fibrosis.[38]

56. In which of the following clinical situations may liver transplantation still be considered, despite potential concerns regarding futility?
a) Patients with evidence of compromised brainstem function
b) Patients with confirmed invasive fungal infection
c) Patients with rapidly escalating inotrope or pressor requirements
d) Patients with severe pancreatitis
e) Patients with severe arterial plaque at the celiac trunk with the majority of hepatic flow through the gastroduodenal artery to the hepatic artery
**Answer: e**
While liver transplantation can be futile in many critical situations (e.g., severe brainstem injury, confirmed systemic fungal infection), patients with significant arterial plaque at the celiac trunk can still be candidates.[39]

57. Evidence shows higher spontaneous survival rates in fulminant hepatic failure patients with acetaminophen toxicity, pregnancy-related conditions, or hepatitis A, compared to those with seronegative hepatitis, idiosyncratic drug reactions, or

Wilson's disease (10–20% survival). Younger patients (30–40 years) and those with rapidly progressive hyperacute liver failure also have better survival outcomes. However, no prognostic model optimally balances sensitivity and specificity to identify patients most likely to benefit from transplantation. Using models with high sensitivity may lead to which consequence?
a) Increased unnecessary transplants
b) Decreased unnecessary transplants
c) Increased avoidable deaths
d) Decreased deaths
e) Increased patient listings
**Answer: a**
High sensitivity may over-identify patients for transplantation, even when their prognosis is better, leading to more unnecessary transplants, resource misallocation, and increased surgical risks.[40]

58. A 45-year-old female patient presents to the clinic with fatigue, pruritus, and jaundice. Laboratory tests reveal elevated ALP levels and positive antimitochondrial antibodies (AMA). Based on these clinical findings and the patient's presentation, which of the following definitions best describes primary biliary cholangitis (PBC)?
a) A chronic autoimmune disease characterized by the destruction of large bile ducts resulting in cholestasis
b) A progressive liver disease marked by the inflammation and obliteration of the medium-sized bile ducts and subsequent fibrosis
c) An autoimmune disorder that leads to the destruction of small and medium-sized bile ducts in the liver, causing progressive cholestasis and portal hypertension
d) A chronic liver disease primarily caused by viral hepatitis leading to inflammation and necrosis of the biliary system
e) A rare autoimmune condition characterized by the inflammation of the liver due to the presence of pathogenic antibodies that target liver tissues
**Answer: c**
PBC is a chronic inflammatory hepatobiliary disease characterized by a T-cell lymphocyte–mediated destruction of the small to medium-sized interlobular bile ducts that can lead to biliary cirrhosis and liver failure if left untreated.[41]

59. The hallmark of primary biliary cholangitis (PBC) is an autoantibody targeting lipoic acids in the dehydrogenase complex of the inner mitochondrial membrane, detected in 90–95% of PBC patients. Which antibody is this?
a) Antimitochondrial antibodies (AMA)
b) Antinuclear antibodies (ANA)
c) Anti-smooth muscle antibodies

d) Anticentromere antibodies
e) Anti-cardiolipin antibodies
**Answer: a**
AMA are the key diagnostic marker for PBC due to their high specificity. A positive AMA test can confirm PBC without a liver biopsy. While antinuclear antibodies (ANA) may also be present, they are less diagnostically significant than AMA.[41]

60. What is the standard medical treatment for primary biliary cholangitis (PBC)?
a) Cholestyramine
b) Ursodeoxycholic acid (UDCA)
c) Omega-3 fatty acids
d) Corticosteroids
e) Colchicine
**Answer: b**
UDCA is the only medication approved by the U.S. Food and Drug Administration for treating PBC. It not only improves LFT but also enhances transplant-free survival in PBC patients and lowers the risk of esophageal varices and cirrhosis.[42]

61. Ursodeoxycholic acid (UDCA) is a cornerstone therapy for primary biliary cholangitis (PBC). Its mechanisms of action include all of the following except:
a) Inhibition of cholangiocyte apoptosis
b) Amelioration of mitochondrial dysfunction by displacing hydrophobic bile salts
c) Suppression of pro-inflammatory cytokine production
d) Stabilization of hepatocyte and cholangiocyte membranes
e) Direct induction of cytochrome P450 enzyme activity
**Answer: e**
UDCA exerts therapeutic effects in PBC by inhibiting apoptosis, displacing toxic hydrophobic bile salts to improve mitochondrial function, reducing cytokine-mediated inflammation, and stabilizing cell membranes.[42]

62. What is the cumulative incidence of recurrent primary biliary cholangitis (PBC) at 10 years following liver transplantation?
a) 5% to 10%
b) 20% to 25%
c) 30% to 35%
d) 40% to 45%
e) Close to 50%
**Answer: b**
Unlike de novo PBC, the clinical and biochemical characteristics associated with recurrent PBC may not be evident. In fact, many cases are identified through protocol

liver biopsies while serum liver biochemistry may remain normal. Additionally, serum anti-mitochondrial antibody levels can vary between positive and negative in patients with or without recurrent PBC.[43]

63. A 60-year-old woman with primary biliary cholangitis (PBC), two years post-liver transplant, suffers a low-impact femur fracture. Given PBC's link to osteoporosis, which statement best describes their relationship and post-transplant care?
a) PBC-related osteoporosis stems from increased bone resorption, best treated with bisphosphonates
b) Osteoporosis risk is lower in PBC patients post-transplant than those awaiting transplant
c) PBC-related osteoporosis results mainly from reduced bone formation, not increased resorption
d) Calcium and vitamin D alone suffice for osteoporosis management in PBC post-transplant patients
e) No specific osteoporosis treatment is supported for PBC patients post-transplant due to unclear causation

**Answer: c**

In PBC, osteoporosis primarily arises from decreased bone formation rather than increased resorption, unlike postmenopausal osteoporosis. Treatments like denosumab are more suitable than bisphosphonates or calcium/vitamin D alone, emphasizing tailored post-transplant care.[44]

64. A 45-year-old man with a 10-year history of ulcerative colitis presents with fatigue, pruritus, and intermittent jaundice for 6 months. Examination shows scleral icterus and scratch marks. Labs indicate elevated ALP and bilirubin. MRCP reveals irregularities and strictures in intrahepatic and extrahepatic bile ducts. What is the most likely diagnosis?
a) Primary sclerosing cholangitis
b) Secondary sclerosing cholangitis from biliary obstruction
c) Cholangiocarcinoma
d) Autoimmune hepatitis
e) Primary biliary cholangitis

**Answer: a**

Primary sclerosing cholangitis (PSC) is a chronic cholestatic liver disease marked by inflammation and fibrosis of intrahepatic and extrahepatic bile ducts. Its strong association with inflammatory bowel disease, particularly ulcerative colitis (prevalence ~70% in PSC), supports the diagnosis in this patient with compatible clinical, laboratory, and imaging findings.[45]

65. Based on the current understanding of the disease's epidemiology, which of the following statements is true regarding primary biliary cholangitis (PBC)?
a) Both incidence and prevalence of PBC are distributed equally geographically
b) PBC is predominantly diagnosed in men, with a male-to-female ratio of 9:1
c) The incidence of PBC increases with age, particularly peaking between 60 and 79 years
d) Over the past 20 years, the female-to-male ratio for PBC has remained constant at 9:1
e) Men with PBC exhibit milder stages of liver disease at the time of diagnosis compared to women

**Answer: c**

Both incidence and prevalence of PBC vary geographically. The disease is predominant in women, and the incidence increases with age, reaching its peak at age 60–79 years. Although the incidence and prevalence remain higher in women than in men, the female-to-male ratio has gradually decreased from 9:1 to 4:1 over the past 20 years. Compared with women, men with primary biliary cholangitis have more advanced stages of liver disease at diagnosis, an increased incidence of HCC, and a worse prognosis.[46]

66. Which statement best reflects the current evidence on medical therapies, including ursodeoxycholic acid (UDCA), for primary sclerosing cholangitis (PSC)?
a) UDCA significantly reduces mortality in PSC
b) UDCA improves symptoms and quality of life in PSC
c) Corticosteroids are effective to slow down PSC progression
d) Corticosteroids significantly reduce mortality in PSC
e) UDCA and immunosuppressants lack clear benefits for PSC outcomes

**Answer: e**

Current evidence shows that UDCA and immunosuppressive therapies do not significantly improve mortality, symptoms, disease progression, or quality of life in PSC. While UDCA may improve liver biochemistry, it lacks impact on clinical outcomes. Corticosteroids are generally ineffective outside overlap syndromes, and liver transplantation remains the main option for advanced PSC.[47]

67. A 57-year-old man with primary sclerosing cholangitis (PSC), cirrhosis (MELD 32), and listed for liver transplantation presents with cholangitis. MRCP shows a 1.5 mm dominant stricture in the common bile duct. What is the most appropriate next step in management?
a) Start IV antibiotics and plan percutaneous biliary drainage
b) Initiate IV antibiotics and supportive care
c) Initiate IV antibiotics and perform ERCP with brush cytology or biopsy

d) Initiate IV antibiotics, perform ERCP with stent placement, and pause transplant listing until cholangitis resolves
e) Initiate IV antibiotics, corticosteroids and high-dose ursodeoxycholic acid
**Answer: c**
In PSC patients with a dominant stricture, cholangiocarcinoma is a concern. Initiating IV antibiotics for cholangitis is critical, but ERCP with brush cytology or biopsy is essential to evaluate for malignancy before interventions like dilation or stenting.[48]

68. A 39-year-old male with a history of primary sclerosing cholangitis (PSC) underwent a successful liver transplantation two years ago. He now presents with new-onset colonic symptoms, including abdominal pain, bloating, and intermittent bloody diarrhea. An infectious workup is negative, including tests for CMV and EBV. Colonoscopy showed diffuse erythema, friable mucosa, numerous small ulcers, and pseudopolyps in a continuous pattern involving rectum. What is the most likely diagnosis?
a) Crohn's disease
b) Ischemic colitis
c) Ulcerative colitis
d) Neutropenic colitis (typhlitis)
e) Infectious colitis
**Answer: c**
It is now recognized that the onset of inflammatory bowel disease (IBD) can occur years after the diagnosis of PSC, and de novo IBD may present after liver transplantation. The colonoscopy findings of continuous mucosal inflammation, ulcers, and pseudopolyps are characteristic of ulcerative colitis, particularly in this context.[49]

69. A 36-year-old female patient with primary sclerosing cholangitis (PSC) presents with MRCP findings of hilar cholangiocarcinoma primarily involving the left hepatic duct. Her laboratory results show a platelet count of 94,000 /μL and bilirubin level of 9 mg/dL. What is the most appropriate management strategy for this patient condition?
a) Neoadjuvant chemotherapy and radiation therapy followed by surgical resection of the tumor
b) Liver transplant followed by adjuvant chemotherapy and radiation therapy
c) Neoadjuvant chemoirradiation followed by liver transplantation
d) Best supportive care with palliative measures, including biliary drain
e) Surgical resection followed by adjuvant chemoirradiation
**Answer: c**

If cholangiocarcinoma is diagnosed, surgical resection is frequently unfeasible in the context of PSC, especially in advanced stages of the disease. Chemotherapy options usually yield poor outcomes; however, transplantation has proven to be lifesaving for carefully selected patients.[50]

70. A 42-year-old man with primary sclerosing cholangitis (PSC) is undergoing liver transplantation. The extrahepatic bile duct appears disease-free and is long enough for anastomosis. What is the best surgical approach?
a) Resect bile duct near hilum, check margins for dysplasia; if negative, do duct-to-duct anastomosis
b) Resect bile duct near duodenum, check margins for dysplasia; if negative, do Roux-en-Y choledochojejunostomy
c) Inspect bile duct; if clear, plan duct-to-duct anastomosis and review explanted liver pathology
d) Inspect bile duct; if clear, plan Roux-en-Y choledochojejunostomy and review explanted liver pathology
e) Resect bile duct near hilum, check margins and portocaval lymph nodes for dysplasia; if malignant, plan liver transplant with Whipple procedure
**Answer: a**
The most appropriate approach is to ensure that any undetected dysplastic or malignant changes can be identified before finalizing the biliary reconstruction. By resecting the bile duct proximal to the hilum and obtaining margins for pathology, the surgical team can make informed decisions based on the biopsy results. If the margins are negative for dysplasia or malignancy, duct-to-duct anastomosis is a suitable method for biliary reconstruction, despite the PSC diagnosis, preserving the natural flow of bile and minimizing complications associated with alternative biliary drainage methods.[51]

71. What is the recurrence rate of primary sclerosing cholangitis after liver transplant in 10 years?
a) Up to 5%
b) Up to 15%
c) Up to 30%
d) Up to 60%
e) Up to 80%
**Answer: c**
The 10-year recurrence rate of PSC after liver transplantation is approximately 20–47%, with most studies suggesting a range of 20–30% in adult populations and potentially higher rates (up to 47%) in pediatric or living donor cohorts. Recurrence

is diagnosed in most individuals within 5 years after transplantation, presenting with symptoms identical to those of the primary disease.[52]

72. A 45-year-old male underwent liver transplantation due to primary sclerosing cholangitis (PSC) complicated by hilar cholangiocarcinoma (CCA) primarily affecting the right hepatic duct. The patient received neoadjuvant chemoradiation therapy, and his CA 19-9 level decreased from 192 U/mL to 40 U/mL. Histopathological examination of the explant revealed the presence of a residual viable tumor within the liver, but the surgical margins were free of malignancy. Recent studies have identified statistically significant predictors of recurrence of CCA following transplantation. What is the patient's most significant risk factor for recurrence?
a) CA 19-9 level of 36 U/mL
b) Presence of residual tumor in the explant liver
c) Age greater than 40
d) Male gender
e) Associated diagnosis of PSC

**Answer: b**
A recent analysis of predictors of recurrence of CCA post-transplantation found a statistically significant association with the presence of a residual tumor in the explant liver, elevated CA 19-9 levels, and portal vein encasement. In this case, the presence of residual tumor is the most critical risk factor for recurrence. Patients with PSC do not have an independent survival advantage over those with de novo tumors but may present with more favorable tumor characteristics.[53]

73. A 53-year-old male underwent liver transplantation for primary sclerosing cholangitis (PSC). The liver graft was obtained from a DBD donor with a cold ischemia time of 5.5 hours. The patient initially recovered well after surgery; however, two months post-operatively, he exhibited elevated bilirubin and ALP levels. A cholangiogram revealed a significant reduction in the number of bile ducts with strictures in the remaining bile ducts, while a triple-phase CT scan demonstrated patent vasculature. Additionally, a liver biopsy showed fibro-obliterative bile duct changes. What is the most likely etiology of these findings?
a) Chronic ductopenic rejection
b) Recurrent PSC
c) Biliary anastomotic stricture
d) Arterial insufficiency
e) Prolonged ischemia time

**Answer: a**
In this case, the presence of fibro-obliterative bile duct changes occurring two months after transplantation is highly suggestive of chronic or ductopenic rejection. Unlike

recurrent PSC, which typically presents later, chronic rejection can cause similar bile duct changes in a shorter time frame and is associated with significant morbidity and mortality for the patient.[54]

74. Which of the following factors is associated with an increased risk of PSC recurrence after liver transplantation?
a) Prolonged cold ischemia time
b) CMV infections
c) Donor-recipient gender mismatch
d) Presence of inflammatory bowel disease
e) Positive lymphocytotoxic crossmatches
**Answer: d**
Recent studies indicate that unlike other potential factors such as cold ischemia time, preservation solutions, and infections, which did not show a significant association with recurrence, inflammatory bowel disease appears to increase the risk of PSC recurrence in liver transplant patients.[55]

75. A 28-year-old female with a BMI of 32 and a past medical history significant for rheumatoid arthritis presents to the clinic with fatigue, jaundice, and right upper quadrant pain. Laboratory tests reveal abnormal LFT, hyperbilirubinemia, and positive antinuclear antibodies and smooth muscle antibodies. A liver biopsy shows interface hepatitis with a predominantly lymphoplasmacytic necroinflammatory infiltrate. Based on these findings, what is the most likely diagnosis for this patient?
a) Primary biliary cholangitis
b) Drug-induced liver injury
c) Autoimmune hepatitis
d) Nonspecific hepatitis
e) Primary sclerosing cholangitis
**Answer: c**
The clinical presentation of fatigue, jaundice, abnormal LFT, and a liver biopsy showing interface hepatitis with lymphocytic infiltration is consistent with autoimmune hepatitis, particularly in a young female patient.[56]

76. Which of the following factors is most likely associated with an increased risk of chronic rejection in patients transplanted for autoimmune hepatitis (AIH)?
a) Advanced age at transplantation
b) Presence of underlying alcoholic liver disease
c) Mild acute rejection on liver biopsy
d) Young age at transplantation
e) History of diabetes

**Answer: d**
Patients transplanted for AIH are predisposed to developing chronic rejection, and significant risk factors identified include young age at transplantation and the occurrence of moderate to severe acute rejection on liver biopsy.[57]

77. A 45-year-old female with no significant past medical history presents to the emergency department with abdominal pain and mild jaundice. The CT scan reveals a well-circumscribed hypervascular lesion in the right lobe of the liver, demonstrating a characteristic "light bulb" appearance due to early arterial enhancement followed by progressive centripetal fill-in of contrast, ultimately leading to a hypodense center. No associated lymphadenopathy or portal vein thrombosis is evident. Based on these findings, which of the following is the most likely diagnosis?
a) Cavernous hemangiomas
b) Focal nodular hyperplasia
c) Hepatic adenoma
d) Focal fatty infiltration
e) HCC

**Answer: a**
The described CT findings—specifically the well-circumscribed hypervascular lesion with characteristic early arterial enhancement and progressive centripetal fill-in—are consistent with cavernous hemangiomas, which are the most common benign vascular tumors of the liver.[58]

78. A 30-year-old female patient with a history of oral contraceptive use presents for evaluation of incidental liver lesions noted during a routine abdominal ultrasound. The CT scan revealing a well-defined, hypervascular mass in the right lobe of the liver measuring 6 cm. The mass shows homogeneous enhancement during the arterial phase and demonstrates washout of contrast in the venous phase. Additionally, the lesion does not exhibit significant surrounding edema or any associated biliary obstruction. Based on these radiological findings, what is the most likely diagnosis?
a) Cavernous hemangiomas
b) Focal nodular hyperplasia
c) Hepatic adenoma
d) Focal fatty infiltration
e) HCC

**Answer: c**
The combination of a well-defined, hypervascular mass that shows homogeneous enhancement during the arterial phase and washout in the venous phase, along with the patient's history of oral contraceptive use, is characteristic of hepatic adenoma, particularly in women. Unlike other hepatic lesions, hepatic adenomas typically exhibit

this pattern without the complications of notable surrounding edema or biliary obstruction.[58]

79. A 62-year-old male with a history of chronic hepatitis C cirrhosis presents with unexplained weight loss and fatigue. The CT scan revealed a 5 cm mass in the right lobe of the liver. The lesion appears heterogeneous, with both hypervascular and hypodense areas. During the arterial phase, the mass demonstrates intense enhancement, which significantly washes out in the portal venous phase, leaving a hypodense appearance. There is surrounding hepatic parenchymal atrophy and mild portal vein thrombosis. Based on these findings, what is the most likely diagnosis?
a) Cavernous hemangiomas
b) Focal nodular hyperplasia
c) Hepatic adenoma
d) Focal fatty infiltration
e) HCC
**Answer: e**
The described CT scan findings—a heterogeneous liver mass with intense arterial phase enhancement and significant washout in the portal venous phase, along with the patient's history of cirrhosis and hepatitis C—are characteristic of HCC. The surrounding parenchymal atrophy and portal vein thrombosis further support the diagnosis of HCC in the context of chronic liver disease.[58]

80. A 40-year-old female patient with a history of oral contraceptive use presents for evaluation of incidental liver lesions noted during a routine abdominal ultrasound. The CT scan revealed a well-defined, hypervascular mass in the left lobe of the liver measuring 4 cm. The lesion exhibits a "central scar" appearance with an accompanying spoke-wheel pattern of peripheral enhancement during the arterial phase. Based on these radiological findings, what is the most likely diagnosis?
a) Cavernous hemangiomas
b) Focal nodular hyperplasia
c) Hepatic adenoma
d) Focal fatty infiltration
e) HCC
**Answer: b**
The CT scan findings—specifically, a well-defined hypervascular mass with a central scar and a spoke-wheel pattern of enhancement—are characteristic of focal nodular hyperplasia.[58]

81. A 70-year-old Asian male with chronic hepatitis B liver cirrhosis presents with localized right upper quadrant abdominal pain, sometimes radiating to the right

shoulder, postprandial fullness, and worsening jaundice. Blood work is significant for a platelet count of 92,000/μL, elevated liver enzymes, and hyperbilirubinemia. The CT scan shows a heterogeneous liver mass in segment 5 measuring 4.2 cm in size, with intense arterial phase enhancement and significant washout in the portal venous phase. AFP is 859 ng/mL. There are no signs of metastatic disease. What is the next step in management?
a) Transjugular biopsy
b) Percutaneous liver biopsy
c) Evaluation for liver transplant
d) Start treatment with sorafenib
e) Surgical resection

**Answer: c**
In this case, the findings are consistent with HCC in the context of chronic hepatitis B and liver cirrhosis. Specifically, the tumor is 4.2 cm in size and the patient has elevated AFP levels (859 ng/mL), which, combined with his cirrhotic background, indicate he may meet criteria for liver transplantation.[59]

82. Routine percutaneous biopsy of lesions suspicious for HCC in patients with liver cirrhosis is generally avoided due to the risk of parietal tumor seeding and bleeding, given HCC's high vascularity. What is the estimated risk of parietal tumor seeding?
a) 0.1% to 0.5%
b) <1%
c) 1% to 5%
d) 5% to 10%
e) Up to 20%

**Answer: c**
The risk of parietal tumor seeding is approximately 1% to 5%, with metastases typically appearing around 17 months post-biopsy and often being challenging to treat.[60]

83. A 70-year-old Asian male with chronic hepatitis B and associated liver disease presents with localized right upper quadrant abdominal pain, sometimes radiating to the right shoulder, and postprandial fullness. Blood work shows a platelet count of 143,000/μL and slightly abnormal LFT. The CT scan reveals a heterogeneous liver mass in segment 2 measuring 3.2 cm, with intense arterial phase enhancement and significant washout in the portal venous phase. There are no signs of portal hypertension on the CT scan. AFP is 780 ng/mL. There are no signs of metastatic disease. What is the next step in management?
a) Transjugular biopsy
b) Transarterial chemoembolization

c) Evaluation for liver transplant
d) Radiofrequency ablation
e) Surgical resection
**Answer: e**
The patient's 3.2 cm liver mass, elevated AFP, and imaging suggest HCC. With no metastatic disease, well-compensated liver disease, and a platelet count above 100,000/µL, surgical resection (left lateral lobectomy) is appropriate. Transplantation would be considered for impaired liver function or multiple lesions.[61]

84. A 71-year-old Asian male with chronic hepatitis B and liver cirrhosis presents with right upper quadrant pain, occasional shoulder radiation, postprandial fullness, and worsening jaundice. Labs show a platelet count of 84,000/µL, elevated liver enzymes, and hyperbilirubinemia. The CT scan reveals a 2.8 cm mass in segment V (LI-RADS 5) and a 1.8 cm mass in segment VI (LI-RADS 4). AFP is 1394 ng/mL. No metastatic disease is noted. What is the next appropriate step in management?
a) Transjugular biopsy of segment VI lesion and locoregional therapy for segment V lesion
b) Surgical resection of segment V lesion and intraoperative biopsy of segment VI lesion
c) Evaluation for liver transplantation and locoregional therapy for both lesions
d) Locoregional therapy for both lesions
e) Chemotherapy with sorafenib
**Answer: c**
Given the multifocal HCC, advanced cirrhosis, and compromised liver function (low platelets, jaundice), surgical resection may not be tolerated. Evaluation for liver transplantation with locoregional therapy to manage both lesions is optimal.[62]

85. A 74-year-old Asian male with chronic hepatitis B, liver cirrhosis, and prior myocardial infarction presents with right upper quadrant pain, shoulder radiation, postprandial fullness, and worsening jaundice and hepatic encephalopathy. He has an ejection fraction of 28%, 70% stenosis of the left anterior descending artery (no revascularization possible), platelet count of 34,000/µL, elevated liver enzymes, hyperbilirubinemia, and a MELD score of 38. The CT scan shows a 4.5 cm mass in segment VIII, suggestive of HCC, with no metastases. AFP is 2130 ng/mL. What is the next appropriate step in management?
a) Transjugular biopsy
b) Locoregional therapy
c) Evaluation for liver transplantation
d) Surgical resection
e) Goals of care discussion and palliative therapy

**Answer: e**
Due to the patient's decompensated liver disease, poor cardiac function, and significant comorbidities, invasive treatments like transplantation, resection, or locoregional therapy are not feasible. A goals of care discussion and palliative therapy are most appropriate to align with the patient's needs and focus on symptom management.[62]

86. A 53-year-old male with end-stage liver disease due to alcohol use is listed for liver transplantation (MELD score 28). A routine liver ultrasound reveals a 1.8 cm mass in the left lobe, classified as LI-RADS 5 on abdominal CT scan. His AFP and CA 19-9 levels are normal. What is the next step in management?
a) Chest X-ray and bone scan
b) CT scan of chest, pelvis, and bone scan
c) CT scan of chest, pelvis, and liver biopsy
d) Chest X-ray and liver biopsy
e) PET scan and bone scan
**Answer: b**
For suspected HCC, extrahepatic staging is required with a CT scan of the chest, abdomen, and pelvis, plus a bone scan to rule out metastasis before transplantation.[63]

87. Which statement accurately describes the Milan criteria for transplant eligibility?
a) Up to three tumors, none larger than 5 cm, or a single tumor up to 7 cm, with no vascular invasion or metastasis
b) A single tumor up to 5 cm or up to three tumors, each up to 3 cm, with no vascular invasion or metastasis
c) Up to five tumors, each up to 3 cm, with no vascular invasion or metastasis
d) A single tumor up to 6 cm or up to two tumors, each up to 4 cm, with no vascular invasion or metastasis
e) Any number of tumors, each up to 3 cm, with no vascular invasion or metastasis
**Answer: b**
The Milan criteria for liver transplantation in HCC are a single tumor ≤5 cm or up to three tumors, each ≤3 cm, with no vascular invasion or extrahepatic metastasis.[64]

88. A 62-year-old female with a history of MASH and compensated cirrhosis is being evaluated for liver transplantation due to a diagnosis of HCC. Imaging reveals three tumors: two in the right lobe measuring 5.2 cm and 3.0 cm in diameter, and a third tumor in segment IV measuring 1.5 cm in diameter. Based on the University of California, San Francisco (UCSF) criteria for liver transplantation, which of the following statements regarding her eligibility is correct?

a) She is eligible for liver transplantation because the largest tumor is less than 6.5 cm
b) She is ineligible for liver transplantation because the total diameter of all tumors exceeds 8 cm
c) She is ineligible for liver transplantation because she has three tumors, with one of them larger than 5.0 cm
d) She is eligible for liver transplantation because the largest tumor is less than 6.5 cm, and the total diameter exceeds 10 cm
e) She is ineligible for liver transplantation due to multifocal disease
**Answer: b**
According to UCSF criteria, liver transplantation is an option for patients with either a single tumor ≤6.5 cm, or up to three tumors with the largest ≤4.5 cm and a total tumor diameter ≤8 cm. This patient has three tumors with a total diameter of 5.2 + 3.0 + 1.5 = 9.7 cm, which exceeds the UCSF limit for multiple tumors, making her ineligible.[65]

89. A 67-year-old Asian male with chronic hepatitis B and cirrhosis undergoes a routine ultrasound, which reveals two HCC lesions: one measuring 4 cm in segment II and another measuring 4.5 cm in segment VII. His MELD score is 24. The diagnosis is confirmed, and metastatic workup is negative. What is the next best step in management?
a) Initiate chemotherapy with sorafenib
b) Proceed with transplant listing and locoregional therapy
c) Surgical resection of the left lobe lesion, locoregional therapy for the right, consider transplant on recurrence
d) Locoregional therapy followed by immune-targeted therapy
e) Recommend palliative therapy due to cirrhosis and advanced cancer
**Answer: b**
The goal is to control tumor growth with locoregional therapy while evaluating for transplant. This strategy can also downstage tumors to meet transplant criteria and avoid disease progression.[66]

90. A 38-year-old female with a history of primary sclerosing cholangitis and HCC, which was treated with radiofrequency ablation 7 months ago, presents for liver transplantation. During the initial exploration, an enlarged portacaval lymph node is noted. What is the next step in management?
a) Proceed with liver transplantation without further evaluation of the lymph node, as the liver is already allocated to the patient, and she has the best chance of survival with a transplant
b) Perform a biopsy of the enlarged portacaval lymph node for frozen section analysis, and abort the transplant if the lymph node is positive for cancer

c) Perform a biopsy of the enlarged portacaval lymph node for permanent analysis, proceed with the liver transplant, and schedule adjuvant therapy with sorafenib if the lymph node contains cancer cells
d) Perform a biopsy of the enlarged portacaval lymph node for permanent analysis, proceed with the liver transplant, and obtain staging CT scans of the chest, pelvis, and bones after the surgery
e) Perform a biopsy of the enlarged portacaval lymph node for permanent analysis, proceed with the liver transplant, minimize postoperative immunosuppression, and schedule adjuvant therapy with sorafenib if the lymph node contains cancer cells

**Answer: b**

If an enlarged lymph node is discovered during liver transplantation surgery, it is vital to perform a biopsy of the lymph node and assess it using frozen section analysis to evaluate for metastatic disease. If the biopsy reveals metastasis, the transplant should be aborted.[67]

91. A 63-year-old male is diagnosed with intrahepatic cholangiocarcinoma (iCCA) measuring 1.5 cm and located in segment V. His right liver volume is 70% to 75% of the total liver volume. He has a history of chronic liver disease that is currently well compensated. Which of the following treatment strategies is the best for this patient is correct?
a) Liver resection
b) Neoadjuvant locoregional therapy followed by liver resection
c) Neoadjuvant systemic chemotherapy followed by radiation
d) Liver transplant
e) Palliative therapy and goals of care

**Answer: d**

The management of iCCA is complex, and while liver resection is the standard treatment, patients like this 63-year-old male with very early iCCA (≤2 cm) and underlying chronic liver disease can be assessed for liver transplantation. This patient is not a surgical candidate for resection given the need for right hepatectomy, chronic liver disease, and insufficient left liver parenchymal volume.[68]

92. Cholangiocarcinoma (CCA) is categorized by its anatomical site in the biliary system. Which of the following statements accurately reflects the classification of CCA types based on their relative frequency?
a) Hilar cholangiocarcinoma (HCCA) is the least common, making up 10% to 15% of cases
b) Intrahepatic cholangiocarcinoma (ICCA) is the most frequent, comprising 50% to 60% of cases

c) Distal cholangiocarcinoma accounts for 40% to 50% of cases, surpassing other types in prevalence
d) Hilar cholangiocarcinoma (HCCA) is the most common, representing 50% to 60% of all cases
e) All CCA types have roughly equal prevalence, each contributing about 25% to 33% of cases

**Answer: d**

CCA is divided into types based on its location in the biliary tree. HCCA is the most common, accounting for 50% to 60% of cases. Distal cholangiocarcinoma represents 20% to 30%, and ICCA constitutes 10% to 20%.[69]

93. A 32-year-old male with a 10-year history of primary sclerosing cholangitis (PSC) presents with progressive jaundice, weight loss, and pruritus over the past two months. Laboratory results show elevated bilirubin (4.5 mg/dL) and ALP (350 IU/L). The CT scan reveals no intrahepatic lesions but shows left-sided hepatic atrophy and dilated intrahepatic bile ducts, raising concern for possible portal vein compromise or biliary obstruction. What is the most appropriate next step in the diagnostic workup?
a) Order serum tumor markers and perform MRCP
b) Order serum tumor markers and arrange a staging CT of the chest, abdomen, and pelvis
c) Schedule an ERCP with brush cytology
d) Repeat the abdominal CT scan in 3 months to monitor for interval changes
e) Perform an ultrasound-guided liver biopsy to evaluate for malignancy

**Answer: a**

In this patient with PSC, progressive jaundice, and imaging findings suggestive of biliary obstruction or vascular compromise (e.g., left-sided hepatic atrophy), the priority is to evaluate for cholangiocarcinoma, a known complication of PSC. Serum tumor markers such as CA 19-9 and CEA can provide supportive evidence, though they lack specificity. MRCP is the most appropriate next imaging modality, as it non-invasively visualizes the biliary tree and vascular structures, helping to identify strictures, bile duct dilation, or tumor-related encasement. This guides further management, such as ERCP for tissue sampling or surgical planning.[70]

94. A 55-year-old woman presents with a 6 cm sigmoid colon cancer causing intermittent abdominal pain and constipation. The CT scan reveals three liver lesions and enlarged para-aortic lymph nodes, with no chest metastases. PET scan is inconclusive for nodal involvement. At a tumor board, the liver metastases are deemed non-resectable due to proximity to major hilar vessels. What is the most appropriate next step in management?
a) Resect colon tumor and start adjuvant chemotherapy

b) Start neoadjuvant chemotherapy, then resect colon tumor
c) Resect colon tumor and sample para-aortic lymph nodes
d) Resect colon tumor and ablate liver lesions
e) Perform diverting ostomy and start chemotherapy
**Answer: c**
In this patient with symptomatic sigmoid colon cancer and non-resectable liver metastases, resecting the primary tumor addresses obstructive symptoms. Sampling enlarged para-aortic lymph nodes is critical, as positive nodes would contraindicate liver transplantation due to systemic disease. If nodes are negative, further systemic therapy could assess tumor biology for transplant candidacy.[71]

95. A 73-year-old woman is diagnosed with sigmoid colon cancer and two metastatic lesions in the right posterior liver segment. A CT scan of the chest shows no lung metastases, and a PET scan confirms the primary tumor and liver lesions. She has well-controlled diabetes and stage 2 chronic kidney disease, with normal LFT. What is the most appropriate treatment approach?
a) Resect the sigmoid colon and liver lesions, then start adjuvant chemotherapy
b) Start neoadjuvant chemotherapy, restage with CT, and if negative, proceed with sigmoid colon and liver resection
c) Perform sigmoid colon resection, followed by chemotherapy and then liver resection
d) Start chemotherapy, restage with CT, and if negative, proceed with colon resection and liver ablation
e) Perform a diverting ostomy and start palliative chemotherapy
**Answer: b**
For this patient with metastatic sigmoid colon cancer and resectable liver metastases, upfront chemotherapy helps reduce tumor burden and assess disease biology. Restaging with CT after chemotherapy guides surgical planning. If the disease remains resectable, resection of the sigmoid colon and liver lesions offers the best chance for complete tumor clearance.[71]

96. In patients with non-resectable colorectal liver metastases, which tumor characteristics are associated with poor survival outcomes and contraindicate eligibility for liver transplantation?
a) Well-differentiated adenocarcinoma
b) Poorly differentiated adenocarcinoma
c) Mucinous adenocarcinoma
d) Signet ring cell carcinoma
e) Extensive lymph node involvement
**Answer: d**

Patients with undifferentiated adenocarcinoma or signet ring cell carcinoma should not be considered for liver transplantation due to poor survival outcomes. Extensive lymph node involvement also indicates a worse prognosis after resection, though its impact may lessen if there's no recurrence over time in cases of late metachronous disease.[72,73]

97. A 62-year-old male patient was diagnosed with partially obstructing right-sided colon cancer, specifically moderately differentiated adenocarcinoma, along with synchronous non-resectable liver metastases. The patient received chemotherapy and subsequently underwent colon resection. A follow-up PET CT scan four months after the colon resection revealed progression of the liver tumor, with no additional metastases identified. Despite undergoing three lines of chemotherapy, a repeat PET scan conducted six months after the initial resection showed continued progression of the liver tumor. What is the next step in the management of this patient?
a) Evaluate the patient for liver transplantation
b) Perform a repeat colonoscopy to assess for recurrence of the primary tumor
c) Modify chemotherapy based on tumor biology and evaluate for a locoregional liver therapy
d) Initiate immunotherapy as a bridge to potential liver transplantation
e) Proceed with liver transplantation followed by immunotherapy
**Answer: c**
The response to any bridging therapy should be monitored for a minimum of six months, and the observation of progressive disease following more than three chemotherapy regimens indicates an aggressive tumor biology that is generally not suitable for consideration of liver transplantation.[71]

98. A 54-year-old male with a history of colon cancer, previously treated with primary colon resection and liver transplantation for non-resectable metastatic disease, presents with a newly identified 8 mm solitary lung lesion on CT imaging. The lesion is suspicious for metastasis but not yet confirmed. What is the most appropriate next step in managing this patient's lung lesion?
a) Initiate systemic chemotherapy to target potential metastatic disease
b) Monitor the lung lesion with serial imaging to assess growth and resectability
c) Proceed with surgical resection of the lung lesion to confirm diagnosis
d) Start radiotherapy to the lung lesion to control local disease
e) Perform a biopsy of the lung lesion to establish a pathological diagnosis
**Answer: b**
Given the potentially slow-growing nature of pulmonary metastases from colon cancer and the opportunity for successful surgical management of isolated lung

metastases, monitoring the lesion with serial imaging to evaluate its growth and suitability for resection is the most appropriate next step.[71]

99. Which of the following criteria is not included in the Milan criteria for assessing eligibility for liver transplantation in patients with metastatic neuroendocrine tumors confined to the liver?
a) Histological confirmation of high-grade neuroendocrine tumor, including small cell carcinoma
b) Complete removal of the primary tumor drained by the portal system
c) Metastatic diffusion to liver parenchyma ≤ 50%
d) Good response or stable disease for at least 6 months during the pretransplantation evaluation period
e) Age ≤ 55 years
**Answer: a**
High-grade neuroendocrine carcinomas, including small cell carcinoma, are considered contraindications for transplantation due to their aggressive behavior and poorer prognosis. These tumors tend to have a higher likelihood of extrahepatic spread and significantly less favorable outcomes following transplantation.[74]

100. A 42-year-old man presents with progressive neuropathy and gastrointestinal symptoms. Genetic testing confirms a transthyretin (TTR) gene mutation, diagnosing familial amyloid polyneuropathy (FAP). He undergoes liver transplantation. Which statement best describes the effects of TTR mutations and the role of liver transplantation in managing FAP?
a) TTR mutations decrease TTR protein solubility, causing amyloid fiber deposits in tissues like nerves and the heart
b) Liver transplantation stops amyloidogenic TTR production, fully reversing neuropathy in all patients
c) Most patients with TTR mutations show amyloidosis symptoms before age 30
d) After liver transplantation, approximately 95% of plasma TTR is wild-type TTR
e) Cardiovascular complications after transplantation are rare, with most patients fully recovering cardiac function
**Answer: d**
FAP, caused by TTR gene mutations such as V30M, follows an autosomal dominant pattern. These mutations lead to amyloid fiber deposition in tissues, causing symptoms like neuropathy and gastrointestinal issues. Liver transplantation replaces the liver producing mutant TTR with one producing mostly wild-type TTR, resulting in about 95% wild-type TTR in plasma. This reduces further amyloid formation, often improving symptoms, though not always completely. Ongoing monitoring for

cardiovascular complications, such as arrhythmias, is necessary, as these can persist post-transplant.[75,76]

101. A 54-year-old man with a history of Budd-Chiari syndrome and liver failure, confirmed to have a JAK2 mutation, presented with portal and hepatic vein thrombosis on CT scan. While on anticoagulation therapy, he experienced severe gastrointestinal bleeding. He underwent a successful liver transplant and portal vein thrombectomy. What is the most appropriate postoperative management strategy for this patient?
a) Start long-term anticoagulation therapy only if portal vein thrombosis recurs
b) Begin anticoagulation therapy and aspirin one week after liver transplant
c) Discontinue all anticoagulation therapy post-transplant, as the liver transplant resolves the thrombotic condition
d) Start anticoagulation therapy when the platelet count exceeds $100,000/\mu L$
e) Administer aspirin alone as immediate antiplatelet therapy, avoiding anticoagulation
**Answer: b**
Postoperatively the patient does not require immediate anticoagulation because recurrent disease thromboses do not occur during the first postoperative week. Despite the risk of severe postoperative bleeding, anticoagulation is crucial for preventing further thrombotic complications after liver transplantation. It is important to note that thrombophilia related to the JAK2 mutation is not corrected by liver transplantation. In contrast, conditions such as protein C deficiency, protein S deficiency, or prothrombin gene mutation can be ameliorated by the transplantation of a liver that synthesizes these coagulation factors normally.[77]

102. A 54-year-old man with Budd-Chiari syndrome, liver failure, and a JAK2 mutation has portal vein thrombosis and suprahepatic vena cava obstruction on CT. During liver transplant surgery, an organized thrombus completely obstructs the suprahepatic vena cava, preventing thrombectomy. What is the next step?
a) Incise the diaphragm, expose the pericardium, and anastomose the hepatic veins to the intrapericardial IVC using veno-venous bypass
b) Consult cardiothoracic surgery for a sternotomy, split the diaphragm, and anastomose the hepatic veins to the right atrium using veno-venous bypass
c) In an emergency setting, perform a sternotomy, split the diaphragm, and anastomose the hepatic veins to the right atrium using veno-venous bypass
d) Perform a sternotomy, access the thoracic IVC, place a vascular clamp higher, and attempt thrombectomy again
e) Abort the transplant, as it is not feasible
**Answer: a**

For suprahepatic vena cava obstruction caused by an organized thrombus, anastomosing the hepatic veins to the intrapericardial IVC through a diaphragmatic incision with veno-venous bypass is a safe and effective approach.[78]

103. A 45-year-old female patient with a history of obesity underwent Roux-en-Y gastric bypass surgery to facilitate weight reduction. Post-operatively, she exhibited marked improvements in metabolic parameters, including complete resolution of metabolic-associated steatotic liver disease (MASLD). During subsequent follow-up evaluations, she reported escalating alcohol consumption and received a diagnosis of alcohol use disorder (AUD). Considering the physiological alterations induced by her bariatric surgery, which of the following represents the most likely risk to her hepatic health?
a) Increased probability of MASLD recurrence due to the high caloric content of alcohol
b) A 2- to 3-fold elevated risk of alcohol-associated liver disease (ALD), including acute alcoholic hepatitis, attributable to altered alcohol metabolism following gastric bypass surgery
c) Reduced hepatic exposure to alcohol due to accelerated elimination from the intestinal lumen secondary to digestive system modifications
d) Decreased likelihood of progression to cirrhosis resulting from significant weight loss achieved through bariatric surgery
e) Enhanced hepatic alcohol metabolism due to prior history of steatotic liver disease, reducing susceptibility to alcohol-related liver injury
**Answer: b**
Roux-en-Y gastric bypass surgery alters the digestive tract, leading to faster alcohol absorption and impaired metabolism, which increases the risk of ALD, including acute hepatitis, by 2- to 3-fold in patients who develop AUD. This heightened risk is due to changes in gastric anatomy and liver processing of alcohol, not caloric intake or recurrence of MASLD.[79,80]

104. Which medication is contraindicated for patients with alcohol-induced liver disease?
a) Acamprosate
b) Disulfiram
c) Gabapentin
d) Naltrexone
e) Topiramate
**Answer: b**

Although disulfiram is approved by the US FDA for the treatment of alcohol use disorder, it is contraindicated for individuals with any degree of liver disease due to its complete metabolism in the liver and its potential hepatotoxic effects.[81]

105. A 52-year-old male with a long history of chronic alcohol consumption presents to the emergency department with confusion, ataxia, and ophthalmoplegia. His family reports that he has been increasingly forgetful and has shown signs of disorientation over the past few weeks. As you consider his differential diagnosis, which condition would most likely account for the acute onset of neurological symptoms?
a) Hepatic encephalopathy
b) Delirium
c) Dementia
d) Sundowning
e) Wernicke's encephalopathy
**Answer: e**
Wernicke's encephalopathy is characterized by a classic triad of symptoms: confusion, ataxia, and ophthalmoplegia, and is most commonly caused by thiamine (vitamin B1) deficiency, often seen in individuals with chronic alcohol use. Wernicke's encephalopathy has a more acute onset of specific neurological signs, identifying the distinct clinical features of Wernicke's encephalopathy is essential for prompt treatment and prevention of progression to Korsakoff syndrome.[82]

106. In the United States, liver transplantation candidates undergo a rigorous multidisciplinary evaluation, integrating clinical, psychological, and psychosocial assessments, with findings presented to the transplant selection committee for review. Which of the following factors is most strongly associated with an elevated risk of relapse to alcohol use following liver transplantation in patients with a history of alcohol use disorder?
a) Critical illness necessitating mechanical ventilation during transplant evaluation
b) Male sex
c) Large extended family with multiple dependents
d) Resumption of a high-stress occupation post-transplantation
e) Absence of structured relapse prevention counseling
**Answer: a**
Critical illness requiring mechanical ventilation during evaluation limits a patient's ability to engage in addiction-focused interventions, increasing the likelihood of relapse to alcohol use post-transplantation. Factors such as male sex, family size, or occupational stress are less consistently associated with relapse risk, while the absence of relapse prevention counseling, though impactful, is not as directly prohibitive as acute critical illness.[83]

107. What is the recidivism rate for alcohol consumption after liver transplantation in patients with alcohol-induced liver disease (ALD)?
a) 5% to 10%
b) 10% to 15%
c) 20% to 25%
d) 45% to 55%
e) 65% to 80%
Answer: c
The recidivism rate for alcohol consumption after liver transplantation in patients with ALD is approximately 20% to 25%.[84]

108. Obesity is linked to several metabolic effects that are significant in the development of hepatic steatosis. These effects include all of the following except:
a) Increased absolute hepatic free fatty acid uptake
b) Increased esterification of hepatic free fatty acids to form triglycerides
c) Increased free fatty acid synthesis from cytosolic substrates
d) Increased apolipoprotein B-100 synthesis
e) Increased beta-oxidation of mitochondrial long-chain fatty acids
Answer: d
There is a decrease in apolipoprotein B-100 synthesis, which adversely affects the export of free fatty acids and triglycerides from the liver. Additionally, there is decreased hydrolysis of triglycerides and reduced export of hepatic triglycerides and free fatty acids. While the exact contribution of these mechanisms to fat accumulation in hepatocytes remains unclear, it is expected that these processes may become more pronounced following liver transplantation.[85]

109. What is the observed pattern of fibrosis progression in patients with recurrent metabolic-associated steatohepatitis MASH compared to those with de novo non-alcoholic fatty liver disease (NAFLD) following liver transplantation?
a) Patients with de novo NAFLD have a significantly higher risk of progressing to advanced fibrosis (≥F3 stage) compared to those with recurrent MASH
b) Both recurrent MASH and de novo NAFLD exhibit rapid progression to advanced fibrosis, typically within 2 years post-transplantation
c) Despite the presence of steatosis and inflammation in both groups, the risk of advancing to severe fibrosis (≥F3 stage) is low
d) Over 50% of patients with recurrent MASH develop advanced fibrosis within 5 years post-transplantation
e) Recurrent MASH leads to a more rapid decline in liver function compared to de novo NAFLD, resulting in earlier graft loss

**Answer: c**
Long-term studies show that both recurrent MASH and de novo NAFLD post-liver transplantation are characterized by steatosis and inflammation, but the progression to advanced fibrosis (≥F3 stage) is uncommon in either group. The risk of severe outcomes, such as decompensated cirrhosis or graft loss, remains low, with fibrosis developing slowly and significant complications being rare.[86]

110. A 53-year-old female patient with obesity and compensated liver cirrhosis, presenting with a MELD score of 12, a BMI of 42, and a platelet count of 136,000/μL, is under evaluation for bariatric surgery as a potential bridge to liver transplantation. Which of the following factors is most likely to adversely affect her eligibility for bariatric surgery and subsequent liver transplantation?
a) History of diabetes mellitus
b) Presence of portal hypertension
c) Age greater than 50 years
d) BMI greater than 40 kg/m²
e) Platelet count less than 150,000/μL
**Answer: b**
Portal hypertension significantly impacts eligibility for bariatric surgery in patients with liver cirrhosis, as it heightens the risk of perioperative complications and postoperative mortality, particularly in those with advanced liver disease. It also complicates liver transplantation candidacy due to increased surgical risks.[87,88]

111. A 54-year-old woman with obesity and liver cirrhosis due to non-alcoholic fatty liver disease (NAFLD) presents for evaluation. She has a sedentary lifestyle, diabetes, and hypertension. Which statement best describes the differences in sarcopenia and frailty between patients with NAFLD and those with alcoholic liver disease (ALD)?
a) Patients with NAFLD have a higher rate of sarcopenia than those with ALD
b) Patients with NAFLD are less likely to have frailty than those with ALD
c) Patients with NAFLD have a lower rate of sarcopenia but a higher rate of frailty compared to those with ALD
d) Patients with NAFLD have better outcomes after liver transplant and a lower risk of delisting compared to those with ALD
e) In patients with NAFLD, sarcopenia is linked to worse outcomes and longer hospital stays
**Answer: c**
Patients with NAFLD exhibit a lower prevalence of sarcopenia (muscle loss) but a higher prevalence of frailty (overall physical decline) compared to patients with ALD at the time of transplant listing. Higher frailty in NAFLD is associated with longer

hospital stays and an increased risk of delisting, while sarcopenia does not significantly correlate with these adverse outcomes in this population.[89]

112. A 25-year-old male presents to the nephrology clinic with progressive renal failure requiring hemodialysis. He has a history of recurrent kidney stones and normal LFT. Upon further evaluation, he is diagnosed with type 1 primary hyperoxaluria (PH1). What is the most appropriate treatment option?
a) Isolated kidney transplant
b) Isolated liver transplant with expected recovery of kidney function
c) Combined liver and kidney transplant
d) Intensive medical therapy with pyridoxine
e) Hyperdialysis and intensive medical therapy

**Answer: c**

PH1 is characterized by a genetic defect leading to a deficiency of the alanine glyoxylate aminotransferase enzyme in the liver, resulting in excessive oxalate production. This condition causes the formation of calcium oxalate crystals, which can lead to nephrocalcinosis and ultimately kidney failure. Isolated kidney transplants have not been effective in treating PH1 because they do not address the underlying metabolic defect, often resulting in graft loss due to the recurrence of disease. Therefore, the best therapeutic approach is a combined liver and kidney transplant. Hyperdialysis and medical therapy should be used in these patients to reduce serum oxalate levels before and after combined kidney and liver transplantation.[90]

113. A 25-year-old male with progressive renal failure and recurrent kidney stones is now requiring hemodialysis, LFT are normal. Upon further evaluation, he is diagnosed with type 1 primary hyperoxaluria (PH1). Following a successful combined liver and kidney transplant, there is a prompt decrease in plasma oxalate concentrations. However, urine oxalate levels remain significantly elevated six months post-transplant. What is the most appropriate next step in management?
a) Continue observation
b) Schedule a renal biopsy
c) Schedule a transjugular liver biopsy
d) Increase hydration and repeat urine test in one week
e) Obtain a renal ultrasound

**Answer: a**

The timeframe for the resolution of hyperoxaluria after liver transplantation can vary significantly. It tends to resolve more rapidly in patients who undergo transplantation within six months of reaching ESRD and who have been on intensive dialysis. Therefore, close observation is the most appropriate approach at this stage.[91]

114. A 67-year-old male patient with a medical history of hepatitis B cirrhosis, HCC, and ESRD has been placed on the waiting list for a combined kidney and liver transplant. A suitable organ offer is received from a 32-year-old male donor who suffered a traumatic accident, resulting in brain death. The donor has a history of chronic kidney disease stage 3 secondary to type 1 primary hyperoxaluria (PH1). The donor's LFT and INR are within normal limits. What is the most appropriate management decision for the transplant team regarding this organ offer?
a) Accept the offer for the liver only and decline the kidney
b) Accept both the kidney and liver, but inform the recipient about the risks of potential kidney dysfunction
c) Accept both organs while preparing for potential complications related to oxalate metabolism
d) Accept the liver offer under condition of a normal liver biopsy results during the procurement
e) Decline both the kidney and liver offers

**Answer: e**

Transplanting a liver from a donor with PH1 carries significant risks, especially the likelihood of early renal failure in the recipient, which may result in a high rate of dialysis dependency shortly after the transplant. Although liver transplants from such donors have been performed, the outcomes have generally been poor. A case report from Europe involving five patients highlighted these concerns, as all recipients required dialysis within the first four weeks despite the liver functioning well. Tragically, four out of the five patients ultimately died.[92]

115. A 45-year-old man with familial hypercholesterolemia (FHH) presents with severe coronary artery disease and ischemic cardiomyopathy. He is scheduled for simultaneous heart-liver transplantation after multidisciplinary evaluation. Which statement accurately describes the management and expected outcomes post-transplantation?
a) Lifelong high-dose statins are required to manage cholesterol post-transplant
b) Simultaneous transplantation has higher complication rates than sequential transplantation
c) Heart graft corrects cardiomyopathy; liver graft normalizes LDL receptor function and cholesterol levels
d) Liver transplantation guarantees cholesterol resolution regardless of pre-transplant levels
e) Post-transplant immunosuppression is sufficient to maintain graft function without additional cholesterol-lowering therapies

**Answer: c**

Simultaneous heart-liver transplantation addresses both ischemic cardiomyopathy and LDL receptor deficiency in FHH. The heart graft resolves cardiac issues, while the liver graft corrects the metabolic defect, often normalizing cholesterol levels long-term. In some cases, statins might still be prescribed post-transplant, but this is typically at lower doses or for specific reasons (e.g., preventing graft vasculopathy in the heart or managing mild residual dyslipidemia).[93,94]

116. A 10-year-old boy is brought to the emergency department after several days of fever, followed by severe vomiting and confusion. His mother reports that he recently had an influenza-like illness and was treated with aspirin to manage his symptoms. Laboratory tests reveal elevated serum ALT and AST, hyperammonemia, and hypoglycemia, while the serum bilirubin level remains normal. A liver biopsy shows microvesicular steatosis without inflammation or necrosis. A hepatic encephalopathy diagnosed and a detoxication of ammonemia with lactulose was started immediately. Based on this clinical presentation, what is the most likely diagnosis and treatment?
a) Viral hepatitis with acute liver failure; continue supportive care
b) Viral hepatitis with acute liver failure; recovery of the liver is not expected; evaluate for a liver transplant
c) Reye's syndrome as a consequence of salicylate therapy associated with a viral illness; continue supportive care
d) Reye's syndrome as a consequence of salicylate therapy associated with a viral illness; evaluate for a liver transplant
e) Wilson's disease presenting with acute liver failure; evaluate for a liver transplant
**Answer: d**
The clinical presentation aligns with Reye's syndrome, which occurs after viral illness in children treated with aspirin. While supportive care is essential for initial management, Reye's syndrome can lead to severe liver failure. In cases of acute liver failure, evaluation for liver transplantation is warranted, particularly if the patient's condition worsens or fails to improve with supportive care.[95]

117. A 6-month-old infant presents with lethargy, vomiting, and irritability. Tests confirm hyperammonemia and ornithine transcarbamylase (OTC) deficiency. Which statement best describes outcomes and management after liver transplantation?
a) Liver transplant corrects hyperammonemia but requires ongoing dietary restrictions
b) Liver transplant ensures normal neurological function without supplementation
c) Liver transplant cures OTC deficiency but requires citrulline or arginine supplements
d) Liver transplant improves enzyme function but has limited impact on survival outcomes

e) Liver transplant provides metabolic control but does not improve quality of life or neurological function

**Answer: c**

Liver transplantation is curative for ornithine transcarbamylase deficiency, but patients will continue to require citrulline or arginine supplements post-transplant. Liver transplantation effectively resolves the hyperammonemia associated with ornithine transcarbamylase deficiency and eliminates the need for dietary restrictions or alternative pathway drugs. However, patients with this deficiency still require supplementation with citrulline or arginine after transplantation due to the persisting low plasma levels of these amino acids, as they primarily derive from intestinal rather than hepatic synthesis.[96]

118. A 32-year-old woman presents to the emergency department with jaundice, abdominal pain, and fatigue. She reports having taken several over-the-counter dietary supplements and antibiotics for a recent respiratory infection. Laboratory tests reveal elevated liver enzymes, with an AST/ALT ratio of 7 times the upper limit of normal. The physician suspects drug-induced liver injury (DILI). Which of the following statements about DILI and its management is correct?
a) DILI is primarily caused by herbal supplement overdose in the majority of cases, necessitating immediate administration of N-acetylcysteine and evaluation for a liver transplant
b) Antibiotics are the least likely class of drugs to cause idiosyncratic drug-induced liver injury compared to herbal supplements
c) The implicated drug should be discontinued immediately, especially with an AST/ALT ratio ≥5 times the upper limit of normal
d) The presence of jaundice in DILI does not typically influence the prognosis or the need for liver transplantation
e) Genetic testing for HLA variants is routinely used to guide treatment decisions in patients suspected of having idiosyncratic DILI

**Answer: c**

The immediate discontinuation of the suspected drug is crucial in managing DILI to prevent further liver damage, particularly in cases with significant transaminitis defined by an AST/ALT ratio of ≥5 times the upper limit of normal. Paracetamol overdose is the primary cause of DILI. Antibiotics are among the most commonly associated drugs with DILI, especially in idiosyncratic cases. Jaundice indicates more severe liver injury and may influence decisions regarding transplantation. While HLA testing can be informative, it is not routinely performed in practice to guide treatment decisions in DILI.[97]

119. A 38-year-old male with no significant past medical history presents with abdominal discomfort and weight loss over the past few months. Imaging studies reveal multiple hepatic lesions, and a liver biopsy confirms a diagnosis of primary hepatic epithelioid hemangioendothelioma (HEH). Which of the following statements about the management and prognosis of HEH is correct?
a) Systemic chemotherapy is the standard first-line treatment for primary HEH with proven efficacy in improving overall survival rates
b) Liver transplantation is the preferred therapeutic option for primary HEH, particularly in patients without macrovascular invasion
c) The presence of lymph node invasion in patients with HEH is a contraindication for liver transplantation
d) Long-term survival rates after liver transplantation for HEH are poor, with a median survival of less than five years
e) Aggressive treatment with local radiotherapy is the most effective management for HEH and should be prioritized over surgical options

**Answer: b**

Liver transplantation has been shown to be the most frequent and effective treatment for primary HEH, particularly in patients without macrovascular invasion. Long-term outcomes following transplantation are favorable, with reported 5- and 10-year survival rates of 83% and 74%, respectively. As of now systemic chemotherapy and local radiotherapy have not demonstrated significant benefits in terms of overall survival. Of note, lymph node invasion is not considered a contraindication for liver transplantation in HEH.[98–100]

120. A 29-year-old female presents to the clinic with abdominal pain and nausea. She has a history of glycogen storage disease type I and has been using oral contraceptives for several years. Imaging studies reveal a large hepatic lesion with signs of central necrosis. Given her symptoms and the characteristics of the lesion, what is the most likely diagnosis?
a) Hepatic adenoma
b) Mesenchymal hamartoma
c) Massive hepatic hemangioma
d) Hepatic lymphangiomatosis
e) Inflammatory pseudotumor of the liver

**Answer: a**

Hepatic adenoma is commonly associated with women who use oral contraceptives and can occur in individuals with glycogen storage disease. The presence of central necrosis in the lesion further supports this diagnosis, as hepatic adenomas, although benign, can undergo hemorrhage and central necrosis, particularly when they are large. Mesenchymal hamartomas usually present in younger patients and have a different composition, massive hepatic hemangiomas tend to be asymptomatic and rarely show signs of necrosis.[101]

121. A 35-year-old woman presents to the emergency department with recurrent fever, abdominal pain, and jaundice. She has a history of cystic kidney disease and prior hospitalizations for cholangitis. MRCP reveals segmental dilatation of intrahepatic bile ducts with multiple cystic lesions in the liver. Based on her clinical presentation and imaging findings, what is the most likely diagnosis?
a) Caroli's disease
b) Congenital hepatic fibrosis
c) Choledochal cyst
d) Polycystic liver disease
e) Primary biliary cholangitis

**Answer: a**

Caroli's disease is a rare congenital condition characterized by non-obstructive segmental dilatation of intrahepatic bile ducts, leading to multiple cystic lesions in the liver. The patient's history of cystic kidney disease and recurrent cholangitis supports this diagnosis, as Caroli's disease is often associated with renal cystic disorders.[102]

# 4. Indications for Liver Transplantation in the Pediatric Population

122. A 3-month-old female infant presents with persistent unconjugated hyperbilirubinemia, with serum bilirubin levels reaching 30 mg/dL despite attempts with phototherapy and phenobarbital. Genetic sequencing reveals mutations in the UGT1A1 gene, confirming a diagnosis of Crigler-Najjar syndrome type I. What is the most appropriate treatment for this infant?
a) Phenobarbital
b) Liver transplantation
c) Long-term phototherapy
d) Exchange transfusion
e) Uridine diphosphate-glucuronosyltransferase enzyme infusion
**Answer: b**
In Crigler-Najjar syndrome type I, there is a complete absence of the UGT1A1 enzyme, leading to unconjugated hyperbilirubinemia and a high risk of bilirubin encephalopathy. The only effective long-term treatment option for these patients is liver transplantation, as it replaces the defective enzyme and greatly reduces bilirubin levels. While phenobarbital can be effective in Crigler-Najjar syndrome type II, it does not work in type I.[103]

123. A 35-year-old male presents with jaundice, abdominal pain, and a history of Langerhans cell histiocytosis (LCH) diagnosed 5 years ago. Imaging reveals biliary tree strictures and dilatation, with laboratory tests showing elevated ALP and GGT. Which of the following is most accurate regarding hepatic involvement in LCH?
a) Surgery resection of the affected bile ducts is curative
b) Recent advances in surgical techniques have significantly improved LCH liver prognosis
c) LCH-related sclerosing cholangitis progresses slower than primary sclerosing cholangitis
d) Endoscopic stenting can prevent progression of secondary sclerosing cholangitis in LCH
e) Secondary sclerosing cholangitis persists despite LCH remission
**Answer: e**
Secondary sclerosing cholangitis (SSC) in LCH results from biliary tree damage by malignant histiocytes, leading to strictures, dilatation, and potential end-stage liver disease. Even after LCH remission, SSC typically progresses, often necessitating liver

transplantation. Advances in surgical techniques have not significantly improved SSC-LCH prognosis, which remains poor without transplant.[104]

124. A 2-year-old child has been diagnosed with hepatoblastoma, and the histology is consistent with the mixed epithelial and mesenchymal type without teratoid features. The child presents with a centrally located tumor that significantly encroaches upon all three hepatic veins. The tumor is deemed unresectable. The child undergoes neoadjuvant chemotherapy, which results in a substantial reduction in tumor size and a significant drop in the AFP level from 900,000 ng/mL to 785 ng/mL. Which of the following factors represents the most unfavorable condition for liver transplantation?
a) Presence of tumor involvement in all four sectors of the liver
b) Initially high AFP level (above 100,000 ng/mL)
c) Evidence of noncontiguous spread of disease in the abdomen
d) Early age of diagnosis (below 3 years old)
e) Tumor histology consistent with mixed epithelial and mesenchymal type without teratoid features

**Answer: c**

The presence of noncontiguous spread of disease in the abdomen is considered the most unfavorable condition for liver transplantation in the context of hepatoblastoma. This condition indicates that the cancer has extended beyond the localized tumor, making it more challenging to achieve complete surgical resection and increasing the risk of recurrence after transplantation. Studies show that unfavorable prognostic factors include small cell undifferentiated tumors, transitional liver cell tumors, AFP levels above 1,000,000 IU/mL and below 100 IU/mL at diagnosis, lung metastases, and local recurrence after initial resection.[105]

125. A 2-year-old child with hepatoblastoma in the right hepatic lobe, involving the right and middle hepatic veins and right portal vein, undergoes neoadjuvant chemotherapy, reducing tumor size and AFP levels, enabling resection. Two weeks post-resection, tumor recurrence occurs, and the child is listed for liver transplantation. What factor most significantly increases the risk of tumor recurrence after transplantation?
a) Initial tumor size before chemotherapy
b) Teratoid features in tumor histology
c) Timing of transplant after resection
d) AFP level at transplant listing
e) Post-transplant chemotherapy

**Answer: c**

In hepatoblastoma, "rescue transplants" performed after tumor recurrence following resection are associated with a significantly higher risk of recurrence and mortality compared to primary liver transplantation. Studies indicate nearly double the risk of recurrence in patients undergoing transplantation post-resection, making the timing of the transplant a critical factor.[105,106]

126. A 4-year-old girl with Wiskott-Aldrich syndrome presents with eczema, recurrent infections, and easy bruising. An abdominal ultrasound reveals an unresectable hepatic hemangioendothelioma, and she is evaluated for liver transplantation. During workup, a patent ductus arteriosus and uterine sarcoma are incidentally found. What is the most significant contraindication to liver transplantation in this patient?
a) Uterine sarcoma
b) Wiskott-Aldrich syndrome
c) Patent ductus arteriosus
d) Recurrent infections
e) Hepatic hemangioendothelioma
**Answer: a**
Active malignancy, such as uterine sarcoma, is a major contraindication to liver transplantation due to the high risk of metastatic spread and recurrence, particularly under post-transplant immunosuppression.[107]

127. A 1-month-old infant diagnosed with biliary atresia undergoes a Kasai portoenterostomy. Thirty days post-surgery, total bilirubin levels remain elevated at 9 mg/dL, raising concerns about the need for liver transplantation. Which of the following is the most critical indicator for predicting the need for liver transplantation in this patient?
a) Age at the time of Kasai portoenterostomy
b) Total bilirubin level 30 days post-portoenterostomy
c) Presence of cirrhosis on liver biopsy at 30 days
d) Delayed growth at the time of transplant evaluation
e) The presence of portal hypertension at the time of evaluation
**Answer: b**
The total bilirubin level 30 days after Kasai portoenterostomy is the most critical prognostic indicator for predicting the need for liver transplantation in infants with biliary atresia. Persistent hyperbilirubinemia indicates inadequate bile drainage, suggesting failure of the portoenterostomy and a high likelihood of progression to end-stage liver disease.[108]

128. A 2-week-old infant with biliary atresia undergoes a Kasai portoenterostomy. In the context of various surgical modifications to the original technique aimed at reducing the risk of ascending cholangitis, it has become evident that some factors may lead to further complications. Which of the following modifications of the

surgery is most strongly associated with adverse outcomes, particularly with post-transplant malabsorption?
a) Use of a longer Roux-en-Y limb (40 to 70 cm in length)
b) Creation of intussuscepted intestinal valves
c) Performance of the procedure at a younger age
d) Use of physiological intestinal valves (i.e., the ileocecal valve)
e) Creation of partial diversion of the biliary drainage limb with the use of various stomas

**Answer: a**

The use of a long biliary limb during a Kasai portoenterostomy is significantly linked to negative outcomes, especially post-transplant malabsorption. Long biliary limbs can interfere with nutrient absorption before transplantation and may contribute to malabsorption after the procedure.[109]

129. A 9-month-old infant with biliary atresia undergoes a Kasai portoenterostomy, but over time, the child develops symptoms indicative of portal hypertension, including splenomegaly. Despite supportive care and monitoring, the child's liver function begins to decline, and there are increasing episodes of intractable cholangitis. When considering the timing for liver transplantation, all of the following factors indicate that the patient needs to be listed for a liver transplant except:
a) Intractable cholangitis
b) Declining liver synthetic function
c) Hepatopulmonary syndrome
d) Development of liver cirrhosis
e) Decrease in growth rate

**Answer: d**

While most older children with biliary atresia will develop progressive cirrhosis, it is not the surgical failure that leads them to require transplantation after 5 to 10 years. Effective medical management and careful surgical approaches can sometimes manage the complications of cirrhosis and prolong life without the need for transplantation. Nonetheless, the presence of end-stage liver disease and growth failure should be regarded as significant indicators to consider moving forward with transplantation.[110]

130. A 3-year-old boy with hepatotoxicity from mushroom poisoning develops fulminant hepatic failure and is listed for liver transplantation. He progresses to Stage IV hepatic encephalopathy, with a GCS score of 4, dilated pupils, and an MRI showing midbrain coning. His mother is prepared as a living donor for transplantation. What is the most appropriate course of action?
a) Proceed with emergent hepatectomy and living-donor liver transplantation

b) Initiate hemodialysis to reduce ammonia levels and reassess in 12 hours
c) Perform an auxiliary partial liver transplantation without hepatectomy
d) Repeat head imaging in 6 hours; if stable, proceed with transplantation
e) Transition to palliative care due to poor prognosis
**Answer: e**
Stage IV hepatic encephalopathy, a GCS score of 4, and midbrain coning on MRI indicate severe cerebral edema and brainstem herniation, which are associated with a dismal prognosis. These findings, particularly midbrain coning, contraindicate liver transplantation due to the high likelihood of irreversible neurological damage and poor post-transplant outcomes.[111]

131. A 4-year-old boy with maple syrup urine disease (MSUD) presents with developmental delays and neurocognitive deficits despite strict dietary management. His parents inquire about the expected neurological outcomes following liver transplantation. Which statement most accurately describes the neurological recovery after liver transplantation in MSUD?
a) Complete neurological recovery is expected due to restored metabolic function
b) Significant improvements in cognitive function and developmental milestones are typical
c) Neurological recovery varies, with partial improvement possible but existing deficits often persist
d) Neurological function remains unchanged, with no impact on existing impairments
e) Transplantation prevents further neurological decline but does not improve existing deficits
**Answer: c**
Liver transplantation in MSUD corrects the metabolic defect by providing functional branched-chain ketoacid dehydrogenase, stabilizing leucine levels and preventing metabolic crises. However, neurological recovery is highly variable. Pre-existing neurocognitive deficits and developmental delays may persist, though some patients experience partial improvement due to metabolic stability.[112]

132. A 3-year-old boy with Alagille syndrome (ALGS) presents with severe pruritus and jaundice due to cholestasis. Which statement most accurately describes liver transplantation in children with ALGS?
a) The primary indication for liver transplantation is complications of cholestasis, such as severe pruritus
b) The most common indication for liver transplantation is portal hypertension with variceal bleeding
c) Most liver transplants occur after age 10 due to progressive liver fibrosis

d) Transplantation is typically delayed until adolescence due to slow disease progression
e) Transplant rates uniform across geographic regions
**Answer: a**
In children with Alagille syndrome, liver transplantation is most commonly indicated for complications of cholestasis, such as intractable pruritus or failure to thrive, rather than advanced liver fibrosis or portal hypertension. Severe pruritus, as seen in this patient, is a frequent driver of early transplantation.[113]

133. A 10-month-old boy with Alagille syndrome (ALGS) presents with persistent jaundice and pruritus. Laboratory tests show a total bilirubin level of 10.5 mg/dL and ALT of 160 U/L. Which statement most accurately describes the child's prognosis?
a) The elevated total bilirubin level indicates a significantly increased risk of requiring liver transplantation due to progressive liver disease
b) The total bilirubin level below 12 mg/dL suggests a low risk of liver transplantation, with likely stabilization of liver function
c) The total bilirubin level is not predictive of liver disease progression in ALGS
d) The elevated ALT level, rather than total bilirubin, is the primary driver of liver failure risk
e) No total bilirubin cutoff exists for predicting liver disease progression in infants under 12 months with ALGS
**Answer: a**
In ALGS, a total bilirubin level of 10.5 mg/dL in a 10-month-old indicates severe cholestasis and is associated with a significantly increased risk (up to 15.6-fold) of requiring liver transplantation compared to total bilirubin levels below 5.0 mg/dL. This reflects progressive liver disease and a poor prognosis for maintaining the native liver, often accompanied by extrahepatic complications like pruritus and failure to thrive.[113]

134. A 3-month-old girl presents with persistent jaundice, dark urine, and pale stools. A liver biopsy shows bile duct paucity, some ductular proliferation, and bile duct plugs, prompting consideration of Alagille syndrome (ALGS) versus biliary atresia. Which statement most accurately guides the clinician's diagnosis and management?
a) Over one-third of infants with ALGS may lack bile duct paucity on biopsy at 3 months of age
b) Bile duct plugs on biopsy definitively indicate biliary atresia and exclude ALGS
c) Bile duct paucity is always present in ALGS infants, regardless of age
d) ALGS can be diagnosed solely based on liver histology without additional testing
e) Repeat biopsies in ALGS always show progressive bile duct paucity over time
**Answer: a**

In infants with ALGS, bile duct paucity is a hallmark feature but is absent in over one-third (approximately 35%) of liver biopsies performed before 3 months of age, as the finding may develop later. This variability complicates the differentiation from biliary atresia, which often shows ductular proliferation and bile duct plugs. Additional testing, such as genetic analysis or imaging, is critical to distinguish ALGS from biliary atresia.[113]

135. A 6-month-old infant presents with persistent jaundice, severe pruritus, chronic watery diarrhea, and failure to thrive. Examination reveals hepatomegaly and excoriations from scratching. Laboratory tests show elevated serum AST and ALP, but a sweat test for cystic fibrosis is negative. Which additional finding would most strongly support a diagnosis of Byler's disease (progressive familial intrahepatic cholestasis type 1, PFIC-1)?
a) Normal or low serum γ-GTP levels
b) Markedly elevated serum cholesterol levels
c) Markedly elevated serum bile acid levels
d) Elevated serum lipase levels
e) Progression to cirrhosis by adolescence
**Answer: a**
Byler's disease (PFIC-1), caused by mutations in the ATP8B1 gene, is characterized by normal or low serum γ-GTP levels despite cholestasis, distinguishing it from other cholestatic liver diseases where γ-GTP is typically elevated. This infant's presentation of jaundice, severe pruritus, diarrhea, and failure to thrive is consistent with PFIC-1. Serum bile acids are markedly elevated in PFIC-1 (C), but this is less specific, as it occurs in other cholestatic disorders. Serum cholesterol is typically normal or mildly elevated, and lipase levels are normal. Progression to cirrhosis often occurs in childhood, not adolescence, and is a long-term outcome, not a diagnostic finding.[114]

136. A 2-year-old boy presents with persistent jaundice and intermittent pruritus. Laboratory tests reveal markedly elevated serum bile acid levels and low serum γ-GTP. He has no significant gastrointestinal symptoms, such as diarrhea or pancreatitis. Which type of progressive familial intrahepatic cholestasis (PFIC) is most likely in this patient?
a) PFIC-1 (Byler's disease, ATP8B1 mutation)
b) PFIC-2 (BSEP defect, ABCB11 mutation)
c) PFIC-3 (MDR3 defect, ABCB4 mutation)
d) PFIC-4 (TJP2 defect)
e) PFIC-5 (NR1H4 defect)
**Answer: b**

PFIC-2, caused by mutations in the ABCB11 gene encoding the bile salt export pump (BSEP), is characterized by persistent jaundice, severe pruritus, markedly elevated serum bile acid levels, and low or normal γ-GTP levels. Unlike PFIC-1, which often includes extrahepatic symptoms like diarrhea or pancreatitis, PFIC-2 primarily affects the liver. PFIC-3 typically presents with elevated γ-GTP due to MDR3 defects. PFIC-4 and PFIC-5 are rarer, with distinct features (e.g., early cirrhosis in PFIC-4, variable γ-GTP in PFIC-5), making them less likely given the low γ-GTP and lack of extrahepatic symptoms. Liver transplantation often corrects cholestasis in PFIC-2.[115,116]

137. A 3-month-old infant presents with persistent jaundice since birth, severe pruritus, and cholestasis. Laboratory tests reveal elevated serum bile acid levels, normal serum γ-GTP, and elevated ALP. Genetic testing is ordered to evaluate for progressive familial intrahepatic cholestasis (PFIC). Mutations in the ABCB11 gene, encoding the bile salt export pump (BSEP), primarily impair which process?
a) Active transport of bile acids into bile canaliculi
b) Synthesis of bile acids in hepatocytes
c) Intestinal absorption of bile acids
d) Uptake of bile acids into hepatocytes
e) Secretion of bile acids into intestinal lumen
**Answer: a**
The ABCB11 gene encodes the BSEP, which actively transports bile acids from hepatocytes into bile canaliculi. Mutations in ABCB11 cause PFIC-2, leading to bile acid accumulation in hepatocytes, elevated serum bile acid levels, cholestasis, and liver injury.[116,117]

138. A 4-year-old boy with progressive familial intrahepatic cholestasis type 2 (PFIC-2) presents with worsening jaundice, hepatomegaly, and elevated serum ALT and AFP levels. Liver imaging shows nodular lesions, and biopsy reveals giant hepatocytes. Despite medical management, his condition is deteriorating, and liver transplantation is being considered. Which complication is most concerning after liver transplantation for PFIC-2?
a) Formation of de novo bile salt export pump (BSEP) antibodies
b) Recurrent cholestasis episodes
c) Development of hepatocellular carcinoma
d) Acute graft rejection
e) Post-transplant lymphoproliferative disorder
**Answer: a**
In PFIC-2, caused by ABCB11 mutations impairing the BSEP, liver transplantation is often required due to progressive liver failure. The most concerning post-transplant

complication is the formation of de novo BSEP antibodies, which can cause alloimmune hepatitis, leading to graft dysfunction or failure requiring retransplantation. Recurrent cholestasis is more typical in PFIC-1.[118]

139. A 5-month-old infant is brought to the pediatric gastroenterology clinic with increasing jaundice and mild pruritus. The mother notes that the infant has been irritable and has had episodes of vomiting. Laparotomy tests show elevated serum bile acids and serum γ-GTP. The infant's abdominal ultrasound reveals patent intrahepatic and extrahepatic bile ducts. A liver biopsy shows portal fibrosis with ductular proliferation and inflammatory infiltrate. Which type of progressive familial intrahepatic cholestasis (PFIC) is most likely in this patient?
a) PFIC type 1 (Byler's disease)
b) PFIC type 2 (canalicular BSEP defect)
c) PFIC type 3 (isolated ATP8B1 defect)
d) PFIC due to mitochondrial dysfunction
e) PFIC associated with cystic fibrosis
**Answer: c**
The presentation of high serum γ-GTP activity, portal fibrosis with ductular proliferation, and patent bile ducts suggests a diagnosis of PFIC type 3. This type is characterized by moderate pruritus, elevated serum bile acids, and an inflammatory infiltrate—even when bile ducts are patent. PFIC type 3 can present in neonates and often mimics biliary atresia, but its distinguishing features include the specific liver histology and the elevated γ-GTP activity.[119]

140. A 6-month-old infant presents with symptoms of jaundice and poor weight gain. Laboratory tests reveal elevated serum γ-GTP. Genetic testing indicates a mutation in the MDR3 (ABCB4) gene. This mutation results in a deficiency of biliary phospholipids. Which of the following best explains how biliary phospholipids protect against the toxicity of bile acids in the liver?
a) Stabilize micelles to block bile acid damage to canalicular membranes
b) Boost CYP450 enzymes to metabolize toxic bile acids
c) Increase bile acid synthesis to dilute cytotoxic bile acids
d) Decreased enterohepatic circulation of bile acids
e) Help transport bile acids into hepatocytes for detoxification
**Answer: a**
Biliary phospholipids, particularly phosphatidylcholine, play a crucial role in protecting the ductular epithelial cells from bile acid toxicity by forming mixed micelles. In patients with MDR3 deficiency (PFIC-3), the absence of these phospholipids leads to destabilization of micelles, which exacerbates the detergent action of bile acids on bile canaliculi and biliary epithelial cells.[120]

141. A 34-year-old woman with intrahepatic cholestasis of pregnancy (IHC) improves on ursodeoxycholic acid (UDCA). However, other IHC patients with MDR3 (PFIC-3) deficiency show no response to UDCA. Why do some patients benefit from UDCA while others do not?
a) Responders make more bile acids, allowing for better management of bile acid levels
b) Non-responders have a complete defect in phospholipid secretion, making any partial replacement of UDCA insufficient to mitigate bile salt toxicity
c) Responders tend to have less severe liver injury, thereby allowing for a more effective response to the medication
d) Non-responders have an additional liver enzyme deficiency that prevents the conversion of UDCA to its active form
e) Patients with complete biliary obstruction are less likely to respond to UDCA, as the drug relies on bile flow for efficacy

**Answer: b**

There is a hypothesis suggesting that patients with a complete defect in phospholipid secretion cannot adequately neutralize bile acid toxicity, regardless of UDCA administration. For these patients, the lack of phospholipids in bile means that the introduction of a partial replacement with UDCA is insufficient to lower bile salt toxicity below a critical threshold. In contrast, patients who retain some phospholipid secretion can benefit from UDCA therapy, as the combination of residual phospholipids and the medication can help protect the liver from damage. This differentiation highlights how MDR3 mutations exhibit significant phenotypic variation, including gallstone formation, biliary fibrosis, and various presentations of IHC.[119]

142. A 2-year-old boy from a North American Indian reservation presents with jaundice, hepatomegaly, and irritability. The jaundice began at around 6 months of age and has progressively worsened. The child has a history of recurrent abdominal pain and has recently experienced a significant episode of upper gastrointestinal bleeding due to variceal hemorrhage. Blood tests reveal elevated LFT and bilirubin levels. Liver biopsy indicates early bile duct proliferation and portal fibrosis. Given the diagnosis consistent with North American Indian childhood cirrhosis (NAIC), what is the most appropriate treatment modality for this child?
a) Oral ursodeoxycholic acid
b) Endoscopic variceal band ligation
c) Portosystemic shunt surgery
d) Liver transplantation
e) Corticosteroid therapy

**Answer: d**
Liver transplantation is currently the only effective therapy for patients with advanced disease like NAIC. The condition typically leads to rapid progression to biliary cirrhosis and necessitates the need for aggressive intervention to prevent complications such as variceal hemorrhage.[121]

143. A 2-year-old Inuit boy from West Greenland presents to the clinic with jaundice, severe pruritus, and growth retardation despite a normal appetite. The boy shows signs of osteodystrophy and marked dwarfism. Laboratory tests indicate low to normal serum cholesterol levels, and a liver biopsy exhibits canalicular cholestasis and rosette formation of hepatocytes. Genetic testing reveals a missense mutation in the FIC1 gene. What is the most likely diagnosis for this patient?
a) PFIC due to mitochondrial dysfunction
b) Cholestasis familiaris groenlandica
c) PFIC associated with cystic fibrosis
d) Biliary atresia
e) Hemochromatosis
**Answer: b**
The clinical presentation and laboratory findings of jaundice, pruritus, growth retardation, and low to normal serum cholesterol levels, combined with the specific demographic context of the Inuit population in Greenland and the identified mutation in the FIC1 gene, point towards cholestasis familiaris groenlandica. This disease is characterized by severe intrahepatic cholestasis and aligns with the patient's symptoms and histological findings.[122]

144. A 15-year-old girl presents to the clinic with a history of recurrent jaundice and intense itching for the past three years. Each episode lasts for several weeks, followed by spontaneous resolution. During these episodes, laboratory tests reveal elevated serum bile acids and mildly elevated aminotransferases, while serum γ-GTP levels remain low. A cholangiogram demonstrates normal intrahepatic and extrahepatic bile ducts, a liver biopsy shows mild bile plugs without significant damage. Her family history is notable for similar episodes occurring in her mother and grandfather. What is the most appropriate treatment option for this patient?
a) Ursodeoxycholic acid
b) Liver transplantation
c) Cholecystectomy
d) Nutritional support and vitamin supplementation
e) Corticosteroids
**Answer: d**

The clinical features and recurrent nature of this patient's cholestasis align with the diagnosis of benign recurrent intrahepatic cholestasis. In this condition, the primary goals of treatment focus on alleviating symptoms, particularly pruritus, and providing nutritional support due to malabsorption concerns. Since benign recurrent intrahepatic cholestasis is characterized by spontaneous remission and does not require liver transplantation or aggressive treatment interventions, the most appropriate management includes ensuring adequate nutrition and supplementing any vitamin deficiencies.[123]

145. A 6-week-old infant presents with a 2-week history of worsening jaundice, dark yellow urine, pale stools, and mild hepatomegaly. The infant was initially gaining weight but is now fussy. Labs show total bilirubin of 12 mg/dL, with conjugated bilirubin at 9 mg/dL. What is the most likely diagnosis and best next step?
a) Breast milk jaundice – start phototherapy
b) Breast milk jaundice – switch to formula and recheck labs
c) Physiologic jaundice – start ursodeoxycholic acid
d) Biliary atresia – refer for liver transplant
e) Biliary atresia – perform Kasai operation
**Answer: e**
The infant has conjugated hyperbilirubinemia (direct bilirubin >2 mg/dL and >20% of total), pale stools, and hepatomegaly—classic signs of biliary atresia. Early surgical intervention with the Kasai procedure (ideally before 2–3 months of age) improves outcomes by restoring bile flow and delaying liver damage.[124]

146. A 9-month-old infant who underwent a Kasai portoenterostomy for biliary atresia at 3 months of age presents for follow-up. The child has had intermittent fever, irritability, increased jaundice, fatigue, and a few episodes of vomiting. What is the most common complication after the Kasai procedure that could explain these symptoms?
a) Liver failure
b) Portal vein thrombosis
c) Ascending cholangitis
d) Hepatic abscess
e) Biliary stricture
**Answer: c**
Ascending cholangitis is the most common complication after a Kasai procedure, occurring in 30–60% of cases. It typically presents with fever, rising bilirubin, irritability, and gastrointestinal symptoms—matching this infant's presentation. Prompt recognition and treatment with IV antibiotics are essential to prevent progression to cirrhosis and liver failure.[125]

147. A 2-month-old infant diagnosed with biliary atresia is being evaluated for surgical intervention. The infant has been experiencing progressive jaundice since birth, with dark urine and acholic stools noted in recent weeks. What is the recommended timing for the Kasai procedure to optimize outcomes, and what is the rationale for this recommendation?
a) At any time before 1 year of age, to minimize surgical risk
b) Before 3 months of age, ideally between 30 to 45 days, to maximize bile flow restoration
c) Between 3 and 6 months of age due to improved postoperative care
d) After 6 months of age, when the child is more stable
e) After 3 months of age, or when the child weighs above 8 kg
**Answer: b**
The optimal timing for the Kasai portoenterostomy is before 3 months of age, particularly between 30 to 45 days, as this timing significantly increases the likelihood of restoring bile flow and reducing the risk of further liver damage. Studies show that survival rates with a native liver decline markedly when surgery is performed after this critical window.[126]

148. A 3-year-old with biliary atresia underwent a successful Kasai procedure but later required a liver transplant using a partial graft from his father. Soon after, he developed jaundice, ascites, lethargy, and abnormal LFT. Imaging shows portal vein thrombosis. What is the most likely cause and best management?
a) Hypoplastic portal vein — consider early reoperation and thrombectomy
b) Technical error — revise venous anastomosis
c) Technical error — start anticoagulation and list for urgent retransplant
d) Graft-related outflow obstruction — revise venocaval anastomosis and perform thrombectomy
e) Hypercoagulable state — start anticoagulation and consult IR
**Answer: a**
Portal vein thrombosis occurs in 6% to 14% of patients with biliary atresia undergoing liver transplantation. The hypoplastic nature of the portal vein in children with biliary atresia increases their vulnerability to such complications. Early postoperative portal vein occlusion can lead to acute liver failure, as evidenced in this child. Timely recognition and intervention through reoperation and thrombectomy are critical to potentially salvage the graft and enhance the child's prognosis.[127]

149. Which of the following is not a metabolic disease typically associated with structural liver damage?
a) Urea cycle defects

b) Alpha-1 antitrypsin deficiency
c) Familial tyrosinemia
d) Wilson's disease
e) Neonatal iron storage disease
**Answer: a**
Urea cycle defects refer to a group of inherited disorders that impair the body's ability to remove ammonia, which leads to hyperammonemia and neurological issues rather than structural liver damage. In contrast, the other listed conditions are characterized by metabolic disruptions that result in direct structural damage to the liver, contributing to the progression towards end-stage liver disease.[128]

150. A 2-year-old boy with lifelong jaundice, pale stools, growth delay, and pruritus is diagnosed with alpha-1 antitrypsin deficiency (PiZZ). Labs show elevated conjugated bilirubin and liver enzymes. What is the most likely prognosis?
a) 50% develop cirrhosis by age 10
b) 25% develop cirrhosis in the first decade; another 25% progress in the second decade
c) Most develop cirrhosis by the second decade
d) Liver fibrosis is usually self-limiting
e) 95% mortality rate without liver transplant by age of 10
**Answer: b**
In children with alpha-1 antitrypsin deficiency (PiZZ phenotype), the prognosis regarding liver disease shows significant variability. Specifically, 25% of PiZZ infants with cholestasis will develop cirrhosis within the first decade, while another 25% may exhibit persistent transaminitis that progresses to cirrhosis during the second decade. Additionally, 25% will experience mild transaminitis without cirrhosis, and the remaining 25% may demonstrate resolution of biochemical abnormalities with only mild fibrosis evident on liver biopsy.[129]

151. A 4-year-old girl with jaundice, abdominal distension, failure to thrive, and recurrent lung infections has elevated liver enzymes and conjugated bilirubin. Liver biopsy shows PAS-positive, diastase-resistant globules in periportal hepatocytes. What is the mechanism of liver injury in alpha-1 antitrypsin deficiency?
a) Elastase-mediated destruction of hepatic tissue
b) Misfolded A1AT protein accumulates in the rough endoplasmic reticulum, causing cell damage
c) Oxidative stress from excess elastase activity
d) Impaired bile acid synthesis and cholestasis
e) Immune-mediated hepatocyte destruction
**Answer: b**

Liver Transplantation and Hepatobiliary Surgery: 500 Practice Questions

In alpha-1 antitrypsin deficiency, particularly in the ZZ genotype, the abnormal folding of the mutant alpha-1 antitrypsin molecule results in accumulation in the rough endoplasmic reticulum of periportal hepatocytes. This accumulation triggers cellular injury due to the buildup of putatively hepatotoxic proteins, as the degradative pathway is impaired. Although the retention of these proteins is initially a protective mechanism aimed at degrading abnormal proteins to prevent further cellular damage, the inability to effectively clear these proteins leads to liver damage and the associated clinical complications.[130]

152. A 6-year-old boy with α1-antitrypsin deficiency presents with jaundice, portal hypertension, and GI bleeding from varices. He is being evaluated for liver transplant. Which factor best predicts his post-transplant prognosis?
a) Duration of jaundice
b) Age at transplantation
c) Liver histology
d) Total bilirubin level at transplantation
e) Disease genotype
**Answer: b**
The prognosis for children with α1-antitrypsin deficiency undergoing liver transplantation is significantly influenced by their age at the time of evaluation and surgery. Generally, older children tend to have better outcomes compared to younger children.[131]

153. A healthy 1-week-old infant has elevated serum copper and liver copper levels similar to those seen in Wilson's disease. What is the most appropriate next step?
a) Abnormal finding; test for genetic mutations
b) Abnormal finding; test and evaluate for transplant
c) Normal for age; repeat copper and ceruloplasmin at 6 months
d) Normal for age; repeat copper and ceruloplasmin at 12 months
e) Diagnostic for Wilson's disease; start treatment
**Answer: c**
High liver copper levels are normal in newborns due to maternal transfer during pregnancy. These levels typically normalize by 6 months. Routine monitoring is appropriate in an otherwise healthy infant. Exact numerical values for copper concentration can vary, but normal hepatic copper levels are generally considered to be less than 250 micrograms of copper per gram of liver tissue in adults.[132]

154. A 14-year-old girl presents with mood swings, irritability, declining school performance, hand tremors, and difficulty speaking. Neurological exam shows

dystonia and dysarthria. Her cousin has Wilson's disease. What best explains her neurological symptoms?
a) Copper buildup in the liver causing encephalopathy
b) Copper redistribution causing peripheral nerves damage
c) Extrapyramidal dysfunction from high ceruloplasmin
d) Mitochondrial damage from copper toxicity
e) Copper accumulation in the brain's extrapyramidal system

**Answer: e**

In Wilson's disease, copper accumulates not only in the liver but also in the extrapyramidal system, which is responsible for coordinating movement. This accumulation leads to various neurological symptoms, including tremors, dystonia, and dysarthria, which are particularly pronounced in adolescents and adults. The patient's subtle personality and behavioral changes, along with the motor findings, reflect the impact of copper toxicity on the neurological system.[133]

155. A 15-year-old boy presents with sudden-onset jaundice, confusion, vomiting, and hepatomegaly. Labs show low ceruloplasmin, normal serum copper, and elevated 24-hour urine copper. No Kayser-Fleischer rings are seen. What is the most likely diagnosis?
a) Acute viral hepatitis
b) Wilson's disease
c) Autoimmune hepatitis
d) Acute cholangitis
e) Drug-induced liver failure

**Answer: b**

Wilson's disease can present with acute liver failure in adolescents. Key findings include low serum ceruloplasmin and high urine copper. Serum copper may be normal. Kayser-Fleischer rings are helpful but not always present, especially early on or in brown-eyed patients. Acute viral hepatitis typically shows an increase in serum copper. Autoimmune hepatitis could present with low ceruloplasmin levels, but it usually has other specific markers. Acute cholangitis would more commonly present with fever, rigors, and elevated ALP levels, while drug-induced acute liver failure would have a known exposure history to a hepatotoxic drug.[134]

156. A 15-year-old patient with Wilson's disease, experiencing severe dysarthria and confined to bed despite maximal medical therapy, develops liver cirrhosis and portal hypertension, necessitating a liver transplant. Based on current evidence regarding neurological outcomes after liver transplantation in Wilson's disease, which statement best describes the potential neurological prognosis for this patient?

a) Most patients achieve complete neurological recovery within a few months post-transplant
b) Significant neurological improvement occurs rapidly, typically within a week post-transplant
c) Neurological symptoms are unaffected by liver transplantation and continue to worsen
d) Neurological recovery varies, with some patients experiencing partial improvement over months
e) Neurological symptoms may persist post-transplant but do not progress further

**Answer: d**

Neurological recovery after liver transplantation in Wilson's disease varies widely. Some patients may experience partial improvement over several months, while others face delayed or incomplete recovery, reflecting diverse outcomes based on individual factors.[135]

157. An 8-week-old infant presents to the emergency department with persistent vomiting, irritability, lethargy, bruising on the arms and legs, and a distended abdomen. Examination reveals hepatomegaly, and labs show elevated tyrosine, methionine, and phenylalanine. Liver biopsy indicates cirrhosis, bile duct proliferation, and steatosis. Given the early onset and findings, which condition is most likely?
a) Wilson's disease
b) Alpha-1 antitrypsin deficiency
c) Tyrosinemia Type I
d) Galactosemia
e) Hemolytic uremic syndrome

**Answer: c**

The infant's early, severe symptoms—vomiting, irritability, lethargy, coagulopathy—and elevated amino acids point to Tyrosinemia Type I. This genetic disorder, caused by fumarylacetoacetate hydrolase deficiency, leads to toxic metabolite accumulation, liver dysfunction, and cirrhosis, typically presenting within the first few months of life.[136]

158. A 2-year-old boy with hereditary tyrosinemia presents to the emergency department with sudden profound weakness, hypertonic posturing, painful dysesthesias, irritability, and seizures. He has respiratory distress, muscle weakness, and elevated δ-aminolevulinic acid levels. How should this neurological crisis be managed?
a) Supportive care with close monitoring
b) Hematin therapy to reduce δ-aminolevulinic acid levels

c) Intubation, supportive care, and hematin therapy
d) Intubation, supportive care, and urgent evaluation for liver transplantation
e) Antiepileptic medication and supportive care
**Answer: d**
In hereditary tyrosinemia, neurological crises can lead to respiratory muscle paralysis and sudden death. Immediate intubation is essential to secure the airway and support ventilation. While hematin may help reduce δ-aminolevulinic acid levels, urgent evaluation for liver transplantation is critical for severe cases to prevent recurrent crises and improve long-term survival.[137]

159. A 5-year-old boy with hereditary tyrosinemia type I, diagnosed at 6 months, has been managed with a strict diet low in aromatic amino acids and methionine. At a recent follow-up, his tyrosine levels are normal, and he shows no signs of liver cirrhosis. Which statement best describes the HCC risk in this patient?
a) Strict dietary control significantly reduces HCC risk to negligible levels
b) HCC risk is elevated, and routine AFP testing is sufficient for monitoring
c) HCC risk is elevated, and liver MRI is recommended only if AFP levels rise
d) HCC risk persists despite controlled liver disease, requiring regular surveillance
e) Strict dietary control eliminates HCC risk by delaying liver disease progression
**Answer: d**
Even with normal tyrosine levels and effective dietary management, the risk of HCC in hereditary tyrosinemia type I remains significant. Regular surveillance is necessary, as serum AFP levels are unreliable for diagnosing HCC in these patients, often being elevated without tumors. Imaging, such as CT or ultrasound, may detect liver nodules early, but these may not always be malignant.[138]

160. A 2-week-old full-term infant boy presents to the emergency department with lethargy, hypotonia, irritability, and feeding difficulties since birth. Testing reveals elevated serum ammonia and low citrulline, confirming ornithine transcarbamylase (OTC) deficiency. Which statement best describes the management of this condition?
a) Liver transplantation is unlikely to improve neurological outcomes after 4 weeks of age
b) Early ammonia-lowering therapies are critical to prevent irreversible neurological damage before transplantation
c) Dietary protein restriction effectively treats OTC deficiency, eliminating the need for transplantation
d) Post-transplantation, patients typically regain normal neurological function
e) Transplantation does not eliminate the need for a protein-restricted diet
**Answer: b**

In OTC deficiency, early diagnosis and aggressive ammonia-lowering therapies are essential to prevent irreversible neurological damage in newborns. While liver transplantation corrects the metabolic defect, neurological outcomes depend heavily on effective ammonia management prior to the procedure.[139]

161. A 4-month-old infant presents to the pediatric clinic with lethargy, poor feeding, irritability, intermittent vomiting, and inadequate weight gain. The parents note a sweet-smelling urine odor. Testing confirms maple syrup urine disease (MSUD). Which finding is most characteristic of MSUD?
a) Elevated serum phenylalanine with normal branched-chain amino acids
b) High levels of branched-chain amino acids (leucine, isoleucine, valine) in urine
c) Elevated serum citrulline and low serum arginine
d) Orotic acid in urine with normal urea cycle metabolites
e) Increased homocysteine with low methionine
**Answer: b**
MSUD results from a deficiency in the branched-chain 2-oxoacid dehydrogenase complex, leading to elevated branched-chain amino acids (leucine, isoleucine, valine) in urine, often causing a sweet, maple syrup-like urine odor. Elevated phenylalanine with normal branched-chain amino acids is typical of phenylketonuria. Elevated citrulline and low arginine suggest urea cycle disorders, like citrullinemia. Orotic acid in urine is associated with urea cycle disorders, such as orotic aciduria. Increased homocysteine with low methionine is characteristic of homocystinuria.[140]

162. A 3-week-old infant presents to the emergency department with vomiting, lethargy, and jaundice after starting milk feeding. Examination shows hepatomegaly, and tests reveal metabolic acidosis, elevated bilirubin, liver dysfunction, and reducing substances in urine. With a family history of consanguinity, galactosemia is suspected. Which statement best describes a key aspect of managing this condition?
a) Early liver transplantation is required to prevent irreversible liver and neurological damage
b) Eliminating milk products resolves acute symptoms and prevents disease progression
c) Lactose-containing formulas are safe with galactose-digesting enzyme supplements
d) Liver transplantation cures galactosemia, as the enzymatic defect is liver-specific
e) Most infants identified via newborn screening require liver transplantation by age one
**Answer: b**
Galactosemia, caused by galactose 1-phosphate uridyltransferase deficiency, is managed by promptly eliminating milk products containing lactose, which resolves acute symptoms and prevents further liver and kidney damage. This dietary

intervention typically avoids the need for liver transplantation, which is reserved for rare cases with complications like cirrhosis. The enzymatic defect affects multiple tissues, not just the liver, and transplantation is not curative. Newborn screening often detects cases early, enabling dietary management without transplantation.[141]

163. A 6-month-old infant is brought to the pediatric clinic due to poor weight gain, intermittent vomiting, and irritability. The parents report that the infant has recently started consuming pureed fruits and fruit juices. Upon examination, the baby shows signs of failure to thrive, and laboratory tests reveal hypoglycemia, hypophosphatemia, and lactic acidosis. The physician is concerned about a possible metabolic disorder. Which of the following statements regarding this infant's condition is the most accurate?
a) Liver transplantation is typically required to prevent long-term complications associated with the disorder
b) The condition is caused by a deficiency in galactose-1-phosphate uridyltransferase, leading to issues with fruit sugar metabolism
c) Symptoms can be effectively managed by eliminating fructose, sucrose, and sorbitol from the diet, resulting in complete recovery
d) Most pediatric patients with this condition will require a liver transplant by the age of ten for liver cirrhosis or HCC
e) The infant's condition is due to maple syrup urine disease, which leads to elevated branched-chain amino acids in the urine
**Answer: c**
In hereditary fructosemia, caused by a deficiency of fructose-1-phosphate aldolase, symptoms typically emerge after the introduction of fruit sugars and sucrose into the diet. The clinical presentation includes failure to thrive, vomiting, hypoglycemia, hypophosphatemia, and lactic acidosis, similar to galactosemia. By completely eliminating fructose, sucrose, and sorbitol from the infant's diet, the symptoms can be resolved, allowing for full recovery, and patients do not require liver transplantation.[141]

164. A 5-year-old child with glycogen storage disease type III, despite strict dietary management, faces progressive liver failure with multiple liver adenomas, recurrent hypoglycemia, and poor growth. The child is evaluated for liver transplantation. Which statement best describes liver transplantation in glycogen storage diseases?
a) It fully cures all metabolic and extrahepatic complications
b) It improves metabolic control in types I and III, but catch-up growth may not always occur
c) It is essential to reverse renal and cardiac damage
d) Type IV patients do not benefit due to cardiac involvement and poor prognosis

e) Dietary therapy alone is sufficient, making transplantation unnecessary

**Answer: b**

Liver transplantation in glycogen storage disease types I and III corrects metabolic abnormalities, improving metabolic control. However, catch-up growth is not guaranteed, and some extrahepatic issues, like neutropenia in type Ib, may persist. Transplantation does not consistently reverse renal or cardiac damage, and while dietary therapy helps, it is often insufficient for severe cases like type III with liver failure. Type IV patients may benefit from transplantation in select cases, despite cardiac involvement.[142]

165. A 10-year-old child with homozygous familial hypercholesterolemia (HoFH) is evaluated for liver transplantation due to severe, refractory hypercholesterolemia and premature atherosclerotic cardiovascular disease (ASCVD), including angina. Cholesterol levels are high but stable. Which statement best describes liver transplantation in pediatric HoFH?
a) It fully resolves all cardiovascular complications
b) HoFH patients face higher in-hospital mortality post-transplant due to cardiovascular disease
c) Post-transplant, cholesterol and LDL levels drop significantly, but some patients may need ongoing lipid-lowering therapy
d) Dietary restrictions must continue indefinitely post-transplant to manage cholesterol
e) It halts ASCVD progression

**Answer: c**

Liver transplantation in pediatric HoFH significantly reduces total cholesterol and LDL cholesterol levels, often allowing dietary restrictions to be lifted. However, some patients may require ongoing lipid-lowering therapy due to persistent suboptimal LDL levels or ASCVD progression. It does not fully resolve all cardiovascular complications, halt ASCVD progression, or inherently increase in-hospital mortality.[143]

166. A 7-year-old girl with Niemann-Pick disease type C presents with hepatosplenomegaly, frequent respiratory infections, progressive neurological decline, and a history of neonatal jaundice and developmental delays. Which statement best describes liver transplantation in Niemann-Pick disease type C?
a) It is life-saving and resolves all neurological and hepatic symptoms
b) It may stabilize patients initially, but neurological decline persists, so it is generally not recommended
c) It is recommended when liver cirrhosis develops

d) It corrects hepatic cholesterol accumulation and partially improves neurological symptoms
e) Bone marrow transplantation is preferred over liver transplantation
**Answer: b**
Liver transplantation in Niemann-Pick disease type C may temporarily stabilize liver function, but progressive neurological deterioration continues due to defective cholesterol transport and storage in cells. As it does not address the underlying disease or halt neurological decline, transplantation is generally not recommended.[144]

167. A 2-week-old newborn presents to the emergency department with worsening jaundice, lethargy, and poor feeding. Initial bilirubin was 15 mg/dL at discharge, now 25 mg/dL (unconjugated), with no hemolysis. Crigler-Najjar syndrome is suspected. Which statement about Crigler-Najjar syndrome is most accurate?
a) Type I is effectively managed with phenobarbital to normalize bilirubin
b) Phototherapy is the mainstay for type I and becomes more effective with age
c) Type I has complete absence of uridine diphosphate glucuronyltransferase (UDPGT) activity, causing severe hyperbilirubinemia and kernicterus risk
d) Type II has a worse prognosis than type I due to severe neurological impairment
e) Prenatal diagnosis is based on elevated conjugated bilirubin in maternal serum
**Answer: c**
Type I Crigler-Najjar syndrome is defined by a complete lack of UDPGT activity, leading to severe unconjugated hyperbilirubinemia and a high risk of kernicterus. Type II has partial UDPGT activity, manageable with phenobarbital. Phototherapy is used for type I but becomes less effective with age due to increased subcutaneous tissue. Type II has a better prognosis, and prenatal diagnosis does not involve maternal conjugated bilirubin.[145,146]

168. A 4-year-old boy with type I Crigler-Najjar syndrome, on phototherapy, presents for follow-up with persistently elevated bilirubin and developmental delays. Which statement about liver transplantation in type I Crigler-Najjar syndrome is most accurate?
a) It restores normal bilirubin but is too risky for children under 10
b) Delaying transplantation past mid-childhood increases risk of irreversible neurological damage
c) It is indicated only for chronic liver disease, not elevated bilirubin alone
d) The risk of HCC remains high even after a liver transplant
e) Most patients develop cirrhosis by their teens, raising HCC risk
**Answer: b**
Type I Crigler-Najjar syndrome, marked by absent uridine diphosphate glucuronyltransferase activity, causes severe unconjugated hyperbilirubinemia.

Delaying liver transplantation beyond mid-childhood heightens the risk of irreversible neurological damage, such as kernicterus. Transplantation corrects the enzyme defect, normalizing bilirubin, and is indicated for high bilirubin levels, not liver disease. It is safe in young children, and cirrhosis or HCC is rare.[147]

169. A 5-year-old boy is diagnosed with primary hyperoxaluria type 1. His initial presentation included recurrent renal stones and signs of renal failure. The child exhibits significant oxalate accumulation, and his renal function shows a GFR of 32 mL/min/1.73 m². Which of the following is considered the most appropriate treatment option for this patient?
a) Kidney transplantation alone
b) Combined liver-kidney transplantation
c) Liver transplantation alone
d) Medical management with increased hydration and dietary modification
e) Dialysis followed by delayed kidney transplant
**Answer: b**
Combined liver-kidney transplantation is the treatment of choice for patients with primary hyperoxaluria who are experiencing renal failure or are at high risk of it. This approach addresses the underlying metabolic defect by replacing both the dysfunctional liver and the failing kidneys, effectively lowering systemic oxalate levels and preventing further oxalate accumulation in the kidneys. In contrast, kidney transplantation alone would not prevent the recurrence of renal failure due to the persistent metabolic abnormality originating from the liver.[148]

170. A 5-year-old boy with hyperoxaluria type 1 underwent combined liver-kidney transplantation. His post-operative monitoring showed an elevated urinary oxalate level of 8,500 μmol/24 hr. Which of the following is the most appropriate management strategy to monitor and assess the patient's post-operative course regarding his elevated urinary oxalate levels?
a) Implement a fluid-restricted diet in order to avoid hemodialysis
b) Perform serial bone mineral density studies to assess improvement in oxalate-associated bone disease
c) Administer high-dose corticosteroids to reduce inflammation
d) Focus on dietary modifications to reduce oxalate intake
e) Obtain a renal biopsy
**Answer: b**
Following transplantation in patients with primary hyperoxaluria, monitoring for elevated urinary oxalate levels is essential due to the significant body stores of oxalate being mobilized. Serial bone mineral density studies are specifically useful in evaluating the improvement in oxalate-associated bone disease, as oxalate

accumulation can lead to osteoarthropathy. In addition, the usual treatment to ensure ongoing depletion of the accumulated oxalate load is to induce high daily urine output with fluid loading. Peritransplant hemodialysis may also be used.[149]

171. A 2-year-old boy presents to the emergency department with an acute onset of lethargy, vomiting, and hypoglycemia following a mild viral illness. He is comatose and exhibits signs of fulminant liver failure, including hyperammonemia and coagulopathy. A liver biopsy reveals microvesicular fat and minimal inflammation. The child's clinical presentation raises suspicion for a mitochondrial disorder that resembles Reye's syndrome. Which of the following tests would provide the most critical information in determining the underlying cause of his acute liver failure and guiding management?
a) Serum ammonia level
b) Liver ultrasound
c) Serum lactate level and lactate-pyruvate ratio
d) Hepatic function panel
e) Accurate history and physical
**Answer: c**
In suspected mitochondrial disease, especially in a comatose child with fulminant liver failure and no clear cause, careful evaluation is critical. The presentation can mimic Reye's syndrome or fatty acid oxidation disorders. Measuring serum lactate and the lactate-pyruvate ratio helps identify mitochondrial dysfunction—elevated levels and a ratio >20:1 suggest impaired mitochondrial respiration. This guides diagnosis and management, including consideration of liver transplant. Definitive diagnosis requires biochemical analysis of liver or muscle tissue.[150]

172. A 1-year-old boy presents with progressive lethargy, failure to thrive, and frequent seizures. He has a history of developmental delay and muscle hypotonia. Examination reveals signs of acute liver failure, including jaundice, coagulopathy, and elevated serum ammonia levels. A thorough workup confirms a diagnosis of mitochondrial disease. Which of the following statements best reflects the treatment option for this child?
a) Liver transplantation is indicated due to end-stage liver disease; neurological recovery will follow liver transplant
b) Liver transplantation is recommended since the liver is primarily affected and can significantly improve overall health
c) Liver transplantation is contraindicated because the presence of extrahepatic disease suggests a poor prognosis
d) Liver transplantation is indicated if metabolic derangements can't be successfully managed by frequent high-carbohydrate feedings and carnitine supplementation

e) Liver transplantation could be performed, but only if accompanied by a thorough evaluation of neurological and cardiac functions
**Answer: c**
In this case, liver transplantation is not indicated due to the presence of extrahepatic disease (neurological involvement) associated with the mitochondrial disorder. Experience with liver transplantation in patients with mitochondrial diseases shows that the survival rate is less than 50%, and the involvement of other organ systems, particularly the neurological system, is linked to poor outcomes.[151]

173. A 2-year-old male is brought to the emergency department with abdominal distention and weight loss. Imaging studies reveal a mass in the liver. A CT scan shows a large heterogeneous mass measuring 8 cm in diameter, located in liver segments IV, V, and VI without vascular invasion, local extension or distant metastases. Considering the PRETEXT staging system for hepatoblastoma, what is the correct PRETEXT stage for this patient?
a) PRETEXT I
b) PRETEXT II
c) PRETEXT III
d) PRETEXT IV
e) PRETEXT V
**Answer: c**
In hepatoblastoma, the PRETEXT staging system categorizes tumors based on their location within the liver's anatomical sectors. In this case, the CT findings indicate the presence of a large mass involving segments IV, V, and VI of the liver. Because the tumor is present in three contiguous sectors (right posterior, right anterior and left medial), it fits the criteria for PRETEXT III, which specifically describes a tumor involving three contiguous sectors or two nonadjoining sectors.[152]

174. A 3-year-old girl diagnosed with hepatoblastoma undergoes a liver transplantation after failing to achieve sufficient tumor reduction with preoperative chemotherapy. Her preoperative AFP levels were initially high and did not decrease significantly during chemotherapy, and cross-sectional imaging showed stable tumor size. Post-transplant, she experiences a recurrence of the tumor 9 months later. Which factor is most predictive of the outcome in this patient's case regarding the recurrence of hepatoblastoma following surgical intervention?
a) Tumor histology
b) The timing of transplantation after initial diagnosis
c) The extent of tumor reduction during preoperative chemotherapy based on changes in AFP levels
d) The age of the patient at the time of surgery

e) The initial AFP levels prior to chemotherapy
**Answer: c**
Recent studies have shown that tumor susceptibility to chemotherapy, as indicated by decreasing AFP levels or a reduction in tumor size, is a good predictor of outcomes. In this case, the lack of significant decrease in AFP levels and stable tumor size during chemotherapy suggest a poor response to treatment.[153]

175. A 5-year-old boy is diagnosed with unresectable HCC after presenting with abdominal pain and elevated AFP. Imaging shows a 6 cm tumor without vascular invasion or extrahepatic spread. He undergoes liver transplantation. Final pathology confirms HCC in the right posterior liver segment, with no tumor in the 4 recovered hilar lymph nodes. Which of the following factors is most predictive of disease recurrence?
a) Tumor size greater than 4 cm
b) Age at the time of transplantation
c) Fewer than 6 hilar lymph nodes recovered
d) Preoperative AFP level
e) Tumor location
**Answer: a**
In HCC, tumor size is a critical prognostic factor that has been shown to correlate with the likelihood of disease recurrence following liver transplantation. A tumor size greater than 4 cm is associated with a higher risk of recurrence and worse overall outcomes.[154]

176. A 12-year-old girl diagnosed with Glycogen Storage Disease Type I (GSD-I) presents to the clinic for her annual follow-up. She was diagnosed at 6 months of age and has been treated for her condition. Despite treatment, her glycemic control has been suboptimal, and she has developed hepatomegaly. Which of the following statements regarding the risk of HCC in patients with GSD-I is most accurate?
a) HCC mostly develops in patients who exhibit symptoms of liver failure
b) Poor glycemic control does not influence the risk of HCC in GSD-I patients
c) The risk of developing HCC is highest in the first decade of life
d) Hepatic adenomas can transform into HCC, especially in patients with poor glycemic control during the second and third decades of life
e) All patients with GSD-I will inevitably develop HCC
**Answer: d**
The risk of developing HCC in patients with GSD-I is closely associated with the formation of hepatic adenomas. These adenomas are more likely to develop in patients with poor glycemic control and have the potential to transform into HCC,

particularly in the second and third decades of life when the prevalence of adenomas increases.[155]

177. A 12-year-old girl presents with fatigue and abdominal discomfort. Evaluation reveals end-stage liver disease due to Alpha-1 Antitrypsin (A1AT) deficiency, PiZZ genotype. Her parents are concerned about the risk of liver cancer. Which of the following statements about HCC risk in A1AT deficiency is most accurate?
a) HCC is common in children with A1AT deficiency, especially before the onset of cirrhosis
b) The risk of HCC increases in A1AT-deficient patients with cirrhosis, especially in older adults and males
c) Nearly all patients with the PiZZ genotype will eventually develop HCC
d) A1AT deficiency is not associated with an increased risk of HCC
e) Only heterozygous genotypes, such as PiMZ, are linked to a higher HCC risk
**Answer: b**
Patients with A1AT deficiency, particularly those with the PiZZ genotype, are at a significant risk for developing HCC. Studies have demonstrated an odds ratio of 5.0 for HCC in individuals with A1AT deficiency compared to the general population. While the risk predominantly increases with age and is more common in older men, it can also occur in younger patients with severe liver disease related to A1AT deficiency.[156]

178. A 9-month-old male presents to the emergency department after being involved in a motor vehicle accident. An abdominal ultrasound reveals a liver lesion, and a subsequent triple-phase CT scan is consistent with an infantile hepatic hemangioma (IHH). The parents report that the child seems generally healthy, is active, and has no signs of distress. What is the most common presentation and clinical course of IHH?
a) Sudden abdominal pain and signs of intra-abdominal hemorrhage; most patients require liver transplantation
b) Most IHHs remain undetected as patients typically stay asymptomatic, with many lesions identified incidentally during imaging for other reasons
c) Common presentations may include congestive heart failure due to arteriovenous shunting, Kasabach-Merritt syndrome.
d) Many patients remain asymptomatic through childhood, with symptoms of liver failure often becoming apparent in adulthood, necessitating liver transplantation
e) IHH typically presents in the first 6 to 12 months of life, usually accompanied by hepatomegaly. It commonly undergoes rapid proliferation postnatally, requiring liver resection or transplantation.
**Answer: b**

IHH is a benign endothelial cell neoplasm typically identified in infants aged 6 to 12 months, often associated with hepatomegaly and sometimes with cutaneous hemangiomas. While IHHs can cause complications such as congestive heart failure, Kasabach-Merritt syndrome, and hypothyroidism, most cases remain asymptomatic and are incidentally discovered during imaging. Only those with significant complications face high risks of morbidity and mortality. Most cases do not require resection or transplant unless severe complications occur, but it typically regresses in infancy or early childhood.[157]

179. A 10-year-old girl is referred to a pediatric specialist after being hospitalized for abdominal pain and rapid weight loss over the past month. Imaging studies reveal a diffuse liver tumor with multiple peripheral lesions, and a biopsy demonstrates factor VIII–related antigen staining consistent with hepatic hemangioendothelioma (HEH). What is the most appropriate management strategy for this patient?
a) Initiate chemotherapy with a doxorubicin-based regimen
b) Perform surgical resection of the tumor
c) Initiate targeted immunotherapy
d) Plan for early liver transplantation
e) Administer radiation therapy to shrink the tumor
**Answer: d**
In cases of HEH, especially in children, early liver transplantation is recommended as the most effective management strategy when surgical resection is not feasible due to multifocal or diffuse disease. The prognosis is improved with transplantation, as evidenced by reported survival rates of 72% at 10 years post-transplantation. Resection, chemotherapy, immunotherapy, and radiation are not effective in this context.[158]

# 5. Special Consideration in Patient Evaluation

180. A 23-year-old man presents with acute liver failure due to an acetaminophen overdose. He is critically ill despite N-acetylcysteine treatment and requires mechanical ventilation. The transplant team is evaluating him for liver transplantation. This was his first suicide attempt, and although he has a past history of alcohol use, he has no ongoing substance abuse. Some team members are concerned about allocating a scarce organ to a patient with this background. What is the most ethical approach in deciding his transplant eligibility?
a) Base eligibility on his current clinical status and urgent need
b) Disqualify him due to his alcohol history, which may affect outcomes
c) Require evidence of rehabilitation and long-term sobriety before proceeding
d) Postpone decision until a full psychiatric evaluation is complete
e) Prioritize another candidate with a better long-term prognosis

**Answer: a**
In this case, the ethical principle of prioritizing urgent medical needs is paramount. The patient is experiencing acute liver failure, which poses an immediate threat to his life. Given his young age, the fact that this is his first suicide attempt, and his current critical condition, the focus should be on his immediate medical status rather than his past history of alcohol abuse.[159]

181. A 32-year-old man with hepatitis C-related cirrhosis is being evaluated for liver transplant. He has a history of drug use but is stable on methadone maintenance and has well-controlled bipolar disorder. What is the most appropriate next step in evaluating his transplant eligibility?
a) Require discontinuation of methadone before listing
b) Approve transplant without further concern
c) Disqualify due to risk of relapse
d) Consult an addiction specialist to assess relapse risk and treatment plan
e) Delay until he completes detoxification

**Answer: d**
The current practice indicates that methadone maintenance therapy is not an absolute contraindication for liver transplantation. With 70% of U.S. transplant programs indicating they would allow patients on methadone maintenance to proceed with transplantation, and with no standardized requirement for discontinuation, this

patient should be considered for transplant eligibility based on his medical status and the stability of his psychiatric condition.[160]

182. A 67-year-old woman with MASH, admitted for esophageal bleeding treated with endoscopic banding, is being evaluated for liver transplantation. Her MELD score is 32, and she has diabetes, hypertension, recent falls, and cognitive decline, with a possible Alzheimer's diagnosis from an outpatient neurologic evaluation. She lives alone but has supportive nieces. Which of the following is the least appropriate next step in determining her transplant eligibility?
a) Conduct an urgent neurological evaluation to differentiate between Alzheimer's disease and liver-related cognitive impairment
b) Perform a multidisciplinary assessment, including neurology, hepatology, and physical therapy, to evaluate cognitive, medical, and mobility status
c) Optimize her medical condition (e.g., manage diabetes, hypertension, and hepatic encephalopathy) and reassess transplant candidacy after stabilization
d) Engage social services to ensure adequate post-transplant support and safety, given her falls and living situation
e) Disqualify her from undergoing liver transplantation due to her new diagnosis of Alzheimer's disease and cognitive impairment
**Answer: e**
Disqualifying her immediately from liver transplantation based on a possible Alzheimer's diagnosis is the least appropriate step. Her cognitive impairment may be reversible (e.g., due to hepatic encephalopathy) rather than Alzheimer's, which requires confirmation through an urgent neurological evaluation. A multidisciplinary assessment, medical optimization, and social support evaluation are essential to determine her transplant eligibility comprehensively.[161]

183. A 54-year-old man with alcohol-related decompensated liver cirrhosis (MELD score 34) is listed for liver transplantation. He has significant coronary artery disease (70% stenosis in the left anterior descending artery, 80% in the right coronary artery) but a preserved left ventricular ejection fraction (60%) and no prior myocardial infarction. What is the most appropriate treatment option?
a) Disqualify him from liver transplantation due to severe coronary artery disease
b) Perform coronary artery bypass grafting (CABG), then delay liver transplant until stabilization
c) Plan simultaneous CABG and liver transplant during the same surgical session
d) Perform liver transplant first, followed by CABG 3–6 months later
e) Perform percutaneous coronary intervention before liver transplant
**Answer: c**

Simultaneous CABG and liver transplant is the most appropriate option. Significant coronary artery disease increases perioperative cardiac risks in liver transplantation, and addressing it in the same surgical session minimizes complications. The preserved ejection fraction supports surgical tolerance, and the disease severity makes percutaneous coronary intervention less suitable.[162]

184. A 47-year-old female with a history of alcohol-induced liver cirrhosis is admitted to the hospital with decompensated liver cirrhosis. She is listed for a liver transplant with a MELD score of 31. Upon admission, a transthoracic echocardiogram reveals a left ventricular ejection fraction of 28%. Concurrently, she receives an offer for a liver transplant organ. How should the transplant team proceed with this patient?
a) Accept the offer and proceed with the liver transplant, expecting cardiac function to improve post-transplant
b) Accept the offer, optimize volume status, and perform the transplant on bypass to reduce cardiac stress
c) Perform simultaneous heart-liver transplantation due to her low ejection fraction and liver disease severity
d) Place the patient on hold, investigate the cause of heart failure, and optimize heart failure therapy before transplantation
e) Accept the offer and proceed with the transplant, monitoring closely for postoperative cardiac decompensation
**Answer: d**
Investigating the cause of heart failure (e.g., cirrhotic cardiomyopathy) and optimizing medical therapy is critical before transplantation. Her low ejection fraction (28%) increases perioperative risks, and liver transplantation is generally avoided with an ejection fraction below 40%. Cardiac function may improve with treatment, but thorough evaluation is needed first.[163]

185. A 54-year-old male with a history of cirrhosis secondary to chronic hepatitis C is admitted to the hospital with worsening dyspnea on exertion and ascites. The process of evaluation for a liver transplant has been initiated. A Doppler evaluation of the tricuspid valve during the echocardiogram reveals an estimated right ventricular systolic pressure of 45 mm Hg. Which of the following is the most appropriate next step in the management of this patient?
a) Initiate treatment with diuretics to manage fluid overload and monitor symptoms
b) Refer the patient for right heart catheterization to confirm the presence of pulmonary hypertension
c) Proceed with the liver transplant evaluation without further cardiac workup, as echocardiographic findings are sufficient

d) Schedule the patient for a pulmonary function test to assess for any underlying pulmonary disease
e) Optimize volume status and initiate sildenafil therapy for suspected pulmonary hypertension based on echocardiographic findings
**Answer: b**
In patients with an estimated right ventricular systolic pressure above 40 mm Hg, further evaluation with right heart catheterization is essential to confirm the presence of pulmonary hypertension. Elevated pulmonary artery pressures, as suggested by the Doppler findings in this patient's echocardiogram, warrant invasive measurement to accurately diagnose and quantify pulmonary hypertension, particularly in the context of potential portopulmonary hypertension. Diuretics and other treatments may be applicable afterward, but confirming the diagnosis first is the priority.[164]

186. A 62-year-old woman with cirrhosis from alcoholic liver disease presents with worsening dyspnea and hypoxemia (SpO2 <85% on room air). She appears cyanotic. An echocardiogram shows mild right ventricular enlargement and a possible patent foramen ovale (PFO) with interatrial shunting. A saline contrast echocardiogram is performed. What finding confirms a PFO?
a) Bubbles in the right ventricle immediately after saline injection
b) Bubbles in the right atrium within the first cardiac cycle after saline injection
c) Bubbles in the left ventricle within the first or second cardiac cycle after saline injection
d) Bubbles in the left ventricle after the fourth or fifth cardiac cycle after saline injection
e) Bubbles in the right atrium after the fourth cardiac cycle after saline injection
**Answer: c**
Bubbles in the left ventricle within the first or second cardiac cycle after saline injection confirm right-to-left shunting through a PFO, indicating increased right atrial pressure. Late bubbles (after the fourth or fifth cycle) suggest intrapulmonary shunting, not PFO.[165]

187. A 58-year-old man with alcoholic liver disease and ascites is admitted for worsening confusion and lethargy. Labs show serum sodium of 124 mEq/L, and he exhibits disorientation and poor concentration. What is the most appropriate management?
a) Give hypertonic saline to rapidly correct sodium levels
b) Restrict fluids and administer tolvaptan to correct hyponatremia gradually
c) Start diuretics to remove fluid and raise sodium levels
d) Restrict fluids and gradually correct sodium with isotonic saline to avoid osmotic demyelination

e) Treat with lactulose to improve cognitive function
**Answer: d**
Gradual correction of hyponatremia is critical in liver disease to prevent osmotic demyelination syndrome. While fluid restriction with tolvaptan (option b) can be part of hyponatremia management, it requires careful monitoring and is less appropriate as the primary approach compared to supportive care and gradual correction. Hypertonic saline risks rapid correction, diuretics may worsen hypovolemia, and lactulose targets hepatic encephalopathy, not hyponatremia.[166]

188. A 65-year-old male with a history of liver cirrhosis secondary to hepatitis B and recent development of hepatorenal syndrome is admitted for a liver transplant. His preoperative laboratory results indicate a serum potassium level of 6.1 mEq/L, a serum creatinine of 2.3 mg/dL, BUN of 45 mg/dL, bicarbonate of 18 mEq/L, and a pH of 7.31. What is the most appropriate management strategy for this patient?
a) Evaluate the patient for a combined liver-kidney transplant
b) Start a continuous infusion of insulin along with dextrose to facilitate potassium uptake into cells
c) Use a β-agonist nebulizer to enhance potassium transport across cell membranes
d) Initiate perioperative dialysis to decrease serum potassium levels prior to reperfusion
e) Administer oral potassium-binding resins to lower serum potassium before surgery
**Answer: d**
In patients with liver cirrhosis and renal dysfunction, especially those diagnosed with hepatorenal syndrome, initiating perioperative dialysis is the most effective strategy to reduce serum potassium levels before liver transplant surgery. A potassium level greater than 5.5 mEq/L poses a significant risk for hyperkalemia during reperfusion, and dialysis can effectively lower the serum potassium concentration. A higher preoperative potassium level is a risk factor for hyperkalemia during reperfusion.[167]

189. What method is regarded as the gold standard for accurately measuring GFR in patients with advanced liver disease, particularly in the context of renal impairment associated with cirrhosis?
a) Creatinine clearance
b) Cystatin C
c) Inulin clearance
d) GFR estimation equations
e) Isotope markers for GFR such as 125 I-iothalamate, 99mTc-DTPA, and 51 Cr-EDTA
**Answer: c**

Inulin clearance is considered the gold standard for determining GFR because it is not influenced by muscle mass, dietary intake, or other factors that can affect serum creatinine levels. While other methods such as creatinine clearance and estimation equations have their utility, they may be less accurate in this patient population. Isotope markers, while precise, are often limited by availability and practicality.[168]

190. A 58-year-old man with alcohol-related cirrhosis presents with severe ascites, 5 kg weight gain in one week, fatigue, and diffuse abdominal tenderness without rebound or guarding. Labs show serum creatinine of 2.3 mg/dL, rising gradually over three months. He has refractory ascites despite diuretics and no proteinuria or hematuria. What is the most likely renal impairment diagnosis?
a) Type 1 hepatorenal syndrome
b) Type 2 hepatorenal syndrome
c) Chronic kidney disease
d) Acute tubular necrosis
e) Pre-renal azotemia
**Answer: b**
The gradual rise in serum creatinine over three months, refractory ascites, and cirrhosis suggest Type 2 hepatorenal syndrome. Unlike chronic kidney disease, Type 2 HRS lacks proteinuria or hematuria and is driven by liver disease severity. Type 1 HRS involves rapid renal decline, acute tubular necrosis requires tubular injury evidence, and pre-renal azotemia is reversible with volume correction.[169]

191. There are known hemodynamic changes that occur in cirrhotic patients as they progress from the preascitic stage to diuretic-sensitive ascites, then to diuretic-resistant ascites, and finally to hepatorenal syndrome. These hemodynamic changes include all of the following except:
a) Splanchnic vasoconstriction
b) Reduced effective arterial blood volume
c) Reduced systemic vascular resistance
d) Vasoconstriction of various extrasplanchnic vascular beds, including the renal and cerebral circulations
e) Increased activity of the renin-angiotensin-aldosterone system
**Answer: a**
In cirrhotic patients, as they progress through various stages of ascites, significant hemodynamic changes occur. One of these changes is actually increased splanchnic vasodilation, which leads to the pooling of blood in the splanchnic circulation and contributes to reduced effective arterial blood volume and increased activity of the renin-angiotensin-aldosterone system.[170]

192. A 62-year-old woman with alcoholic cirrhosis presents with abdominal pain and fever. Imaging shows large-volume ascites, and diagnostic paracentesis confirms spontaneous bacterial peritonitis. Despite antibiotics treatment, her serum creatinine rises from 1.2 mg/dL to 2.3 mg/dL in days, with new oliguria. What is the most likely precipitating factor for her hepatorenal syndrome (HRS)?
a) Aggressive diuretic therapy
b) Prolonged hypotension
c) Bacterial infection
d) Diagnostic paracentesis
e) Acute tubular necrosis
**Answer: c**
SBP is the most likely precipitant of HRS in this patient. The inflammatory response from the bacterial infection causes renal vasoconstriction and impaired renal blood flow in cirrhosis. Aggressive diuretics or large-volume paracentesis (without albumin) could contribute, but diagnostic paracentesis involves minimal fluid removal. Hypotension and acute tubular necrosis are less likely without specific evidence.[171]

193. A 54-year-old man with alcoholic cirrhosis and hepatorenal syndrome (HRS) undergoes liver transplantation after 10 weeks of hemodialysis for renal failure. Post-transplant, he shows some kidney recovery with increased urine output but still requires hemodialysis. What is the most significant predictor of his post-transplant renal recovery?
a) Transfusion needs during surgery
b) Recipient age
c) Serum creatinine on day 7 post-transplant
d) Pre-transplant hemodialysis duration
e) Post-transplant complications
**Answer: d**
The duration of pre-transplant hemodialysis, especially over 8 weeks, is the most significant predictor of post-transplant renal recovery in HRS patients. Prolonged dialysis increases the risk of persistent renal impairment post-transplant, outweighing other factors.[172]

194. A 60-year-old woman with decompensated MASH cirrhosis is evaluated for liver transplantation. She has a MELD score of 30, recurrent ascites, and has been on hemodialysis for 9 weeks due to hepatorenal syndrome (HRS). Labs show total bilirubin 6.1 mg/dL and INR 2.5, with no active infections. What is the most appropriate transplant recommendation?
a) List for liver transplant only, expecting HRS to resolve post-transplant

b) List for simultaneous liver-kidney transplantation (SLKT) due to prolonged hemodialysis
c) List for liver transplant and use the kidney transplant safety net if renal function does not recover within 4 months after liver transplant
d) List for liver transplant only and plan for a living donor kidney transplant later to optimize the outcome
e) List for liver transplant only and continue dialysis for renal failure

**Answer: b**

SLKT is the most appropriate due to prolonged hemodialysis (>8 weeks) and advanced liver disease (MELD 30), indicating irreversible renal failure. HRS is unlikely to resolve post-liver transplant alone. Option c (safety net) is less optimal, as prolonged dialysis suggests low renal recovery likelihood, making SLKT the preferred choice to address both organ failures concurrently.[172]

195. A 58-year-old woman with alcoholic cirrhosis, recently treated for spontaneous bacterial peritonitis (SBP), is listed for liver transplantation with a MELD score of 22. She undergoes a complex liver transplant due to adhesions and requires revisional surgery within a year post-transplant. Which statement about her pre- and post-transplant condition is most accurate?
a) SBP significantly increases post-transplant mortality compared to patients without SBP
b) Treated SBP before transplant does not affect postoperative complication rates
c) MELD score reliably predicts post-transplant outcomes, regardless of SBP history
d) SBP increases the likelihood of abdominal surgical interventions within a year post-transplant
e) The incidence of SBP and its associated complications post-transplant is found to be higher in females

**Answer: d**

Patients with SBP have an increased likelihood of requiring surgical interventions post-transplant due to complications such as hernias and other issues tied to their advanced liver disease. While SBP does not significantly affect post-transplant mortality, it does lead to a higher incidence of surgical needs in the postoperative period.[173]

196. A 54-year-old male with end-stage liver disease from alcoholic cirrhosis is offered a liver transplant from a 62-year-old Black female donor with a history of hypertension, type 2 diabetes, and positive blood cultures for Enterobacter species diagnosed 48 hours ago, treatment with antibiotics initiated. How should the transplant team respond to this donor organ offer?
a) Decline the organ due to high sepsis and mortality risk from positive blood cultures

b) Accept the organ but withhold immunosuppressive therapy post-transplant to reduce infection risk
c) Accept the organ, as graft survival rates are not significantly affected by positive blood cultures
d) Delay the transplant until the donor's bacteremia is treated and blood cultures are negative to ensure an infection-free liver
e) Accept the organ and treat the recipient with antibiotics if infection signs develop

**Answer: c**

Research indicates that accepting organs from donors with positive blood cultures is feasible, as graft survival rates are only slightly lower, with negligible clinical impact on overall patient outcomes. Given the critical need for organs and the donor's ongoing antibiotic treatment, proceeding with the transplant is reasonable, balancing infection risks with the potential for favorable long-term results.[174]

197. A 47-year-old female with end-stage liver disease secondary to primary biliary cholangitis presents for a liver transplant. A 48-year-old male donor, who recently immigrated from Uzbekistan, experienced a motor vehicle accident and was pronounced brain dead. The donor's family has consented to organ donation. However, prior to organ procurement, the OPO alerts the transplant team that the donor has been found to have active pulmonary tuberculosis. How should the transplant team respond to the offer of the liver organ from this donor?
a) Accept the liver for transplantation, as the risk of transmission is low with proper pre-operative antibiotic coverage
b) Decline the liver organ offer due to the high risk of transmission of tuberculosis, as it poses a significant risk to the recipient
c) Accept the liver organ but initiate a course of anti-tubercular therapy for the recipient immediately after the transplant
d) Consult with infectious disease specialists before deciding whether to accept the liver organ
e) Delay the transplant until the donor's understanding of communicable diseases can be fully evaluated

**Answer: b**

Transplantation of an organ from a donor with an active tuberculosis infection poses a significant risk of transmission to both the transplant recipient and the entire care team. Tuberculosis can be spread through aerosolized particles, and the recipient's immunocompromised state post-transplant heightens the risk of developing active tuberculosis. Therefore, the standard protocol is to decline such organ offers to protect the recipient's health.[175]

198. A 55-year-old female with end-stage liver disease from hepatitis C and alcohol-related injury, MELD score 24, is listed for liver transplantation. She lacks varicella and measles antibodies and received the measles, mumps, rubella (MMR) vaccine one week ago. With a 6-month estimated wait time in the area, a liver offer suddenly becomes available. How should the transplant team respond?
a) Accept the liver, as the MMR vaccine does not affect transplant eligibility
b) Decline the liver, as the MMR vaccine was given only one week ago, and live vaccines require a 4-week wait before transplantation
c) Accept the liver and start antiviral prophylaxis to mitigate vaccine-related risks
d) Decline the liver temporarily to evaluate the donor's infectious disease history
e) Accept the liver and monitor closely for vaccine-related complications post-transplant
**Answer: b**
Receiving a live virus vaccine like MMR shortly before transplantation poses risks, as the immune system needs at least 4 weeks to respond safely. Declining the liver offer is prudent to ensure patient safety and optimal transplant outcomes.[176]

199. A 62-year-old male with end-stage liver disease from autoimmune hepatitis, MELD score 35, is in the ICU after stabilizing from esophageal bleeding. The patient is listed for liver transplant. He lacks measles immunity. How should the transplant team proceed with vaccination?
a) Vaccinate immediately with the measles vaccine to establish immunity before transplantation
b) Vaccinate after ICU discharge, before transplantation, to ensure immunity
c) Avoid vaccination during hospitalization, as live virus vaccines are risky for urgent transplant candidates
d) Delay vaccination until after transplantation for better immunity establishment
e) Start with inactivated measles vaccines for immediate protection
**Answer: c**
Live virus vaccines like measles are risky for critically ill patients with high MELD scores awaiting urgent transplantation, due to potential vaccine-induced complications. Vaccination should be avoided during hospitalization, and live vaccines are contraindicated post-transplant. No inactivated measles vaccine exists.[176]

200. A 68-year-old female patient with a history of autoimmune hepatitis is listed for liver transplantation with a MELD score of 32. She undergoes routine liver ultrasounds every 6 to 12 months for cancer surveillance. Recent ultrasound findings were abnormal, prompting a triple-phase CT scan that revealed hepatic cirrhosis and an enhancement pattern in the right anterior lobe measuring 2.4 cm. This

enhancement showed hyperattenuation in the arterial phase and hypoisodensity in the portal phase. What is the most likely diagnosis?
a) Hemangioma
b) Atypical dysplastic nodule
c) Liver cell adenoma
d) Focal nodular hyperplasia
e) HCC
**Answer: e**
This question stem presents a clinical scenario involving a patient with significant risk factors for liver cancer, including autoimmune hepatitis and cirrhosis. In patients with hepatic cirrhosis an enhancement pattern consisting of hyperattenuation in the arterial phase and hypoisodensity in the portal phase is virtually diagnostic of HCC.[58]

201. A 65-year-old male with a history of alcohol-induced cirrhosis presents for routine imaging and surveillance for HCC. A recent MRI scan with Gd-EOB-DTPA (gadoxetate disodium) shows a 2.5 cm hepatic lesion in segment 7. During the hepatocyte phase, the lesion exhibits signal intensity similar to the surrounding liver parenchyma, while the surrounding liver demonstrates normal enhancement. The patient has no history of weight loss or abdominal pain. Which of the following is the most likely diagnosis for the hepatic lesion observed in this patient?
a) HCC
b) Regenerative nodule
c) Dysplastic nodule
d) Focal nodular hyperplasia (FNH)
e) Liver adenoma
**Answer: b**
In patients with cirrhosis, regenerative nodules retain the ability to take up and excrete Gd-EOB-DTPA, showing similar signal intensity to the surrounding liver tissue during the hepatocyte phase. This contrasts with HCC, which typically appears as a hypointense area due to its inability to take up the contrast agent effectively.
Dysplastic nodules can have variable imaging characteristics. While they may retain the ability to uptake contrast agents, they typically do not present with signal intensity similar to surrounding liver parenchyma in the hepatocyte phase because they often reflect some alteration in liver function.
FNH typically displays a characteristic "central scar" and may enhance differently compared to surrounding liver tissue. In the hepatocyte phase of Gd-EOB-DTPA imaging, FNH can show variable enhancement, but it usually does not demonstrate a similar signal intensity to the surrounding liver like a regenerative nodule does. Additionally, FNH is less common in cirrhotic livers than regenerative nodules.

Liver adenomas are usually hypervascular lesions that typically appear hyperintense during the arterial phase but may not retain similar contrast uptake to the surrounding liver tissue during the hepatocyte phase. Moreover, these lesions are often more associated with younger patients and have specific associations, such as oral contraceptive use.[177]

202. A 27-year-old male with a history of alcohol-induced liver cirrhosis and a MELD score of 31 has been transferred from a community hospital to a transplant center for advanced management and potential liver transplantation. Previously, the patient underwent an exploratory laparotomy and cholecystectomy due to gangrenous cholecystitis but experienced diffuse bleeding. Despite aggressive resuscitation, including numerous blood product transfusions, he underwent two reoperations without achieving hemostasis. The patient arrived intubated with an open abdomen, two laparotomy sponges still in place from the last surgical intervention two days prior, and a temporary Abthera dressing. Laboratory results indicate a hemoglobin level of 8.7 g/dL (stable from this morning), an INR of 4.3, and a fibrinogen level of 97 mg/dL. How should the transplant team proceed?
a) Correct coagulopathy and proceed with TIPS before taking patient to the operating room for washout, hemostasis, and closure
b) Correct coagulopathy and take the patient to the operating room immediately for washout, hemostasis, and possible closure
c) Correct coagulopathy and take the patient to the operating room for washout, hemostasis, and possible closure in a couple of days when he is clinically stable
d) Correct coagulopathy and obtain a CT triple phase to evaluate for active bleeding with possible interventional radiology consult for embolization
e) Take the patient to the operating room immediately for total hepatectomy and plan for an anhepatic state until liver transplantation
**Answer: a**
This clinical scenario involves a critically ill patient with severe coagulopathy and ongoing bleeding after multiple surgical interventions. The correct approach would be to correct the coagulopathy first and then consider TIPS before returning to the operating room. TIPS can reduce portal pressure, improve blood flow, and facilitate hemostasis.[178]

203. A 52-year-old female liver transplant recipient presents for routine follow-up six months post-transplant. She has been stable but now complains of fatigue and moderate jaundice. A HIDA scan is conducted to evaluate graft function. The scan reveals larger photopenic areas in the right posterior segment with decreased radiotracer uptake, along with significant retention of the HIDA compound in the

blood pool. Given these findings, all of the following may be reasons for this radiographic appearance, except:
a) Large hepatic cyst
b) Hepatic abscess
c) Right hepatic artery thrombosis
d) Stenosis at the anastomosis of the right hepatic artery reconstruction to the gastroduodenal artery
e) Systemic hyperbilirubinemia from graft cholestasis, where elevated bilirubin competes with the contrast for hepatocyte uptake

**Answer: e**

Elevated bilirubin levels can impair the transport of technetium Tc 99m IDA compounds, resulting in lower radionuclide uptake independent of hepatocyte function. This is important to recognize, as it necessitates caution when interpreting imaging results in hyperbilirubinemia, which typically leads to generalized decreased contrast uptake. Additionally, scintigraphic appearances of graft rejection and infections (bacterial, viral, or fungal) are similar, showing high retention of the HIDA compound in the blood pool and poor graft uptake. Photopenic regions on HIDA studies may also indicate abscesses, hepatic cysts, or thrombosis, although these usually produce focal findings.[179]

204. A 35-year-old female underwent a liver transplant due to autoimmune disease. During the procedure, her native anatomy revealed a replacement of the right hepatic artery. The donor liver graft exhibited Type 1 anatomy, and the arterial anastomosis was performed by connecting the donor celiac trunk to the recipient's small common hepatic artery using running 7-0 Prolene sutures. The patient initially recovered without complications; however, on postoperative day 3, she experienced an acute rise in LFT. The CT angiogram of the abdomen revealed significant stenosis at the level of the arterial anastomosis. What is the most appropriate treatment option?
a) Treat with percutaneous transluminal angioplasty using a small-caliber, low-profile balloon at the site of stenosis
b) Treat with percutaneous transluminal angioplasty with the placement of a small-caliber stent at the site of stenosis
c) Initiate a heparin drip and perform an operative revision of the anastomosis using interrupted 8-0 Prolene sutures
d) Initiate a heparin drip and perform an operative revision of the anastomosis, planning to install an infrarenal aortic conduit utilizing third-party cadaveric iliac vessels
e) Initiate a heparin drip and perform an operative revision of the anastomosis, planning to install an infrarenal aortic conduit utilizing a polytetrafluoroethylene graft

**Answer: d**

This clinical scenario illustrates an inflow problem shortly after surgery, suggesting a technical error in the anastomosis. Given the small size of the recipient's native hepatic artery secondary to the replacement of the right hepatic artery, the common hepatic artery's size and flow may not be adequate to sustain graft perfusion. In this context, performing an arterial conduit utilizing third-party vessels is preferred to avoid the use of prosthetic material.[180]

205. Hepatic artery thrombosis is a significant complication following liver transplantation. Which of the following options accurately provides the incidence ranges for hepatic artery thrombosis in pediatric, adult, and living donor liver transplantation?
a) 1% to 2%, 0.1% to 0.5%, and 5% to 10%
b) 25% to 35%, 5% to 15%, and 10% to 20%
c) 5% to 25%, 1% to 5%, and 5% to 10%
d) 15% to 40%, 0.1% to 1%, and 20% to 30%
e) 3% to 5%, 1% to 2%, and 1% to 5%
**Answer: c**
The incidence of hepatic artery thrombosis in pediatric liver transplant recipients ranges from approximately 5% to 25%. In adult liver transplant recipients, the rate is generally lower, approximately 1% to 5%. The rates for hepatic artery thrombosis in living donor transplants can be slightly higher than in deceased donor transplants, typically ranging from about 5% to 10%.[181,182]

206. What is the incidence of portal vein thrombosis following adult liver transplantation?
a) 0.5% to 1%
b) 1% to 3%
c) 5% to 7%
d) 10% to 15%
e) 10% to 25%
**Answer: b**
Portal vein stenosis is rare, and portal vein thrombosis occurs in only 1% to 2.2% of liver transplant recipients.[183]

207. A 55-year-old male undergoes liver transplantation due to end-stage liver disease secondary to hepatitis C and HCC, treated with transarterial chemoembolization and Yttrium-90 (Y-90) radioembolization. The surgery is complicated by extensive hilar adhesions, scarring, and a short length of the common bile duct. To perform a choledochocholedochostomy, the donor bile duct is intentionally left longer. Postoperatively, the patient experiences elevated bilirubin levels and signs of biliary

obstruction. A CT angiogram shows a patent artery. He is found to have an anastomotic bile leak. What is the most likely pathophysiology of this complication, and what is the preferred treatment option?
a) The anastomotic bile leak is likely due to ischemic injury of the donor bile duct, necessitating a Roux-en-Y hepatojejunostomy for proper bile drainage
b) The anastomotic bile leak is likely due to ischemic necrosis of the recipient bile duct, requiring surgical revision of the anastomosis
c) The complication arises from mechanical tension at the anastomosis; therefore, the bile leak should be addressed using endoscopic stenting of the bile duct
d) The anastomotic leak is caused by a failure in the anastomotic technique, necessitating operative re-exploration and repair of the anastomosis
e) The bile leak results from localized infection around the anastomosis, best managed with antibiotics and supportive care

**Answer: a**

The preferred treatment option is that the bile leak likely resulted from ischemic injury to the donor bile duct, which is more susceptible to ischemic injury due to the division of its primary blood supply from the gastroduodenal artery and retroportal artery during the transplantation procedure. This risk is compounded by the short length of the common bile duct, making it challenging to create a tension-free anastomosis. As a result, the Roux-en-Y hepatojejunostomy is indicated to bypass the compromised area and ensure proper bile drainage, helping to prevent further complications associated with biliary obstruction and leaks.[184]

208. A 60-year-old female patient undergoes liver transplantation due to decompensated cirrhosis from MASH. During the postoperative period, she develops fever, tachycardia, and elevated LFT. An MRCP reveals leakage of contrast material from the donor biliary tree at nonanastomotic sites, particularly in the hilar region. What is the most likely pathophysiology underlying this complication, and what is the recommended management strategy?
a) Bile duct strictures; manage with ERCP and balloon dilation
b) Ischemic bile duct necrosis from hepatic artery occlusion; manage with retransplantation
c) Surgical trauma during anastomosis; manage with ERCP and follow-up imaging
d) Benign bilomas from hepatic artery occlusion; manage with antibiotics and IR drainage
e) Downstream bile flow obstruction; manage with reoperation and Roux-en-Y conversion

**Answer: b**

The leakage of contrast material from the donor biliary tree at nonanastomotic sites is suggestive of ischemic necrosis of the bile duct due to hepatic artery occlusion. This complication commonly occurs in the hilar region and is associated with poor outcomes. When biliary complications arise from hepatic artery occlusion, the prognosis is often grim, and retransplantation is usually warranted to address the necrosis and related complications effectively.[185]

209. A 54-year-old female patient with a history of liver transplantation due to cirrhosis secondary to hepatitis C four months ago presents for routine follow-up. She reports recent episodes of mild abdominal pain and intermittent jaundice. An ultrasound showed normal intrahepatic and extrahepatic bile ducts without any notable dilation. Which of the following statements accurately describes the findings and what the next step in treatment should be?
a) The absence of intrahepatic and extrahepatic ductal dilation indicates that there is no ductal obstruction; consider investigating for sphincter of Oddi dysfunction
b) Ultrasound findings of normal-appearing ducts can reliably rule out significant biliary stricture or obstruction; consider investigating for intrahepatic cholestasis
c) In the setting of biliary obstruction, normal-appearing bile ducts on ultrasound may still signify significant underlying pathology; proceed with MRCP
d) The presence of jaundice and abdominal pain typically correlates with visible ductal dilation on ultrasound in post-transplant patients; repeat the liver ultrasound
e) Normal findings on ultrasound in this context suggest that further evaluation may be unnecessary; however, monitoring LFT should continue
**Answer: c**
Ultrasound may not always reveal ductal dilation in cases of biliary obstruction. The patient's symptoms, including jaundice and abdominal pain, coupled with the normal ultrasound findings, warrant further evaluation using MRCP. MRCP is more sensitive for identifying biliary strictures or obstructions, even when ultrasound results appear normal. Prolonged biliary obstruction can result in inflammatory changes and fibrosis within the biliary tract, meaning that even extended periods of obstruction might not cause noticeable proximal dilation.[186]

210. A 50-year-old Asian male with a history of hepatitis B, advanced cirrhosis, and HCC undergoes a liver transplantation. Two months post-surgery, he presents to the emergency department with persistent abdominal pain, fever, and elevated bilirubin levels. Imaging studies suggest the possibility of a biliary obstruction. What is the most appropriate next step in the management of this patient?
a) Initiate pretreatment with high-dose corticosteroids to reduce inflammation
b) Urgent liver biopsy to rule out rejection
c) Start broad-spectrum antibiotics while awaiting further treatment
d) ERCP to diagnose and possibly treat biliary obstruction
e) Full viral workup including hepatitis B and CMV testing

**Answer: c**

In a liver transplant recipient presenting with fever, abdominal pain, and suspected biliary obstruction, early initiation of broad-spectrum antibiotics is the most appropriate next step. This approach addresses the potential for ascending cholangitis or sepsis, which can rapidly worsen. While ERCP is the definitive diagnostic and therapeutic tool for biliary complications, it should follow initial stabilization with antibiotics.[187]

211. A 45-year-old man with alcohol-related liver disease undergoes liver transplantation. Two months later, he develops cholestasis, jaundice, and abdominal discomfort, and is diagnosed with a biliary complication. Which of the following statements is most accurate regarding biliary complications after liver transplantation?
a) Occur in 2–5% of adult liver transplants
b) Non-anastomotic strictures are most common
c) Rare but often lead to retransplant in 40% of cases
d) Occur in 5–32%, mostly anastomotic strictures and leaks
e) Mainly linked to pre-op liver disease severity

**Answer: d**

The incidence of biliary complications after liver transplantation varies and is indeed estimated to be between 5% and 32%. The most common complications are strictures and bile leaks. Prompt recognition and management of these complications are essential, as they are associated with a mortality rate of up to 20% and may require retransplantation in approximately 13% of cases.[188]

212. A 58-year-old female with chronic hepatitis C presents with decompensated cirrhosis, and her calculated MELD score is 18. She is being evaluated for liver transplantation. Given her clinical status, the transplantation team is considering antiviral therapy. Which of the following treatment strategies would be the most appropriate for this patient?
a) A 12-week course of direct-acting antiviral therapy prior to transplantation
b) A 4-week course of direct-acting antiviral therapy starting at the time of transplantation
c) A 12-week course of direct-acting antiviral therapy administered at disease recurrence post-transplant
d) No antiviral therapy, as it is not indicated for patients with MELD scores below 20
e) A short course of direct-acting antiviral therapy paired with aggressive management of her cirrhosis symptoms immediately prior to transplantation

**Answer: a**

For patients with decompensated cirrhosis and a MELD score of 16-20 who do not have HCC, the strategy of administering a 12-week course of direct-acting antiviral therapy before transplantation. This approach is regarded as both dominant (providing better outcomes at lower costs) and cost-effective. It helps mitigate the risk of hepatitis C recurrence post-transplant and improves overall liver transplant success rates.[189]

213. A 55-year-old woman presents to your clinic with a history of fatigue and pruritus. Following a comprehensive evaluation, she is diagnosed with primary biliary cholangitis (PBC). All of the following statements regarding the management and complications of PBC are false except for:
a) Currently, there is a genetic therapy that is considered curative treatment for PBC
b) Treatment with ursodeoxycholic acid is controversial, since the impact on disease progression, survival, or the need for liver transplant is undetermined
c) Osteopenia, with progression to osteoporosis, is a well-known complication of PBC, but the relative risk remains low, less than 2.0
d) Both decreased osteoblastic activity and increased osteoclastic activity contribute to the development of osteoporosis in PBC patients
e) Patients with PBC should have bone mineral density testing at the time of diagnosis and every 5 to 10 years thereafter
**Answer: d**
There is currently no curative genetic therapy for PBC, however, treatment with ursodeoxycholic acid does improve disease progression and survival. Osteopenia, with progression to osteoporosis, is a well-known complication of PBC, with a relative risk of 4.4. Both decreased osteoblastic activity and increased osteoclastic activity contribute to the development of osteoporosis in PBC patients. Bone mineral density testing is recommended at diagnosis and every 5 to 10 years.[190]

214. A 38-year-old woman presents to the gastroenterology clinic with fatigue, intermittent abdominal pain, and jaundice. She is diagnosed with primary sclerosing cholangitis (PSC) and has no history of inflammatory bowel disease (IBD). What is the most appropriate recommendation for colorectal cancer (CRC) surveillance?
a) Perform colonoscopy with random biopsies to rule out IBD and assess CRC risk, repeating annually
b) Perform colonoscopy with random biopsies to rule out IBD and assess CRC risk, repeating every 10 years
c) Defer colonoscopy with biopsies for 10 years, as CRC risk is negligible in PSC without IBD
d) If IBD is ruled out, repeat colonoscopy every 10 years for CRC surveillance
e) Perform colonoscopy with random biopsies to rule out IBD; if IBD is absent, repeat every 5 years or with new clinical suspicion
**Answer: e**

Patients with newly diagnosed PSC require a colonoscopy with random biopsies to exclude IBD, which is strongly associated with PSC and increases CRC risk. If IBD is absent, surveillance colonoscopy every 5 years is recommended due to elevated CRC risk in PSC, even without IBD, or sooner if new symptoms arise.[191]

215. A 50-year-old man with newly diagnosed primary sclerosing cholangitis (PSC) and elevated ALP is evaluated in the gastroenterology clinic. Based on current guidelines for ursodeoxycholic acid (UDCA) use in PSC, which statement is most accurate?
a) High-dose UDCA (>30 mg/kg/day) improves liver function and survival
b) UDCA consistently improves ALP and histological outcomes, making it first-line therapy
c) Low to moderate-dose UDCA (13–23 mg/kg/day) may be continued if ALP normalizes or significantly decreases within 12 months.
d) UDCA should be avoided due to lack of benefit and significant side effects
e) ALP reduction to <3× upper limit of normal reduces liver decompensation and transplantation risk but not liver-related mortality
**Answer: c**
Guidelines support low to moderate-dose UDCA (13–23 mg/kg/day) in PSC if ALP normalizes or significantly improves within 12 months, as this is associated with reduced risk of liver decompensation, transplantation, and liver-related death. High-dose UDCA is not recommended due to limited benefit and potential harm.[191]

216. A 60-year-old man with cirrhosis due to alcoholic liver disease is found to have large esophageal varices with red wale marks, indicating high bleeding risk. Which statement about nonselective β-blocker therapy for this patient is most accurate?
a) Titrate β-blockers to achieve systolic blood pressure <90 mm Hg
b) β-blockers prevent variceal bleeding by directly constricting esophageal varices
c) Titrate β-blockers to reduce resting heart rate by ≥50% from baseline
d) β-blockers reduce portal pressure by decreasing cardiac output and promoting splanchnic vasoconstriction
e) Titrate β-blockers to achieve a resting heart rate ≤60 beats/min
**Answer: d**
Nonselective β-blockers (e.g., propranolol, nadolol) reduce portal pressure by decreasing cardiac output (β1-blockade) and promoting unopposed α-mediated splanchnic vasoconstriction (β2-blockade), lowering portal blood flow. Titration targets a 20–25% reduction in resting heart rate or a hepatic venous pressure gradient (HVPG) <12 mmHg, while maintaining systolic blood pressure ≥90 mm Hg.[192]

217. A 60-year-old male patient with a history of cirrhosis secondary to alcoholic liver disease and esophageal varices was initiated on propranolol as prophylaxis against bleeding. However, the patient did not tolerate beta-blockers due to hypotension and subsequently underwent band ligation of the esophageal varices. Despite these interventions, he presented to the hospital with massive gastrointestinal bleeding secondary to bleeding from esophageal varices four weeks later. The gastroenterologist performed an endoscopy but was unable to control the bleeding. What is the next step in treatment?
a) Obtain a CT angiogram and consult interventional radiology for embolization
b) Place a Blakemore tube and consult interventional radiology for TIPS
c) Place a Blakemore tube and repeat endoscopy in 8 to 12 hours
d) Place a Blakemore tube and plan for open surgical intervention to control the bleeding
e) Transfuse, continue supportive care, and repeat endoscopy in 4 to 8 hours
**Answer: b**
Rebleeding is a common occurrence, with recurrence reported as high as 70% in patients who have had at least one prior bleeding episode. Generally this occurs within 6 weeks of the index episode. The appropriate next step is placing a Blakemore tube can help control bleeding from esophageal varices, while consultation with interventional radiology for TIPS. TIPS remains a valid rescue method for those patients in whom pharmacological, endoscopic, or combined measures have failed.[193]

218. A 60-year-old male patient with a history of cirrhosis secondary to alcoholic liver disease and esophageal varices underwent esophageal band ligation and subsequently had TIPS four weeks later due to recurrent bleeding. He is now being admitted to the hospital for the third time for hepatic encephalopathy (HE), despite compliance with lactulose and rifaximin. Given that he has experienced multiple episodes of HE since the TIPS procedure six months ago, what is the next appropriate step in his management?
a) Optimize lactulose dosage and increase rifaximin therapy
b) Perform the TIPS reduction or occlusion
c) Consult interventional radiology to assess the patency of the TIPS, as it appears to be occluded
d) Consult a family member regarding medical noncompliance
e) Continue current therapy and perform a workup for infectious sources of encephalopathy, such as urinary tract infection or bacterial peritonitis
**Answer: b**
The most appropriate next step is to perform the TIPS reduction or occlusion, because the patient has had recurrent episodes of hepatic encephalopathy despite

adherence to medical management with lactulose and rifaximin. TIPS reduction or occlusion can help alleviate symptoms of TIPS-induced HE by decreasing portosystemic shunting, particularly in patients who have significant HE, thus improving overall clinical outcomes.[194]

219. A 56-year-old man with cirrhosis due to chronic alcohol use presents to the emergency department with hematemesis and hypotension. After initial resuscitation, octreotide is started for acute esophageal variceal bleeding. Which mechanism best explains how octreotide controls variceal bleeding?
a) Inhibits gastrointestinal hormone release, reducing splanchnic blood flow and portal pressure
b) Stimulates splanchnic vasodilation, increasing portal vein blood flow
c) Enhances gastric mucosal protection by increasing gastrointestinal hormone release
d) Directly constricts esophageal varices, reducing local blood flow
e) Blocks nitric oxide (NO) production, causing splanchnic vasoconstriction
**Answer: a**
Octreotide, a somatostatin analog, inhibits the release of vasodilatory gastrointestinal hormones (e.g., glucagon), leading to splanchnic vasoconstriction, reduced portal blood flow, and lower portal pressure, thereby controlling variceal bleeding. While NO is a vasodilator and its inhibition could theoretically cause vasoconstriction, octreotide's primary effect is not through direct blockade of NO production. There is no significant evidence that octreotide modulates NO pathways in the context of acute variceal bleeding. Instead, its effect is mediated through hormonal regulation and subsequent splanchnic vasoconstriction.[195]

220. A 54-year-old male with end-stage liver disease due to chronic alcohol abuse presents with fatigue and ascites despite adhering to a sodium and fluid restriction regimen. The hepatologist has initiated treatment with spironolactone and furosemide; however, the patient experiences side effects related to spironolactone. Which of the following is not an antiandrogenic effect of spironolactone?
a) Hyperkalemia
b) Decreased libido
c) Impotence
d) Gynecomastia
e) Reduced conversion of testosterone to dihydrotestosterone
**Answer: a**
Hyperkalemia, or elevated potassium levels, is a side effect associated with spironolactone but does not fall under its antiandrogenic effects. The other options listed, such as decreased libido, impotence, gynecomastia, and reduced conversion of testosterone to dihydrotestosterone, are recognized antiandrogenic effects of the

medication. The primary management of ascites in patients involves educating them about dietary sodium restriction (typically 2000 mg per day or 88 mmol per day) and the use of oral diuretic therapy. Symptoms related to hyponatremia typically do not arise until sodium levels drop below 110 mmol/L or in cases of a rapid decline.[196]

221. A 63-year-old female with a known history of cirrhosis secondary to hepatitis C presents to the emergency department with progressive dyspnea. Imaging reveals a large right-sided pleural effusion consistent with hepatic hydrothorax. She has been previously treated for ascites with diuretics, but her symptoms persist despite medical management. Which of the following is considered the most effective management strategy for her condition?
a) Chemical pleurodesis with talc
b) Therapeutic paracentesis
c) TIPS
d) Antibiotic therapy for potential infection
e) Chemical pleurodesis with chemotherapeutic agent
**Answer: c**
The most effective management strategy for this patient's hepatic hydrothorax, particularly in the presence of significant ascites, is TIPS. It can effectively reduce portal hypertension, leading to a decrease in ascitic fluid production and subsequently relieving symptoms associated with hepatic hydrothorax. While therapeutic paracentesis may alleviate immediate shortness of breath, it is not a long-term solution, and chemical pleurodesis is often unsuccessful in these patients.[197]

222. A 68-year-old male with a history of hepatic encephalopathy secondary to cirrhosis is admitted to the hospital due to an acute exacerbation of his condition. He exhibits signs of confusion and altered mental status. The medical team suspects spontaneous bacterial peritonitis as the underlying cause for the worsening encephalopathy. Laboratory results reveal a blood ammonia level of 154 μmol/L. The CT scan of the abdomen demonstrates diffuse dilation of both the small and large intestines, consistent with ileus. What is the optimal treatment strategy for managing this patient's encephalopathy?
a) Increase the lactulose dose to 15 to 30 mL four times daily and continue rifaximin
b) Insert a nasogastric tube for decompression, initiate rectal lactulose, and discontinue oral rifaximin
c) Insert a nasogastric tube for decompression, hold lactulose, and continue oral rifaximin
d) Insert a nasogastric tube for decompression, discontinue lactulose and oral rifaximin
e) Initiate hemodialysis to decrease ammonia levels

**Answer: c**
In the context of ileus, administration of lactulose may exacerbate abdominal distension and increase flatus, complicating the clinical presentation. Therefore, all forms of lactulose should be withheld to avoid worsening the ileus. Decompression of the gastrointestinal tract via a nasogastric tube is essential to relieve pressure and improve patient comfort. Meanwhile, continuing oral rifaximin is appropriate to help lower blood ammonia levels. Although hemodialysis can reduce ammonia, it is not indicated as an immediate intervention in this scenario.[198]

223. A 38-year-old female with a diagnosis of autoimmune hepatitis leading to liver cirrhosis is undergoing evaluation for liver transplantation. During the initial assessment, she presents with hypoxia, digital clubbing, and orthodeoxia, raising concern for hepatopulmonary syndrome. Which of the following criteria is not required for the diagnosis of hepatopulmonary syndrome?
a) The patient must have chronic liver disease, typically associated with portal hypertension
b) A reduced PaO2 must be present
c) An increased alveolar-arterial gradient in partial pressure of oxygen (AaDO2) must be observed
d) Evidence of intrapulmonary vascular dilatation must be documented
e) Persistent elevated pulmonary artery pressure must be demonstrated
**Answer: e**
Hepatopulmonary syndrome is characterized by a triad consisting of chronic liver disease, pulmonary gas exchange abnormalities leading to arterial hypoxemia, and widespread pulmonary vascular dilatation. The diagnosis is confirmed when specific criteria are satisfied. First, there must be evidence of chronic liver disease, often complicated by portal hypertension. Second, arterial hypoxemia is indicated by either a reduced PaO2 or, more precisely, an increased AaDO2. Finally, there must be documentation of intrapulmonary vascular dilatation, which can be detected using two-dimensional contrast echocardiography or a macroaggregated albumin lung perfusion scan. However, persistent elevation of pulmonary artery pressure is not necessary for the diagnosis of hepatopulmonary syndrome.[199]

224. A 32-year-old man with primary biliary cholangitis presents with severe pruritus, significantly affecting his quality of life. His physician starts cholestyramine, but the patient, who has been on a stable selective serotonin reuptake inhibitor (SSRI) for anxiety for two years, reports worsening anxiety and insomnia. What best explains the worsening psychiatric symptoms?
a) Cholestyramine increases SSRI metabolism, reducing its efficacy
b) Cholestyramine binds the SSRI in the gut, decreasing its absorption

c) Cholestyramine causes heightened alertness, exacerbating anxiety
d) Cholestyramine competes with the SSRI for receptor binding, lowering its effect
e) The patient has developed SSRI tolerance, requiring alternative psychiatric treatment
**Answer: b**
Cholestyramine, a bile acid sequestrant, binds to medications like SSRIs in the gastrointestinal tract, reducing their absorption and efficacy. This likely explains the patient's worsened anxiety and insomnia. Administering cholestyramine and the SSRI at least 4 hours apart can minimize this interaction.[200]

225. A 27-year-old male with a history of chronic alcohol use presents with decompensated liver disease secondary to spontaneous bacterial peritonitis. He is 175 cm tall and weighs 60 kg, appearing severely malnourished. He is listed for liver transplantation. Given his clinical condition and normal kidney function, what is his daily protein requirement?
a) 50 grams of protein per day
b) 75 grams of protein per day
c) 120 grams of protein per day
d) 150 grams of protein per day
e) 180 grams of protein per day
**Answer: c**
For patients with decompensated liver disease who are severely malnourished, the protein requirement is calculated at a rate of 1.5 to 2.0 grams of protein per kilogram of dry weight. In this case, the patient's weight is 60 kg, so applying the higher end of the protein requirement calculation (2.0 g/kg), we get:
60 kg × 2.0 g/kg = 120 grams of protein per day.[201]

226. A 27-year-old male with a history of chronic alcohol use presents with decompensated liver disease secondary to spontaneous bacterial peritonitis. He is 175 cm tall and weighs 60 kg, appearing severely malnourished. He is listed for liver transplantation. Given that his caloric needs are estimated at 40 kcal/kg of dry weight, what is the appropriate daily fat intake in grams?
a) 18 grams of fat per day.
b) 40 grams of fat per day.
c) 80 grams of fat per day.
d) 120 grams of fat per day.
e) 180 grams of fat per day.
**Answer: c**
First, we calculate the daily caloric needs for the patient based on the weight:
60 kg × 40 kcal/kg = 2400 kcal per day.

Now, to determine the appropriate fat intake, we calculate 30% of this total caloric intake.
At 30%: 0.3 × 2400 kcal = 720 kcal from fat.
Next, we convert calories from fat to grams (since there are 9 calories per gram of fat):
720 kcal ÷ 9 kcal/g ≈ 80 grams of fat.[201]

227. A 27-year-old male who recently recovered from a liver transplant is being evaluated for his post-transplant nutritional requirements. He is 175 cm tall and weighs 70 kg. Given his weight, what is his recommended daily carbohydrate intake in grams?
a) 120 grams of carbohydrates per day.
b) 180 grams of carbohydrates per day.
c) 260 grams of carbohydrates per day.
d) 320 grams of carbohydrates per day.
e) 400 grams of carbohydrates per day.
**Answer: c**
First, we calculate the daily caloric needs for the patient using a moderate caloric intake recommendation of 25 kcal/kg, aiming for the midpoint:
70 kg × 30 kcal/kg = 2100 kcal per day.
Next, to determine the carbohydrate intake as 50% of total calories:
0.50 × 2100 kcal =1050 kcal from carbohydrates.
Now, converting calories from carbohydrates to grams (since there are 4 calories per gram of carbohydrate):
1050 kcal ÷ 4 kcal/g = 262 grams of carbohydrates.[202]

228. A 27-year-old male who recently recovered from a liver transplant is being assessed for his long-term nutritional needs. He is 175 cm tall and weighs 70 kg. According to the long-term nutritional guidelines, what is his daily protein requirement?
a) 20 grams of protein per day.
b) 50 grams of protein per day.
c) 70 grams of protein per day.
d) 100 grams of protein per day.
e) 120 grams of protein per day.
**Answer: c**
The long-term nutritional recommendation for protein intake after liver transplantation is to consume 1 gram of protein per kilogram of body weight. Given this patient's weight of 70 kg, the calculation for daily protein needs is as follows:
70 kg × 1 g/kg = 70 grams of protein per day.[202]

229. A 54-year-old female with MASH leading to cirrhosis presents to the emergency department with massive bleeding from esophageal varices. She appears pale and diaphoretic, showing signs of hemorrhagic shock. The medical team promptly initiates resuscitation protocols, which include airway protection and establishing large-bore IV access. Given her critical condition, which of the following management steps is not part of the medical management?
a) Initiation of IV proton pump inhibitor drip
b) Initiation of octreotide drip
c) Initiation of broad-spectrum IV antibiotics with ceftriaxone
d) Administering blood products and albumin to maintain central venous pressure above 10 mm Hg
e) Transfusing blood products to maintain hemoglobin levels between 7 to 8 g/dL
**Answer: d**
In the setting of severe acute variceal hemorrhage, prompt and aggressive resuscitation is critical for managing patients in hemorrhagic shock. This management includes airway protection, large-bore IV access, and the infusion of crystalloid and colloid products to stabilize hemodynamics. However, the goal for central venous pressure should be to keep it less than 10 mm Hg, rather than above 10 mm Hg, in order to manage fluid status effectively and avoid exacerbating portal hypertension.[203]

230. A 62-year-old Asian male with cirrhosis from chronic hepatitis B is being evaluated for liver transplantation. Although previously hesitant, he became interested after a recent episode of massive esophageal variceal bleeding, treated with endoscopic band ligation. He currently has no major symptoms but is anxious about the risk of rebleeding while awaiting transplant. What is his estimated risk of variceal rebleeding within the first year?
a) 1–2%
b) 3–5%
c) 5–10%
d) 10–12%
e) 12–50%
**Answer: e**
Variceal bleeding is a severe consequence of portal hypertension in cirrhotic patients. Following an initial bleed, the risk of rebleeding can be as high as 50% within the first year, with associated mortality reaching up to 33%. This underscores the importance of transplant evaluation and timely intervention.[204]

231. A 64-year-old female with MASH is being evaluated for liver transplantation. During the physical examination, a decrease in the PaO2 by 7% is noted upon the patient standing. Given these findings, you suspect the presence of hepatopulmonary syndrome. What is the term used to describe this phenomenon?
a) Platypnea
b) Orthostatic hypoxia
c) Orthodeoxia
d) Orthopnea
e) Orthohypoxia

**Answer: c**

The term "orthodeoxia" refers to a decrease in the PaO2 by 5% or more, or 4 mm Hg or more, that occurs when the patient stands up. This finding is characteristic of hepatopulmonary syndrome and is attributed to preferential perfusion of the lung bases when in an upright position. Although platypnea is also associated with worsened breathlessness while sitting, orthodeoxia is more specific to the decline in oxygen levels in such patients. While this phenomenon can present in other conditions, it is particularly indicative of hepatopulmonary syndrome in those with liver disease.[205]

232. A 52-year-old woman with a 20-year history of alcoholism and liver cirrhosis is evaluated for increased shortness of breath. She mentions that her symptoms have worsened significantly over the past month and that she experiences dizziness when standing. On examination, you find her oxygen saturation to be 88% on room air, and she has a slight cyanosis of the lips. A chest X-ray shows clear lung fields, and hepatopulmonary syndrome is suspected. Which of the following best explains the respiratory impairment observed in this patient?
a) Increased resistance in the pulmonary vasculature
b) Inability of red blood cells to pass through pulmonary capillaries
c) Dilation of pulmonary capillaries, impeding oxygenation
d) Shunting of blood directly from pulmonary arteries to veins
e) Alveolar consolidation due to inflammation

**Answer: c**

In the context of intrapulmonary vascular dilatations observed in hepatopulmonary syndrome, the excessive dilation of the pulmonary capillaries reduces the effective surface area available for gas exchange. This impaired oxygen transfer leads to hypoxemia, as the red blood cells are unable to effectively load oxygen in the distended capillary network, therefore limiting the amount of oxygen that can enter the bloodstream. Occasionally a single large shunt may be found that bypasses the pulmonary vasculature; this may be amenable to coiling by the interventional radiologist.[199]

233. What is the normal range for the A-a pulmonary gradient in a healthy individual at sea level?
a) 1-2 mmHg
b) 2-4 mmHg
c) 5-10 mmHg
d) 13-17 mmHg
e) 20-25 mmHg
**Answer: c**
The normal A-a pulmonary gradient in healthy individuals at sea level typically ranges from 5 to 10 mmHg. This gradient reflects the difference between the amount of oxygen in the alveoli and the amount that reaches the arterial blood, and an elevated A-a gradient can indicate issues such as diffusion limitation, shunt, or ventilation-perfusion mismatch. Normally, the A–a gradient increases with age. For every decade a person has lived, their A–a gradient is expected to increase by 1 mmHg.[206]

234. A 58-year-old woman with a long-standing history of alcoholic liver disease presents with worsening shortness of breath. She has progressive hypoxemia with a $PaO_2$ of 48 mm Hg, along with digital clubbing and cyanosis. She is on the liver transplant list, but her MELD score is too low to qualify for early transplantation. Based on clinical findings, she is diagnosed with hepatopulmonary syndrome (HPS). Which of the following statements best reflects the prognosis and management of HPS?
a) Liver transplant is not advised if liver dysfunction is mild, as it won't improve HPS
b) Early transplant has no impact on HPS outcomes
c) Noninvasive ventilation is ineffective post-transplant
d) Medical therapy (e.g., methylene blue, garlic) is recommended for long-term benefit
e) Without transplant, 5-year mortality is 77% vs. 24% with transplant
**Answer: e**
Hepatopulmonary syndrome is a serious complication of liver disease characterized by intrapulmonary vasodilation and hypoxemia. Liver transplantation is the only definitive treatment, and outcomes significantly improve when performed before severe hypoxemia develops. Without transplant, 5-year mortality is as high as 77%, while patients who undergo transplant have a significantly better prognosis (~24% mortality). Post-transplant improvement in oxygenation is common but may take time.[207]

235. A 62-year-old female with a history of liver cirrhosis presents to the cardiology clinic complaining of increasing exertional dyspnea and decreased exercise tolerance. On examination, she exhibits signs of portal hypertension, including splenomegaly

and ascites. The physician suspects portopulmonary hypertension (POPH) and plans to conduct a thorough evaluation, including right heart catheterization. Which of the following is not included in the diagnostic criteria for POPH?
a) Mean pulmonary artery pressure >20 mm Hg
b) Pulmonary arterial wedge pressure ≤ 15 mm Hg
c) Pulmonary vascular resistance > 2 WU
d) Presence of portal hypertension
e) Presence of high cardiac output

**Answer: e**

POPH is a serious condition characterized by elevated mean pulmonary artery pressure due to pulmonary vascular resistance changes, occurring in the setting of portal hypertension. The diagnosis of POPH requires careful consideration of hemodynamic criteria and the exclusion of other causes of pulmonary hypertension. Key diagnostic criteria include elevated mean pulmonary artery pressure and pulmonary vascular resistance, as well as the presence of portal hypertension. However, the presence of high cardiac output is not a diagnostic criterion for POPH.[208]

236. A 55-year-old man with a long-standing history of MASH presents to the emergency department with worsening dyspnea on exertion and fatigue. He is diagnosed with portopulmonary hypertension (POPH). Right heart catheterization reveals a mean pulmonary artery pressure of 22 mm Hg and pulmonary vascular resistance of 3 WU. Which of the following statements about his condition is correct?
a) Severity of POPH directly correlates with liver disease severity
b) POPH occurs only in patients with cirrhosis and portal hypertension
c) Right heart catheterization is unnecessary; symptoms are sufficient for diagnosis
d) POPH requires portal hypertension, but its severity is independent of portal hypertension severity
e) Liver transplantation is not beneficial in patients with non-cirrhotic POPH

**Answer: d**

POPH is characterized by elevated pulmonary artery pressures in the presence of portal hypertension, whether or not cirrhosis is present. While portal hypertension is necessary for diagnosis, the severity of POPH does not directly correlate with the degree of liver dysfunction or portal hypertension. Right heart catheterization is essential for diagnosis and staging, as clinical symptoms alone are insufficient. Additionally, patients with non-cirrhotic portal hypertension can still benefit from both targeted medical therapies and liver transplantation, when appropriate. The presence of non-cirrhotic portal hypertension does not exclude a patient from transplant consideration or therapeutic benefit.[209]

237. A 60-year-old woman with autoimmune hepatitis and cirrhosis presents with progressive dyspnea, orthopnea, fatigue, ascites, and peripheral edema. Echocardiography shows elevated left atrial pressure. Right heart catheterization reveals the following: mean pulmonary artery pressure of 24 mm Hg, pulmonary capillary wedge pressure (PCWP) of 22 mm Hg, pulmonary vascular resistance (PVR) of 4 WU, and cardiac output of 8 L/min. What is the most likely diagnosis, and the most appropriate initial management?
a) Portopulmonary hypertension – start pulmonary vasodilator therapy
b) Volume overload–initiate diuretics and reassess after fluid removal
c) Arteriovenous shunting – order CT angiogram and consider embolization
d) Congestive pneumonia –initiate broad coverage antibiotics
e) Portopulmonary hypertension – refer for liver transplantation
**Answer: b**
This patient's elevated PCWP and high cardiac output suggest pulmonary hypertension due to volume overload, not portopulmonary hypertension. Portopulmonary hypertension typically presents with normal or low PCWP and elevated PVR. Starting vasodilators in volume overload can worsen symptoms. The first step should be diuresis, followed by reassessment of hemodynamics.[208]

238. A 52-year-old man with alcohol-related cirrhosis and portopulmonary hypertension (POPH) presents with fatigue, confusion, and reduced exercise capacity. He is on a calcium channel blocker for POPH, non-selective β-blocker for variceal prophylaxis, and diuretics for ascites. He now has hepatic encephalopathy and elevated right atrial pressure. What is the most appropriate treatment adjustment?
a) Increase calcium channel blocker
b) Stop β-blocker and consider variceal ligation
c) Start epoprostenol
d) Add endothelin receptor antagonist
e) Arrange TIPS for ascites
**Answer: b**
In POPH, non-selective β-blockers reduce cardiac output and worsen symptoms like fatigue and exercise intolerance. They should be avoided, especially with hepatic encephalopathy. Calcium channel blockers are also not recommended. TIPS is contraindicated due to the risk of worsening pulmonary pressures. The best approach is to discontinue the β-blocker and manage varices with ligation.[210]

239. A 54-year-old woman with portopulmonary hypertension (POPH) secondary to autoimmune hepatitis–related cirrhosis presents for liver transplant evaluation. She has been stable on oral vasodilators and is asymptomatic. Her latest hemodynamics show a mean pulmonary artery pressure (mPAP) of 42 mm Hg, pulmonary vascular

resistance (PVR) of 2.5 WU, and normal right ventricular function. What is the most accurate statement regarding her transplant eligibility?
a) mPAP and PVR meet criteria for MELD exception
b) Elevated mPAP disqualifies her from transplant
c) Monthly right heart catheterization is required
d) She can be listed but is not MELD-exception eligible
e) mPAP must be <35 mm Hg for transplant eligibility

**Answer: a**

Patients with mPAP 35–45 mm Hg and PVR <3 WU are eligible for MELD exception if RV function is preserved. This patient meets all criteria and can be prioritized for transplant. While ongoing monitoring is needed, catheterization every 3 months is standard to maintain exception status.[211]

240. A 60-year-old man with alcohol-related cirrhosis presents for liver transplant evaluation. He has a history of portal hypertension, ascites, and hepatic encephalopathy, but has been sober for 2 years and has a strong support system. Right heart catheterization reveals a mean pulmonary artery pressure (mPAP) of 52 mm Hg and pulmonary vascular resistance (PVR) of 5 WU. He is clinically stable at the time of assessment. What is the most accurate statement regarding his transplant eligibility?
a) Eligible due to sobriety and strong support
b) Eligible despite high PVR since mPAP is acceptable
c) Eligible—elevated pressure likely from fluid overload
d) Not eligible due to severely elevated mPAP and PVR
e) Should be listed immediately due to liver decompensation

**Answer: d**

Patients with mPAP >50 mm Hg and PVR >3 WU are considered high-risk for liver transplantation, with near 100% perioperative mortality. Despite his sobriety and clinical stability, his hemodynamics contraindicate transplant until pulmonary pressures are better controlled. He must first achieve safer thresholds (typically mPAP <35 mm Hg, PVR <3 WU) with medical therapy before being reconsidered for listing.[208]

241. A 49-year-old man with portopulmonary hypertension (POPH) due to alcohol induced liver cirrhosis undergoes liver transplantation. Before transplant, he was on prostacyclin therapy and had limited exercise capacity. What is the expected outcome regarding his pulmonary hypertension after transplant?
a) Most patients experience complete resolution of pulmonary hypertension and can gradually discontinue all pulmonary arterial hypertension therapy

b) Approximately one-half of patients will experience improvement or resolution of pulmonary hypertension, but some may require ongoing pulmonary arterial hypertension therapy
c) Most patients will experience worsening pulmonary hypertension during the first 6 months following liver transplantation
d) To improve outcomes, initial postoperative fluid management should maintain a positive fluid balance to prevent rapid right ventricular dysfunction due to decreased preload
e) All patients experience consistent improvement in symptoms and pulmonary hemodynamics after transplant

**Answer: b**

Liver transplant can improve or resolve POPH in ~50% of patients, potentially allowing discontinuation of pulmonary arterial hypertension therapy. However, many still need long-term treatment, and outcomes are variable. Close hemodynamic monitoring is essential. Postoperative fluid balance should also be managed cautiously to avoid right ventricular strain, but this was not the primary focus of the question.[208]

# 6. Organ Donation and Technical Aspects of Liver Transplantation

242. A 42-year-old man, pronounced brain dead after a fentanyl overdose, is evaluated for multi-organ donation. His BMI is 37, with no history of obesity-related conditions or hypertension. Liver biopsy shows 30% macrosteatosis, 60% microvesicular steatosis, and no fibrosis or necrosis. Which statement best reflects the suitability of this liver for transplantation?
a) The liver is unsuitable due to moderate macrosteatosis, risking primary nonfunction
b) The liver is unsuitable due to 60% microvesicular steatosis
c) The liver is suitable, as 30% macrosteatosis is acceptable without other risk factors
d) The liver is suitable if cold ischemia time is <8 hours, biopsy findings
e) The liver is suitable if normothermic machine perfusion is used, given 30% macrosteatosis
**Answer: c**
A liver with 30% macrosteatosis is generally acceptable for transplantation, especially without fibrosis, necrosis, or other donor risk factors. While 60% microvesicular steatosis raises caution, it is less concerning than macrosteatosis and does not preclude transplantation when liver function is preserved. Normothermic machine perfusion may optimize outcomes but is not mandatory.[212]

243. A 55-year-old man with end-stage liver disease from alcohol abuse (MELD score 34) is listed for liver transplantation. He has antibodies to hepatitis B surface antigen (anti-HBs) only. He has no other significant comorbidities. The transplant team considers a liver graft from a donor positive for hepatitis B core antibody (anti-HBc+) but negative for hepatitis B surface antigen (HBsAg). What is the most appropriate management for this graft?
a) Use the graft with indefinite antiviral prophylaxis to prevent HBV transmission
b) Use the graft without prophylaxis, as the recipient's vaccination ensures immunity
c) Reject the graft due to the recipient's lack of prior hepatitis B infection
d) Use the graft with antiviral prophylaxis for 6 months
e) Use the graft with hepatitis B immunoglobulin (HBIG) at transplant and monitor without routine antiviral prophylaxis
**Answer: e**
The recipient's anti-HBs positivity from vaccination and low-risk profile (no comorbidities, no prior HBV infection) indicate a low risk of HBV transmission from an anti-HBc+, HBsAg– donor graft. Per current guidelines, administering HBIG at

transplant mitigates this risk. Routine antiviral prophylaxis is not required in vaccinated, low-risk recipients, but monitoring for HBV reactivation is recommended.[213]

244. A 50-year-old female patient with a history of well-controlled human immunodeficiency virus (HIV) infection and liver cirrhosis secondary to hepatitis C virus (HCV) is being evaluated for liver transplantation. The transplant team has received an offer for a liver from an HIV-positive donor who is on antiviral medication and has an undetectable viral load. How should the team proceed?
a) Organs from HIV-positive donors should not be considered for transplantation due to the high risk of complications
b) Transplantation of organs from HIV-positive donors can be performed safely, provided that the recipient is also HIV-positive and receiving effective antiretroviral therapy
c) Transplantation of organs from HIV-positive donors should not be considered due to the high risk of viral transmission to the medical team
d) The use of organs from HIV-positive donors is discouraged, as they are associated with significantly poorer outcomes compared to organs from HIV-negative donors
e) Organs from HIV-positive donors can be utilized in recipients who are HIV-negative, but only in exceptional cases where all other donor options have been exhausted

**Answer: b**

The evolving landscape of organ transplantation now permits the use of organs from HIV-positive donors, particularly given the advancements in antiretroviral therapies that effectively manage the virus. Organs from HIV-positive donors can be utilized without significantly compromising outcomes, especially when the recipient is also living with HIV and adheres to an effective treatment regimen.[214]

245. A 72-year-old male DBD liver donor, previously healthy except for hypertension, has normal pre-donation LFTs and a liver with 7% macrovesicular steatosis on biopsy. Cold ischemia time during retrieval is 10 hours. The recipient is a 50-year-old man with decompensated cirrhosis. Which factor is most critical in assessing the suitability of this liver graft for transplantation?
a) Donor age >70, increasing risk of arterial thrombosis
b) Degree of macrovesicular steatosis in the donor liver
c) Total cold ischemia time
d) Donor's history of hypertension
e) Donor age >70, increasing long-term graft loss and mortality

**Answer: c**

Cold ischemia time is the most critical factor, as prolonged times (>8–12 hours) increase the risk of primary nonfunction and poor graft outcomes. The donor's age (>70) and mild steatosis (7%) are acceptable in the absence of other risk factors, and hypertension has minimal impact on graft suitability.[215]

246. A transplant team is reviewing potential organ donors to determine if they meet the criteria for being classified as high-risk donors by the Centers for Disease Control and Prevention (CDC). Among the following options, which scenario does not qualify as a CDC high-risk donor?
a) A 28-year-old male who recently had sex with a person with suspected human immunodeficiency virus (HIV)
b) A 45-year-old female with a history of diabetes, who recently traveled to a region with high endemic rates of malaria but has never had a positive malaria test
c) A 30-year-old female who had sex in exchange for money in the preceding 7 months
d) A 21-year-old female who is a college student and had been locked up in jail for 5 days in the preceding 3 months
e) A 50-year-old female who has been diagnosed with treatment-resistant hypertension and I drug use in the preceding 5 months

**Answer: b**

The criteria defined by the CDC for high-risk donors generally include individuals with the following risk factors:
1. Men who have sex with men in the past 12 months.
2. IV drug users or individuals who have used drugs in a manner that is not socially acceptable, including sharing needles.
3. People with known positive tests for HIV, viral hepatitis (such as Hepatitis B and Hepatitis C), or other sexually transmitted infections.
4. People who have engaged in transactional sex or those who have had sex with persons diagnosed with or at high risk for HIV, in the preceding 12 months.
5. People who have been in lockup, jail, prison, or a juvenile correctional facility for more than 72 consecutive hours in the preceding 12 months
6. People who have had certain medical procedures in settings with less stringent screening for blood-borne pathogens.
7. A child who is 18 months of age and born to a mother known to be infected with, or at increased risk for, HIV, hepatitis B virus and hepatitis C virus infection.
8. A child who has been breast-fed within the preceding 12 months and the mother is known to be infected with, or at increased risk for, HIV infection.[216]

247. A 55-year-old female, whose past medical history is not well known, was declared brain dead after a hemorrhagic stroke. Which of the following pieces of information from her donor history is considered a contraindication for organ donation?
a) History of low-grade CNS tumor treated with ablation 1 year ago
b) History of squamous cell carcinoma of the lower lip 2 years ago, treated with resection
c) History of basal cell carcinoma of the upper lip 2 years ago, treated with resection
d) History of upper back melanoma 6 years ago with one lymph node positive, treated with resection
e) History of right-sided ductal cell carcinoma of the breast, treated with bilateral mastectomy 6 years ago
**Answer: d**
Melanoma is associated with a higher risk of metastatic disease and transmission to organ recipients, particularly when lymph nodes are affected. This raises concerns about malignancy transmission during transplantation. Overall, liver allografts from donors with low-grade CNS tumors or a distant history (>5 years) of treated low-grade malignancies (e.g., nonmelanoma skin cancers) may be considered for transplantation.[217]

248. What is the most important consideration for a patient receiving a domino liver transplant from a donor with familial amyloid polyneuropathy (FAP)?
a) Long-term graft function is slightly reduced compared to deceased donor liver transplantation
b) The risk of developing amyloid polyneuropathy from the donor liver is negligible
c) Transmission of the metabolic defect varies, and many recipients never develop variant transthyretin
d) Reconstructing the venous outflow of the graft is technically challenging
e) Domino liver transplants are rare due to both metabolic and structural liver abnormalities
**Answer: d**
Domino liver transplantation is a specialized procedure used primarily for patients with metabolic diseases, including FAP. This condition is caused by a genetic mutation that leads to the abnormal production of the transthyretin protein, resulting in amyloid fibrils that deposit in various organs, including the heart and nervous system. Liver transplantation is curative for this disorder, as over 95% of transthyretin is synthesized in the liver.
While domino transplants can provide outcomes comparable to those of deceased donor liver transplants, they present specific technical challenges. The major difficulty lies in reconstructing the venous outflow of the graft, which is crucial for maintaining normal liver function. The use of cava-sparing techniques and interposition grafts has

been developed to address this issue. Furthermore, patients receiving a domino liver transplant carry a risk of developing de novo metabolic disease due to the persistent presence of variant transthyretin, and continuous surveillance post-transplant is advised.[218]

249. A 65-year-old male patient with end-stage liver disease is being evaluated for liver transplantation and is considered for a graft from an older DCD donor. Which statement regarding the transplantation outcomes of older DCD donors is most accurate?
a) Graft and patient survival rates for older DCD donors have consistently remained lower than those of younger DCD donors
b) Despite advancements in normothermic machine perfusion technology, graft loss in older DCD remains statistically significant
c) Graft survival rates from older DCD donors have become comparable to those from younger donors due to improved management of ischemic times
d) The use of older DCD donors has declined significantly over the past decade as the risks associated with their grafts have heightened
e) The use of machine perfusion in liver transplantation increased rates of liver utilization but did not improve DCD graft survival
**Answer: c**
Recent advancements in surgical techniques and better management of ischemic times have resulted in graft survival rates from older DCD donors becoming comparable to those from younger donors. The use of machine perfusion in liver transplantation increased rates of liver utilization and improved graft survival after DCD.[219]

250. A 63-year-old woman with autoimmune hepatitis and a previous liver transplant 20 years ago is now listed for a second transplant. She is in the ICU on low-dose norepinephrine for recurrent cholangitis, with a MELD score of 37. The transplant team receives an offer from a 43-year-old DCD donor. What is the most appropriate next step?
a) Place the patient on hold; she is currently too ill for surgery
b) Decline the DCD offer and wait for a DBD offer for this patient
c) Accept the DCD offer, use ice-cold preservation, and have a backup patient ready
d) Accept the DCD offer and use normothermic machine perfusion
e) Accept the DCD offer only if warm ischemia time is under 20 minutes
**Answer: d**
In high-risk cases like redo liver transplants, especially in critically ill patients, normothermic machine perfusion improves outcomes by reducing ischemic injury and allowing real-time assessment of graft function. This is especially important for DCD livers, which are more vulnerable to cold ischemia damage. Normothermic

machine perfusion offers better preservation and is preferred in complex surgical cases to optimize graft viability and patient survival.[220]

251. In liver transplantation from DCD donors, warm ischemia time includes phases like hypotension, hypoxia, and circulatory arrest. These phases may impact graft outcomes differently. Which statement best describes the risk factors for post-reperfusion syndrome (PRS), a condition marked by severe hemodynamic instability after graft reperfusion?
a) Total warm ischemia time (including hypotension and hypoxia) is the main predictor of PRS
b) Prolonged total ischemia time increases PRS risk but does not affect 1-year graft survival
c) Asystolic warm ischemia time is more strongly associated with PRS than total warm ischemia time
d) PRS is primarily influenced by cold ischemia time and is not significantly affected by asystolic warm ischemia time
e) PRS is mainly influenced by recipient factors such as age and comorbidities
**Answer: c**
Among the phases of donor warm ischemia, asystolic time (no cardiac activity) has the strongest link to post-reperfusion syndrome (PRS). When asystolic time exceeds 10 minutes, the risk of severe ischemic reperfusion injury increases, leading to complications like renal failure, hyperbilirubinemia, and longer hospital stays. Unlike total warm ischemia, asystolic time more accurately predicts both PRS risk and poorer graft outcomes, including reduced 1-year graft survival.[221]

252. A 57-year-old man with hepatitis B–related cirrhosis and HCC (segments 6 and 7) is listed for liver transplant (MELD 28). He has undergone transarterial chemoembolization and selective internal radiation therapy with Yttrium-90. He has mild portal hypertension, no ascites, and a partially occlusive portal vein thrombus. Imaging shows a liver anteroposterior (AP) dimension of 15.7 cm and a portocaval space of 4.8 cm. He receives an offer from a 62-year-old DCD donor (AP dimension 15.5 cm, portocaval space 7.4 cm). What is the best course of action?
a) Accept based on AP dimension only; portocaval measurement is unreliable due to portal vein thrombus
b) Accept based on compatible AP and portocaval dimensions
c) Decline due to donor age
d) Decline due to mismatched AP and portocaval dimensions
e) Decline due to significant portocaval mismatch, despite acceptable AP dimension
**Answer: d**

In recipients with prior radiation or interventions, scar tissue and limited abdominal space increase the risk of graft compression or poor fit. A donor liver with a significantly larger portocaval dimension may lead to technical complications like portal vein kinking or thrombosis, especially when the recipient's portocaval space is small. In this case, both AP and portocaval dimensions suggest size mismatch, and the offer should be declined.[222]

253. A 45-year-old male, weighing 120 kg, is undergoing liver transplantation due to end-stage liver disease secondary to MASH. The donor is a 30-year-old female, significantly smaller than the recipient, weighing 50 kg. During the transplantation procedure, the surgical team intends to employ the bicaval technique for implantation. Following portal vein and arterial reconstruction, the liver appears well-perfused but is positioned loosely within the spacious abdominal cavity. Which of the following statements is the most accurate regarding the management approach in this scenario?
a) Utilizing the piggyback technique is preferable because the increased space will facilitate easier anastomosis
b) Firm fixation of the falciform ligament to the diaphragm aids in minimizing the risk of liver torsion
c) The smaller size of the donor liver eliminates the risk of vascular complications, allowing for a straightforward implantation process
d) The risk of liver torsion is generally negligible, even in the scenario where the donor liver being substantially smaller than the recipient's abdominal cavity
e) With this graft size mismatch, portal vein and bile duct reconstructions are typically more technically straightforward
**Answer: b**
In this scenario, the significant size disparity between the donor liver and the recipient necessitates the use of techniques aimed at reducing the potential for complications. Firm fixation of the falciform ligament to the diaphragm is important in reducing the risk of liver torsion. Difficulty may occur during portal and bile duct anastomosis due to wide gap between donor and recipient structures if the liver is implanted using piggyback technique.[222]

254. During a donor kidney procurement, a transplant surgeon is teaching a surgical fellow about retroperitoneal dissection. The surgeon emphasizes the importance of identifying the upper limit of dissection to avoid injury to surrounding structures. Which anatomical structure marks the cephalic limit of retroperitoneal dissection?
a) Right renal vein
b) Right renal artery
c) Left renal vein
d) Duodenum

e) Splenic vein
**Answer: c**
The left renal vein marks the cephalic limit of retroperitoneal dissection during kidney procurement. Dissection beyond this point increases the risk of damaging critical structures such as the superior mesenteric artery, left renal artery, pancreas, or the left kidney. Over-dissection may also lead to vascular torsion or bleeding, particularly from manipulation near the superior mesenteric artery.[223]

255. A surgical team is preparing for multi-organ procurement from a 50-year-old DBD male donor, who is scheduled to donate his heart, lungs, liver, and kidneys. At which point in the surgical procedure should the heparin be administered, and what is the correct dosage to be used?
a) Before induction of anesthesia; 10,000 units
b) Immediately after the abdominal aorta cannulation; 30,000 units
c) At least 3 minutes before the cannulation of the abdominal aorta; 30,000 units
d) Immediately after cross clamp; 20,000 units
e) During the incision of the abdominal cavity; 50,000 units
**Answer: c**
In the context of multi-organ donation, the administration of 30,000 units of heparin, calculated at 300 units/kg of the donor's body weight, should be administered, preferably via a central line, and circulated for at least 3 minutes. This timing is critical as an adequate anticoagulation effect is necessary prior to starting the harvesting of the organs to prevent thrombus formation within the vascular system, ensuring that the donated organs remain perfused and viable for transplantation.[223]

256. A surgical team is preparing for multi-organ procurement from a 50-year-old DBD male donor, scheduled to donate lungs, liver, and kidneys. After administering heparin and inserting the abdominal aortic cannula, cross-clamping and cold flush begin. The liver is being monitored, but the effluent from the suprahepatic IVC remains bloody. Upon checking the cannula placement, the catheter appears correctly positioned but is leaking significant fluid. What should the surgical team do next?
a) Remove the aortic cannula to access the vessel for dissection. If extensive dissection is found, cannulate the thoracic aorta and clamp the abdominal aorta
b) Remove the aortic cannula to access the vessel for dissection. If extensive dissection is found, reinsert a larger cannula deeper into the right lumen
c) Continue flushing the liver with more fluid; if it doesn't flush well, consider the liver non-viable for transplantation
d) Apply manual compression to the aorta around the cannula and infuse more fluid, hoping to achieve a sufficient liver flush

e) Perform all liver flushing through the portal vein by inserting a 14Fr cannula into the inferior mesenteric vein and flush each kidney separately

**Answer: a**

In this scenario, removing the aortic cannula to access the vessel for further dissection is crucial, especially if extensive dissection is evident. Inserting a larger cannula into the dissected aorta can exacerbate the dissection and increase the risk of complications. Cannulating the thoracic aorta and clamping the abdominal aorta allows for better management of the vascular structures while ensuring adequate perfusion to the liver and other organs. This approach promotes safe surgical techniques in multi-organ procurement.[224]

257. A surgical team is preparing for multi-organ procurement from a 45-year-old DBD male donor who is scheduled to donate his liver and kidneys. Upon entering the abdominal cavity, the organs are inspected, and no abnormalities are identified. The organ retrieval surgery is completed successfully, with all organs procured intact and without surgical damage. However, during a close inspection of the right kidney on the backtable, an abnormal mass measuring 7 mm in size is discovered on the superior pole. A biopsy confirms the presence of renal cell carcinoma (RCC). A potential recipient for the liver graft is a 68-year-old male with hepatitis C liver cirrhosis complicated by HCC. How should the surgical team proceed regarding the liver and kidney grafts?
a) Discard both kidneys and liver grafts from this donor to avoid any risk of cancer transmission
b) Discard both kidneys but accept the liver graft from this donor, as the risk of cancer transmission with liver transplant is negligible
c) Accept the liver graft on the condition of full disclosure with the recipient and his full understanding of potential risks
d) Discard the right kidney and accept the left kidney and liver grafts, given the risk of RCC transmission can be as high as 3%
e) The liver and kidney grafts should be utilized for research only

**Answer: c**

This case presents a potential dilemma regarding the risk of RCC transmission to the recipient. Given the small size of the tumor and the absence of transmission in similar cases, the surgical team could consider accepting the liver graft while also evaluating the possibility of accepting the remaining kidney after excising the tumor or discarding the affected kidney while utilizing the unaffected one. This careful selection process will help balance the benefits of transplantation against the risks involved.[225]

258. A 48-year-old male donor is being prepared for liver and kidneys donation after suffering a severe traumatic brain injury. The family has agreed to withdraw life

support and proceed with organ donation through the DCD pathway. Upon evaluation, it is noted that the donor has a history of a previous median sternotomy for coronary artery bypass grafting. Which of the following techniques should the surgical team prioritize for the organ procurement procedure in this scenario?
a) Perform a median sternotomy before withdrawal of life support to ensure direct access to the heart and major vessels
b) Access the thoracic cavity using a left lateral thoracotomy while avoiding manipulation of the cardiac structures
c) Conduct the entire retrieval procedure solely through the abdominal cavity by venting through the IVC
d) The patient is not a candidate for DCD donation given the need for rapid chest access to vent the IVC at the junction with the right atrium
e) Before aortic cross-clamping, proceed with splitting the diaphragm, opening the pericardium, and dividing the caval-atrial junction to facilitate venting of perfusate
**Answer: c**
Given the donor's history of a prior median sternotomy, rapid chest access for DCD procurement is challenging. Therefore, the preferred approach is to perform the entire organ retrieval through the abdominal cavity, utilizing techniques that avoid direct thoracic access. Venting through the IVC ensures adequate perfusion and preservation of the organs, improving the chances of successful transplantation. The last answer choice would be accurate if splitting the diaphragm, opening the pericardium, and dividing the caval-atrial junction were done after cross-clamping.[226]

259. During liver transplantation, a harvested liver is preserved using static cold preservation techniques, with the liver core temperature reaching equilibrium near 0°C. Given that the metabolic rate significantly decreases with cooling and that temperature affects enzymatic activity differently, which enzyme's activity would most likely be completely inhibited at temperatures around 5°C during the preservation period?
a) LDH
b) Na+, K+-adenosine triphosphatase (ATPase)
c) ALT
d) AST
e) Glucose-6-phosphatase
**Answer: b**
Na+, K+-adenosine triphosphatase (ATPase) is almost completely inhibited at temperatures around 5°C, with its activity dropping to about 0.35%. In contrast, enzymes like LDH remain partially active at low temperatures, retaining roughly 10% of their function.[227]

260. Which accurately describes hypothermia-induced cell swelling during liver preservation?
a) Decreased extracellular potassium causing membrane hyperpolarization
b) Increased intracellular sodium leading to passive water influx and cell swelling
c) Suppressed ATP production reducing intracellular sodium and causing swelling
d) Intracellular potassium accumulation triggering swelling and apoptosis
e) Prolonged cold ischemia reducing K+, Ca+-ATPase activity, causing swelling with calcium influx upon reperfusion
**Answer: b**
During liver preservation, hypothermia impairs Na+, K+-ATPase function due to reduced enzyme activity and ATP depletion. This leads to increased intracellular sodium concentration, creating an osmotic imbalance that drives passive water influx, resulting in cell swelling.[228]

261. Which property is undesirable for an effective organ preservation solution?
a) Prevention of hypothermia-induced cell swelling and interstitial edema
b) Prevention of electrolyte imbalance
c) Prevention of intracellular acidosis
d) Reduction of oxidative damage by reactive oxygen species
e) Induction of toll-like receptor 4 activation
**Answer: e**
An effective organ preservation solution should minimize cellular damage and maintain homeostasis during cold storage. Preventing cell swelling, electrolyte imbalances, intracellular acidosis, and oxidative damage is beneficial. However, inducing toll-like receptor 4 activation is undesirable, as it triggers pro-inflammatory cytokine release, worsening inflammation and potentially harming graft function.[229]

262. The UW (University of Wisconsin) preservation solution was developed by the surgeon Folkert Belzer and the basic scientist James Southard at the University of Wisconsin in the 1980. This solution safely allowed extended preservation of human liver grafts to more than 15 hours. Which of the following components of the UW preservation solution is primarily responsible for preventing intracellular edema and promoting cellular protection during cold preservation?
a) Lactobionic acid
b) Adenosine
c) Hydroxyethyl starch
d) Glucose
e) Sodium bicarbonate
**Answer: a**

Lactobionic acid serves as a crucial component of the UW solution; it helps to maintain osmotic balance and prevents intracellular edema by stabilizing cell membranes during the cold storage period. Additionally, it has antioxidant properties that contribute to cellular protection. The UW preservation solution does not contain glucose.[230]

263. All of the following statements accurately describe characteristics of the UW (University of Wisconsin) preservation solution, except:
a) Osmolarity of 320 mOsm/L
b) pH of 7.4
c) Viscosity of 5.70 cp
d) Mannitol concentration of 60 g/L
e) High potassium concentration ranging from 125 to 130 mmol/L
**Answer: d**
Mannitol is not a component of the UW preservation solution, which typically includes other formulations aimed at preserving organ viability during transplantation.[230]

264. Which of the following antioxidant qualities of the University of Wisconsin (UW) preservation solution specifically aids in mitigating oxidative stress during reoxygenation following transplantation?
a) Inclusion of lactobionic acid to enhance cellular membrane stability
b) Presence of hydroxyethyl starch to reduce extracellular edema
c) Addition of allopurinol to inhibit xanthine oxidase
d) Integration of raffinose to provide osmotic balance
e) Omission of calcium to prevent intracellular accumulation
**Answer: c**
The UW preservation solution contains allopurinol, an antioxidant that inhibits xanthine oxidase, blocking reactive oxygen species production in the hypoxanthine-xanthine-uric acid pathway. This reduces oxidative stress during reperfusion, protecting the graft from cellular damage.[230]

265. During liver transplantation, both parenchymal and non-parenchymal cells undergo loss through various death signaling pathways due to ischemia/reperfusion injury. Within the first hour after reperfusion, necrosis is the primary mode of cell death in the liver graft resulting from cold preservation, followed by subsequent apoptosis. The influence of necroptosis is significantly heightened in steatotic grafts. In this context, iron-overload-dependent cell death, known as ferroptosis, is predominantly observed in the steatotic liver due to which of the following mechanisms?

a) Excessive ATP production
b) Increased mitochondrial activity
c) Exaggerated lipid peroxidation
d) Upregulation of antioxidant enzymes
e) Depletion of intracellular iron
**Answer: c**
In steatotic liver grafts, ferroptosis is driven by exaggerated lipid peroxidation, fueled by iron overload and accumulated fatty acids. This process generates reactive lipid species, triggering iron-dependent cell death.[229]

266. Which medication is administered to an organ donor to reduce the inflammatory response during organ recovery?
a) Insulin
b) Methylprednisolone
c) Bicarbonate
d) Epinephrine
e) Albumin
**Answer: b**
Administering methylprednisolone to the donor reduces inflammation and improves organ function post-transplantation.[231]

267. What is a key strategy to reduce the risk of hepatic artery dissection during hepatectomy in liver transplant surgery?
a) Minimize use of LigaSure and Bovie in the hilum; use sharp dissection and double-ligate vessels with ties
b) Mobilize the right hepatic lobe before hilar dissection to avoid excess tension on exposed vessels
c) Obtain early control of hepatic artery inflow
d) Skeletonize and divide the left, middle, and right hepatic arteries to preserve maximal recipient arterial length
e) Routinely release the median arcuate ligament to augment hepatic flow and minimize aortic conduit use
**Answer: c**
Early control of hepatic artery inflow during hepatectomy reduces the risk of hepatic artery dissection by minimizing trauma to arterial walls. This strategy decreases complications like arterial thrombosis and dissection, preserving vascular integrity and improving surgical outcomes.[232]

268. In liver disease-related encephalopathy, diminished liver function impairs protein metabolism, where the liver combines two ammonia molecules with which molecule to form urea?
a) Nitrous oxide
b) Water
c) Carbon dioxide
d) Carbon
e) Nitrate
**Answer: c**
The liver combines two ammonia molecules with carbon dioxide to form urea, a process impaired in liver disease, contributing to encephalopathy.[233]

269. The pathogenesis of the hepatic encephalopathy has been linked to changes levels of which neurotransmitter in the brain?
a) Increased level of dopamine
b) Decreased level of dopamine
c) Increased level of serotonin
d) Increased level of GABA
e) Decreased level of GABA
**Answer: d**
Increased level of GABA neurotransmitter, which is a potent inhibitory neurotransmitter in the brain, can be potentiated by benzodiazepine drugs and may contribute to the development of hepatic coma.[234]

270. What is the reversal agent for hepatic encephalopathy exacerbated by diazepam?
a) Narcan
b) Flumazenil
c) Rifaximin
d) Lactulose
e) Sodium benzoate
**Answer: b**
Flumazenil reverses the effects of diazepam, a benzodiazepine that can worsen hepatic encephalopathy by enhancing GABA-mediated sedation.[235]

271. A 44-year-old male with end-stage liver disease secondary to alcohol abuse presents for liver transplant surgery. Preoperative blood work is significant for sodium 128 mEq/L, creatinine 2.1 mg/dL (with a baseline creatinine of 1.3 mg/dL on blood work conducted 3 months prior), and BUN of 44 mg/dL. Further urine studies reveal a urine osmolality 534 mOsm/kg and a fractional excretion of sodium (FENa) of

<1%. Due to worsening ascites, the furosemide dose was increased 3 weeks ago, and he was started on propranolol. What is the most likely cause of acute kidney injury?
a) Prerenal
b) Intrinsic renal
c) Postrenal
d) Exogenous, drug induced

Answer: a

The patient likely has pre-renal azotemia, which is related to the increased dose of diuretics. Pre-renal azotemia is characterized by elevated serum creatinine and BUN, with a BUN to creatinine ratio greater than 20:1, low urine sodium concentration, high urine osmolality (>500 mOsm/kg), and low FENa (<1%). Pre-renal azotemia is treated by volume expansion.[236]

272. In hepatorenal syndrome, characterized by increased serum creatinine, cirrhosis with ascites, no identifiable kidney injury, no improvement after 48 hours of albumin volume expansion, absence of shock or nephrotoxic drugs, what additional laboratory parameter is diagnostic?
a) Increased urinary sediment
b) High urinary sodium level (>10 mEq/L)
c) No significant proteinuria (<500 mg/dL)
d) High urinary output (>2 L/day)
e) Hematuria (>50 RBC/HPF)

Answer: c

Hepatorenal syndrome is marked by no significant proteinuria (<500 mg/dL), indicating the absence of parenchymal kidney disease.[237]

273. A patient who is currently taking selective serotonin reuptake inhibitor (SSRI) is undergoing liver transplantation and has developed refractory hypotension that is not responsive to increasing doses of vasopressors. The anesthesiologist administered a third agent that resulted in severe serotonin toxicity. What medication was likely given?
a) Norepinephrine
b) Epinephrine
c) Vasopressin
d) Angiotensin II (Ang II)
e) Methylene blue

Answer: e

Methylene blue can produce severe serotonin syndrome when administered to patients taking SSRI.[238]

274. Since the liver participates in the formation of procoagulant, anticoagulant and fibrinolytic factors, patients with liver disease often suffer from extensive coagulopathy. A useful tool for resuscitation in these patients is thromboelastography (TEG). In a cirrhotic patient with a decreased maximal amplitude (MA) value below 50 mm, the appropriate product for resuscitation should be which of the following?
a) FFP
b) Cryoprecipitate
c) Fibrinogen
d) Platelets
e) Thromboxane
**Answer: d**
R Time (Reaction Time): This measures the time taken for the initial fibrin formation, with normal values between 6-8 minutes. Prolonged R time indicates coagulation factor deficiencies, for which FFP or protamine may be administered.
K Time (Kinetics Time): This measures the time taken to reach a certain amplitude of clot firmness (usually 20 mm). Normal values range from 1 to 5 minutes. Prolonged K time suggests a deficiency in fibrinogen and should be corrected with fibrinogen or cryoprecipitate.
Alpha Angle (α Angle): This measures the rate at which fibrin cross-linking occurs, with normal values ranging from 50 to 70 degrees. A decreased alpha angle suggests impaired platelet function or reduced fibrinogen levels, which should be addressed with cryoprecipitate or fibrinogen products.
MA: This identifies the maximum strength of the clot, with normal values ranging from 50 to 70 mm. A decreased MA indicates thrombocytopenia (low platelet count) or functional defects in platelets. To correct this, platelet transfusions (or desmopressin, DDAVP) may be indicated.
Lysis at 30 minutes (LY30): This indicates the percentage of clot breakdown that occurs 30 minutes after reaching maximum amplitude, with normal values ranging from 0 to 10%. Increased LY30 may be indicative of excessive fibrinolysis, although treatment typically focuses on addressing any underlying coagulopathy rather than thromboxane administration specifically.
In summary, Hypocoagulability is characterized by prolonged R time, prolonged K time, low MA, and increased LY30. Hypercoagulability is indicated by shortened R time, shortened K time, high MA, and decreased LY30. And platelet dysfunction is suggested by a low MA coupled with normal R and K times.[239]

275. After liver transplantation, a patient with pre-surgical hyponatremia (serum sodium 120 mEq/L) experiences rapid sodium correction and develops central pontine myelinolysis. Which symptoms characterize this condition?
a) Myoclonus, hyperreflexia, tremor

b) Agitation, sweating, hyperthermia
c) Nausea, vomiting, tachycardia
d) Confusion, dysarthria, flaccid quadriparesis
e) Myoclonus, hyperthermia, agitation
**Answer: d**
Central pontine myelinolysis, triggered by rapid correction of hyponatremia, presents with confusion, dysarthria, and flaccid quadriparesis.[240]

276. During liver transplantation, the use of a cell saver device is considered safe in most patients. However, in which of the following conditions is its use contraindicated?
a) Active HCC
b) Hypothermia
c) Severe peritonitis
d) Need for rapid blood transfusion
e) Hyperkalemia
**Answer: c**
The use of cell saver technology is controversial in patients with active malignancy. However, recent studies, including systematic reviews and meta-analyses, show that the use of cell savers in patients with HCC does not result in impaired disease-free survival, an increase in HCC recurrence, or impaired overall survival. Hypothermia is not a contraindication for cell saver use. In emergency situations, the cell saver can be directly connected to a rapid infusion device. A cell saver system washes the red blood cells before transfusion and eliminates ammonia, lactate, and potassium. However, the system does not possess antibacterial properties, which raises the potential for bacterial contamination.[241,242]

277. At which phase of the orthotopic liver transplant is a large dose of steroids administered?
a) Preanhepatic
b) Anhepatic
c) Neohepatic
d) Posthepatic
**Answer: b**
Steroids are administered during the anhepatic phase of liver transplantation to suppress the immune response. They work by preventing macrophages from releasing interleukin-1, which helps inhibit the initiation of a strong immunogenic response.[243]

278. Which patient would benefit the most from the use of venovenous bypass during liver transplantation?
a) A patient with active bleeding from superior rectal hemorrhoids
b) A patient with active HCC
c) A patient in whom the piggyback technique is utilized
d) A patient who is volume depleted
e) A patient with extensive portal vein clot

**Answer: a**

Venovenous bypass during liver transplantation improves venous return to the heart and reduces congestion in the intestine. It should be strongly considered for use in patients experiencing bleeding due to portal hypertension. In these cases, performing a bicaval liver transplant with full occlusion of the IVC can increase venous pressure and exacerbate bleeding. Additionally, venovenous bypass enhances renal perfusion and can delay the development of metabolic acidosis. Therefore, it should also be considered for patients with significant fluid overload, renal dysfunction, or those who might not tolerate total IVC occlusion well.

There is no specific benefit from using venovenous bypass in patients with HCC. For patients undergoing the piggyback technique, the IVC is only partially occluded, and most patients tolerate the liver transplant procedure well without the need for bypass. In patients with extensive portal vein clots, significant collateral flow typically allows them to tolerate IVC clamping adequately.[244]

# 7. Split and Living Donor Transplantation

279. A 35-year-old female is being evaluated for partial liver donation to her 9-year-old son, who has liver cirrhosis secondary to biliary atresia. A pre-operative CT scan revealed a liver attenuation index (LAI) greater that 5 HU. How should this findings be interpreted?
a) The value indicates severe macrovesicular steatosis (>30%); therefore, the patient is not a surgical candidate for donation
b) The value indicates mild to moderate macrovesicular steatosis (5% to 30%); thus, the patient is not an optimal candidate for donation
c) The value suggests subclinical liver steatosis; a liver biopsy should be undertaken for confirmation
d) The value suggests the absence of liver steatosis; proceed with the liver donation
e) The value is inconclusive; a liver biopsy is warranted for further evaluation

**Answer: d**
The LAI is defined as the difference between the mean hepatic CT attenuation and the mean splenic CT attenuation measured on a non-contrast CT scan, expressed in HU. The formula for calculating LAI is as follows:
LAI = Mean Hepatic Attenuation (HU) − Mean Splenic Attenuation (HU).
LAI > 5 HU: No significant histological macrovesicular steatosis.
LAI between -10 HU and 5 HU: Moderate macrovesicular steatosis (5% to 30%).
LAI < -10HU: Moderate to severe macrovesicular steatosis (>30%).[245]

280. A 40-year-old male presents for evaluation as a potential partial liver donor for his 7-year-old daughter, who has been diagnosed with the urea cycle disorder. During the pre-operative workup, the donor undergoes extensive laboratory testing, imaging studies, and a multidisciplinary assessment to determine eligibility. The results indicate that the donor has normal LFT and an adequate volume of healthy liver tissue, but the arterial anatomy classified as type 3. What correlates with this description?
a) Proper hepatic artery arises from the common hepatic artery and divides distally to form the right and left hepatic arteries (75%)
b) Replaced or accessory left hepatic artery arising from the left gastric artery (10%)
c) Replaced or accessory right hepatic artery arising from the superior mesenteric artery (10%)
d) Replaced or accessory left hepatic artery plus replaced or accessory right hepatic artery (2.3%)
e) Common hepatic artery arising from the superior mesenteric artery (1.5%)
f) Common hepatic artery arising from the aorta (0.2%)

**Answer: c**
In the context of liver anatomy, the classification of arterial supply is critical for surgical planning, especially during living donor liver transplantation. Michels classification describes various anatomical variations of the hepatic artery. In Type 3 of Michels classification, replaced or accessory right hepatic artery arising from the superior mesenteric artery (10%).[246]

281. A 38-year-old mother presents to the transplant center for evaluation as a potential partial liver donor for her 6-year-old daughter, who has been diagnosed with Alagille syndrome. During the evaluation, it is noted that the mother has a history of recurrent jaundice but without liver test abnormalities. She reports a family history of cholestatic liver disease but was previously unaware of any personal diagnosis. Genetic testing reveals mutations in the JAGGED1 gene, confirming a diagnosis of subclinical Alagille syndrome in the mother. MRI of the abdomen shows a reduction in the extrahepatic biliary ducts. How does this diagnosis affect donor candidacy?
a) Complete the evaluation and plan to proceed with donation with caution
b) Complete the evaluation and plan for Roux-en-Y biliary reconstruction for the biliary system to minimize biliary complications
c) The mother needs additional testing, including ERCP, before her candidacy can be determined
d) Obtain a liver biopsy to confirm subclinical Alagille syndrome and exclude other pathologies contraindicating donation
e) Exclude the mother candidacy for donation

**Answer: e**
Alagille syndrome is a congenital autosomal dominant disorder characterized by variable penetrance. Caution is essential in the selection of living related donors, as approximately 40% of parents may carry the JAGGED1 mutation, and even asymptomatic individuals can exhibit normal LFT but moderate to severe hypoplastic biliary ducts. While a subclinical form of the disease with preserved hepatic integrity and absence of biliary abnormalities does not constitute an absolute contraindication for donation, a significant reduction in interlobular bile ducts and extrahepatic biliary ducts is deemed an absolute contraindication.[247]

282. A 41-year-old male is being evaluated as a potential partial liver donor for his 1-month-old son, who has been diagnosed with hepatoblastoma. The donor has no significant medical history, and his laboratory results are within normal limits. A CT scan shows a normal liver with patent vasculature and Type 1 arterial anatomy. The calculated graft weight of the left lateral segment is 300 grams, and the recipient weighs 5 kilograms. Which of the following statements is correct?

a) The graft-to-recipient weight ratio is 6%; the graft size is considered adequate for a pediatric recipient
b) The graft-to-recipient weight ratio is 6%; the graft is oversized, and further reduction procedures are needed
c) The graft-to-recipient weight ratio is 6%; the graft is too small, and the left lobe should be used instead
d) The graft-to-recipient weight ratio is 0.6%; the graft is too small, and the left lobe should be used instead
e) The graft-to-recipient weight ratio is 0.6%; the graft size is considered adequate for a pediatric recipient

**Answer: b**

The ratio of graft weight to the recipient's body weight (calculated as graft weight divided by recipient body weight, multiplied by 100%) is used to determine the appropriate graft size in relation to the potential volume of the graft and the recipient's size. A graft-to-recipient body weight ratio between 1% and 3% is generally considered an appropriate size match. If the ratio exceeds 4%, there is a risk of developing large for size syndrome, which can be life-threatening and result in poor graft perfusion and primary non-function.[248]

283. A 32-year-old female is being evaluated as a potential partial liver donor for her 3-year-old son with liver failure from biliary atresia. Her medical history is negative, and she has favorable liver anatomy for left lobe donation. Serological typing showed that there is a donor dominant one-way HLA matching in the 3 loci of HLA-A, -B, and -DR. The recipient of this graft has higher probability of developing what?
a) Increased risk of humoral rejection
b) Increased risk of cellular rejection
c) Increased risk of malignancy
d) Increased risk of graft-versus-host disease
e) Increased likelihood of developing graft tolerance

**Answer: d**

Donor-dominant one-way HLA matching in three loci (HLA-A, -B, and -DR) has been associated with a significantly elevated risk of fatal graft-versus-host disease (GVHD) following liver transplantation. Research findings indicate that a greater number of matched loci correlates with a higher risk of GVHD.[249]

284. A 2-year-old child with biliary atresia is scheduled for a living donor liver transplantation (LDLT). Preoperative imaging shows a sclerotic and underdeveloped portal vein. During surgery, minimal portal vein flow is observed, along with significant narrowing just beyond the confluence of the superior mesenteric and

splenic veins. Which of the following interventions is most effective for improving portal vein flow before graft implantation?
a) Ligation of dominant collaterals
b) Obliteration of small retrosplenic venous collaterals
c) Placement of an interposition graft in the narrowed segment of the portal vein
d) Use of curved forceps to align the anastomotic axis
e) Abort the procedure, as nothing can be done
**Answer: c**
In pediatric LDLT, especially in biliary atresia, adequate portal vein flow is essential. When significant narrowing of the portal vein is present, the most effective way to restore flow is to insert an interposition graft to bypass the narrowed segment. This directly improves portal circulation and optimizes graft function. Other options may assist in improving venous drainage or surgical exposure but do not effectively resolve the primary issue of reduced portal inflow.[250]

285. A 7-month-old infant with biliary atresia is experiencing worsening liver function and is listed as Status 1A for urgent liver transplantation. The child has blood type A. A liver becomes available from a 7-month-old deceased donor with blood type B. What is the most appropriate next step?
a) Decline the offer due to ABO incompatibility and continue searching for a compatible donor
b) Proceed with the transplant using preoperative desensitization therapy to reduce anti-isohemagglutinin antibodies
c) Discuss the offer with the parents, highlighting the risks of ABO-incompatible transplantation
d) Decline the offer; the patient can only receive a liver from type A or O donors
e) Initiate a three-way crossmatch protocol to assess compatibility despite ABO mismatch
**Answer: b**
In critically ill infants listed as Status 1A, ABO-incompatible liver transplantation can be life-saving. Although traditionally associated with higher complication risks, outcomes have significantly improved with the use of preoperative desensitization protocols that reduce anti-isohemagglutinin antibodies. In this case, proceeding with the transplant and appropriate immunologic management offers the best chance of survival.[251]

286. A 22-year-old woman with a history of bipolar disorder presents for evaluation as a potential partial liver donor for her boyfriend, who has alcohol-induced liver cirrhosis. Her psychiatric condition is well controlled, with no history of hospitalizations or recent relapses. She is a current smoker, unemployed, and

considering returning to college. She reports having met her boyfriend just two weeks ago but states she "knew right away he was the one." She also mentions that his parents fully support her decision and have offered to buy her a brand-new BMW car as a token of appreciation to help with transportation. What is the absolute contraindication to donation?
a) Psychiatric disorder
b) Unemployment
c) Smoking
d) Financial gain from the donation
e) Lack of stable social support
**Answer: d**
In living organ donation, one of the primary ethical considerations is that donors should not be motivated by financial gain. In this scenario, the promise of a brand-new BMW car as financial support for her decision to donate raises concerns about coercion and the potential for undue influence. This could compromise the integrity of the donation process, making financial gain an absolute contraindication to donation regardless of the donor's other medical or psychological factors. While the patient has a manageable psychiatric history, is unemployed, and is a smoker, these factors alone do not automatically disqualify her from being a donor as long as they are adequately addressed.[252]

287. A 37-year-old woman with hepatitis B-related cirrhosis, who underwent a prior liver transplant that developed chronic graft dysfunction complicated by Budd-Chiari syndrome, is now evaluated for living donor liver transplantation (LDLT) from her husband. Her imaging shows portal vein thrombosis extending into the superior mesenteric vein. The transplant team is concerned about vascular reconstruction challenges for right liver LDLT and debates her suitability for retransplantation. Which of the following statement is the most accurate?
a) Her age and health status preclude her from retransplantation
b) Portal vein thrombosis is an absolute contraindication to LDLT
c) Advanced surgical techniques can manage vascular reconstruction challenges in LDLT
d) Retransplantation requires a full liver graft
e) Budd-Chiari syndrome is an absolute contraindication to LDLT
**Answer: c**
Advanced surgical techniques enable effective management of vascular reconstruction challenges in LDLT. Despite historical concerns about Budd-Chiari syndrome, retransplantation, and portal vein thrombosis as contraindications, modern surgical advancements allow safe LDLT in complex cases.[253]

288. When assessing a candidate for living liver donation, it is important to evaluate the effect of the recipient's disease severity on the necessary size of the graft and the overall success of adult-to-adult liver transplants. Which of the following factors would least likely necessitate an increase in graft size?
a) Significant portal hypertension in the recipient
b) Older donor age
c) Fatty liver changes in the donor
d) Recipient with a higher MELD score
e) Recipient with a portal vein thrombus
**Answer: e**
In adult-to-adult living donor liver transplantation, the recipient's condition significantly impacts graft size requirements and postoperative outcomes. Factors such as significant portal hypertension, older donor age, fatty liver changes in the donor, and a higher MELD score typically indicate a need for a larger graft to ensure adequate function and minimize the risk of complications. However, the presence of a portal vein thrombus in the recipient does not automatically correlate with the necessity for a larger graft size, as it may still be managed without affecting the graft volume required.[254]

289. Which statement about the CUSA and liver parenchyma transection is most accurate?
a) The CUSA should be set to high amplitude to maximize liver parenchymal disruption
b) High suction settings are needed to maintain clear visualization of the operative field
c) Electrocautery cannot be used simultaneously with the CUSA to control bleeding
d) Coagulation occurs primarily through parenchymal disruption rather than electrical current
e) Powerful hemostatic devices are preferred to visualize vessels and biliary radicles during transection
**Answer: d**
The CUSA device uses ultrasonic energy (typically at 32 kHz, 60–70% amplitude) and saline irrigation (4–6 mL/min) to disrupt liver parenchyma, enabling visualization of vascular structures. Coagulation of small vessels (<1 mm) is achieved primarily through ultrasonic disruption rather than thermal electrocautery. High-amplitude settings, excessive suction, or powerful hemostatic devices that obscure vessels and biliary radicles are not preferred, as they hinder precise transection.[255]

290. A 50-year-old woman is undergoing a living donor right liver transplant due to end-stage liver disease secondary to autoimmune hepatitis. Which of the following

considerations is most critical during recipient hepatectomy and preparation for transplantation in this specific scenario?
a) Allow excessive skeletonization of the common hepatic duct to ensure maximum length for anastomosis
b) Use diathermy coagulation liberally on the bile duct to control any minor bleeding
c) Preserve the recipient's IVC during the procedure to maintain venous return
d) Control the proximal ends of the hepatic arteries only after the distal ends have been ligated
e) Dissection of the common hepatic duct should start at the superior border of the duodenum and continue until it merges with the cystic duct, where it should be transected.

**Answer: c**

In living donor right liver transplantation, one crucial aspect is to preserve the recipient's IVC, which is distinct from procedures involving deceased donor grafts. Careful mobilization of the caudate lobe and division of the short hepatic veins are required to facilitate this process. The other options either describe inappropriate techniques or disregard the necessary precautions, such as excessive skeletonization of the bile duct or inappropriate coagulation techniques, which can compromise blood supply or increase the risk of complications. Dissection of the common hepatic duct should start high up at the hilum.[256]

291. A 45-year-old man is undergoing living donor liver transplantation using the piggyback technique. After hepatectomy, the recipient's IVC is partially clamped to facilitate hepatic vein anastomosis. Upon completing the suprahepatic anastomosis, the patient exhibits hemodynamic instability, with his heart rate rising to 140 bpm and blood pressure dropping to 75/50 mmHg. What should the surgical team prioritize to address the patient's instability?
a) Proceed with the portal vein anastomosis as quickly as possible to perfuse the graft and release the IVC clamp
b) Immediately restore blood flow through the IVC by repositioning the clamp distal to the anastomosis, occluding the donor hepatic vein
c) Initiate venovenous bypass to effectively restore venous return
d) Maintain the IVC clamp and administer aggressive fluid resuscitation and epinephrine
e) Delay the portal vein anastomosis, focus on improving the patient's blood pressure, and prepare for cardiac arrest

**Answer: b**

The patient's hemodynamic instability results from intolerance to partial IVC clamping, which reduces venous return. The best course of action is to immediately restore IVC blood flow by repositioning the clamp distal to the anastomosis, occluding the donor hepatic vein. This step stabilizes hemodynamics without the complications of venovenous bypass, such as hypothermia and bleeding diathesis, which is time-consuming due to cannula insertion and bypass initiation. Rapid restoration of IVC blood flow improves cardiac output and blood pressure, enabling safer progression to portal vein anastomosis and better overall outcomes.[257]

292. A 38-year-old female is undergoing liver transplantation from a living donor, who is donating a left lobe combined with the caudate lobe. The surgical team is preparing to perform the portal vein anastomosis between the graft's left portal vein and the recipient's main portal vein. Which of the following practices should the surgical team prioritize to ensure the success of the portal vein anastomosis?
a) Keep the anastomosis as tight as possible to minimize potential redundancy in the graft
b) Use a larger suture, such as 4-0 Prolene, for the anastomosis to strengthen the connection given the extra tension on the anastomosis in a smaller partial graft
c) Aim for a slightly longer and redundant portal vein anastomosis to accommodate graft regeneration
d) Mark the posterior walls of the graft and recipient portal branches to ensure proper alignment
e) To maximize the length of the portal vein, ligate a portal vein branch leading to the caudate lobe
**Answer: c**
The best practice is to aim for a slightly longer and redundant anastomosis to allow for anticipated changes during rapid graft regeneration and rotation. If the anastomosis is too short, it can lead to complications such as tension on the vessel, which can impair blood flow and result in graft failure. The first stitch is started with the adjustment of the marked anterior walls of the graft and recipient left portal branches. An isolated caudate portal vein originating from the left-sided wall of the portal branches of the caudate lobe is sometimes observed. It is advisable to undertake a reconstruction that ensures full graft function of the caudate lobe. The portal vein anastomosis is performed with 6-0 Prolene.[258]

293. A 40-year-old woman with end-stage liver disease secondary to MASH is evaluated for living donor liver transplantation (LDLT). During the preoperative planning, the surgical team faces a dilemma regarding whether to select a right or left liver graft from a living donor, her 25-year-old brother. Given that the right liver is often preferred for its larger volume and anatomical features, which of the following considerations should be prioritized when deciding between a right or left liver graft for this patient?

a) The presence of a larger hepatic artery in the right liver graft, which is crucial for perfusion
b) The ability to procure the middle hepatic vein with the right liver graft for improved venous drainage
c) The need to preserve inflow and outflow for both the resected liver and the remaining liver to prevent congestion
d) The donor's willingness to provide a graft of any size, regardless of anatomical considerations
e) The fact that the left liver graft alone is adequate due to the patient's body size and condition
**Answer: c**
In the context of living donor liver transplantation, it is essential to prioritize the preservation of inflow and outflow for both the resected graft and the remaining liver segments. This consideration helps prevent potential congestion and ensures adequate blood flow to the transplanted and remaining liver tissues. While the right liver graft's larger volume and the presence of the middle hepatic vein are important, maintaining proper vascular anatomy to support both the donor and recipient livers is critical. The other options either focus on aspects that are secondary to the primary goal of maintaining vascular integrity or overlook the complexities of donor safety and surgical planning.[258]

294. A 7-month-old boy with end-stage liver disease due to biliary atresia, weighing 6 kg, is on the waiting list for a liver transplant. A split-liver transplantation (SLT) offer from a deceased donor has become available, and the boy is being evaluated for this option. His parents are concerned about the risks of SLT compared to waiting for a whole-liver transplant (WLT). What should the medical team recommend?
a) Advise declining the SLT offer in favor of waiting for a WLT, as WLT yields superior surgical outcomes
b) Recommend accepting the SLT offer, as it reduces mortality by 63% for candidates weighing ≤7 kg
c) Recommend accepting the SLT offer despite higher risks of arterial and biliary complications
d) Suggest waiting for a WLT or accepting a living donor partial graft, due to the increased risk of ischemic cholangiopathy with split deceased donor grafts
e) Inform the family that SLT offers no survival benefit and should be declined for safety reasons
**Answer: b**
For a 7-month-old with end-stage liver disease weighing 6 kg, accepting a split-liver transplant significantly reduces mortality by 63% compared to waiting for a whole-liver transplant. The medical team should recommend accepting the SLT offer, as it

provides a critical survival advantage during this vulnerable period. Modern outcomes of SLT are comparable to WLT in pediatric recipients, making it a safe and effective option despite historical concerns about complications.[259]

295. A 23-year-old male, previously healthy with a BMI of 32, is involved in a severe car accident and is declared brain dead 2 days later while in the ICU. His family expresses a desire to donate his organs. During the evaluation process, the transplant team reviews the donor's clinical history and imaging results, considering the possibility of split liver transplantation. The patient's initial ALT was 34 U/L, but subsequent tests show that the ALT levels have increased to 234 U/L and continue to trend upward. Total bilirubin has also increased to 2.4 mg/dL from 1.0 mg/dL on admission. The INR is 1.2. The CT scan of the abdomen reveals no evidence of liver injury or trauma. How should the transplant team proceed?
a) Accept the offer and split the liver for pediatric and adult recipients
b) Decline the split liver offer based on BMI being above 30
c) Decline the split liver offer secondary to the cause of death being trauma
d) Decline the split liver offer, given that his ALT is 3 times the upper limit of normal and continues to trend upward
e) Decline the split liver offer secondary to prolonged ICU stay
**Answer: d**
In this scenario, the rising ALT levels, which have increased to 234 U/L, indicate potential liver dysfunction. The total bilirubin level has also increased, suggesting the possibility of cholestasis or impaired liver function despite no visible injuries on CT scan. ALT levels exceeding three times the upper limit of normal and continuing to trend upward are concerning for potential graft viability and predict poor outcomes if the organ were to be split for transplant.[260]

296. A 21-year-old male, weighing 70 kg and with a BMI of 23, is evaluated for organ donation after being declared brain dead following a car accident. The surgical team is planning to split his liver for transplantation into two adult recipients. What is the estimated weight of this donor's liver?
a) 210 g
b) 400 g
c) 800 g
d) 1400 g
e) 2100 g
**Answer: d**
The liver typically weighs about 2% of total body weight. In this case, the donor weighs 70 kg. To estimate the liver weight, we calculate 2% of 70 kg:
Estimated liver weight = 70 kg x 0.02 = 1.4 kg = 1400 g.[261]

297. A 50-year-old man, designated as the primary recipient for a split-liver transplant from a deceased donor, is informed that the donor liver may be divided to benefit another patient. After considering his options, he asks whether he can decline the split and receive the entire liver graft instead. According to current OPTN guidelines, what is the appropriate response to his inquiry?
a) He may decline the split and automatically receive the entire liver graft
b) Declining the split will result in his removal from the transplant list
c) He should understand that declining the split may jeopardize the organ's availability for his transplant
d) He must accept the split-liver arrangement without any choice
e) He should be assured that the right liver lobe offers outcomes equivalent to a whole liver graft
**Answer: c**
Under current OPTN guidelines, while the primary recipient has the right to decline the option for splitting the liver, it is essential for them to understand that this decision could impact the availability of the organ for their transplant. If they refuse to participate in the split, they may not receive any graft at all if the transplant center decides to proceed with the split donor liver for another recipient. In addition, even though the right lobe can provide a larger graft, outcomes can depend on various factors including the individual recipient's health, underlying conditions, and compatibility. The assessment of which lobe is "better" is made during the surgical procedure based on the anatomy of the donor liver and the specific needs of the recipients. Therefore, it is incorrect to guarantee that a recipient will receive a better liver or that a split yields an inherently similar outcome.[262]

298. A 32-year-old man is undergoing right lobe hepatectomy to donate to his older brother for liver transplantation. During the procedure, Doppler ultrasonography reveals hepatofugal flow in the anterior branch of the portal vein, and temporary clamping of the right hepatic artery shows a dark red surface in a liver segment. The surgical team must decide whether reconstruction of the middle hepatic vein (MHV) tributaries is necessary. Which statement best indicates the need for MHV tributary reconstruction?
a) Reconstruction is required due to a congested area insufficient for the recipient's metabolic demands
b) Reconstruction is unnecessary, as the area drained by the right hepatic vein meets the recipient's metabolic demands
c) Reconstruction is unnecessary, as functional communication veins between the right hepatic vein and MHV tributaries provide adequate drainage

d) Reconstruction is not required, as adequate portal vein flow was observed during hepatectomy
e) Reconstruction is mandatory, as the dark red surface indicates irreversible ischemia
**Answer: a**
The hepatofugal flow in the portal vein and the dark red surface after clamping the right hepatic artery indicate a congested liver segment, insufficient to meet the recipient's metabolic demands. Reconstruction of the MHV tributaries is necessary to ensure adequate blood flow and graft function. Doppler ultrasonography confirms congestion, and the congested area's color change suggests inadequate inflow, resolvable with reconstruction. Although communication veins between the right hepatic vein and MHV tributaries exist in 20–30% of donors and may reduce the need for reconstruction if functional, the observed congestion in this case necessitates reconstruction to support the graft's viability.[263]

299. During bench surgery for a right liver graft from a living donor, intended for liver transplantation, the surgical team notes that the right anterior and posterior portal vein branches are too widely separated for venoplasty. What is the optimal strategy for reconstructing the portal venous inflow?
a) Direct anastomosis of the right anterior and posterior branches to the recipient's corresponding branches to ensure immediate vascular continuity
b) Directly anastomose the graft's right anterior branch to the recipient's right portal vein and the posterior branch to the left portal vein for vascular continuity.
c) Dissect the graft parenchyma to align the anterior and posterior branches, then perform venoplasty to create a single portal orifice if the branches are suitably positioned
d) Use a cryopreserved vein graft, such as a bifurcated iliac vein, for interposition between the graft's anterior and posterior branches due to its availability
e) Use an autologous vein graft from the recipient for interposition between the graft's anterior and posterior branches to ensure long-term patency
**Answer: e**
Given the significant distance between the graft's right anterior and posterior portal vein branches, which precludes venoplasty, the optimal strategy is to use an autologous vein graft from the recipient for interposition. Autologous grafts offer superior long-term patency compared to cryopreserved vein grafts. Direct anastomosis to the recipient's portal vein branches risks misalignment and is complicated by challenges in preserving recipient branches during hilar dissection, making it less favorable.[264]

300. During a left hepatectomy for partial liver donation, the donor's left hepatic artery is found to originate from the left gastric artery. What is the best method to determine whether this is the main or an accessory left hepatic artery?
a) Use intraoperative Doppler ultrasonography, temporary clamping of the left hepatic artery, and back-table saline flush to assess arterial flow and communication
b) Rely solely on preoperative CT angiography to define the arterial anatomy and its dominance
c) Perform a back-table saline flush into the left hepatic artery stump to observe backflow from the middle hepatic artery
d) Proceed with graft harvesting without further assessment, assuming the left gastric artery origin indicates an accessory artery
e) Temporarily ligate the left gastric artery and visually assess liver perfusion intraoperatively

**Answer: a**

Combining intraoperative Doppler ultrasonography, temporary clamping of the left hepatic artery, and back-table saline flush provides a comprehensive assessment of whether the left hepatic artery is the main or an accessory artery. Doppler ultrasonography evaluates flow dynamics, temporary clamping isolates the artery's contribution to the left liver, and back-table saline flush confirms intragraft arterial communication, ensuring accurate determination of arterial dominance.[265]

301. A 47-year-old woman with end-stage liver disease undergoes living donor liver transplantation with a right segment graft. Postoperatively, she develops persistent hyperbilirubinemia and ascites exceeding 1 liter per day. Despite stable prothrombin time and no severe encephalopathy, her bilirubin levels rise steadily by the third week, with minimal transaminase elevation. Which condition best explains her clinical presentation?
a) Acute rejection
b) Primary graft nonfunction
c) Small-for-size syndrome
d) Sepsis-related liver dysfunction
e) Graft-versus-host disease

**Answer: c**

The patient's presentation, with prolonged hyperbilirubinemia, intractable ascites, stable prothrombin time, and minimal transaminase elevation, is consistent with small-for-size syndrome (SFSS). SFSS reflects delayed hepatic recovery due to an undersized graft, typically without severe encephalopathy or significant transaminase spikes, distinguishing it from acute rejection, primary nonfunction, encephalopathy, or graft-versus-host disease.[266]

302. A 60-year-old male patient with end-stage liver disease undergoes liver transplantation using a small graft from a living donor. One week post-surgery, he develops increasing jaundice and abdominal distension despite receiving appropriate immunosuppressive therapy. A follow-up liver biopsy is performed due to concerns of small for size syndrome (SFSS). Which of the following pathological findings would most likely be associated with SFSS?
a) Centrilobular hepatocyte ballooning and cholestasis
b) Centrilobular ballooning accompanied by portal vein thrombosis and extensive necrosis of hepatocytes
c) Portal hyperperfusion with sinusoidal endothelial denudation and zone 1 hepatocyte necrosis
d) Diffuse ischemic changes without any signs of cholestasis or vascular congestion
e) Patchy necrosis accompanied by inflammation, predominantly lymphocytic infiltrates in portal areas
**Answer: a**
Pathological features of SFSS include portal hyperperfusion that causes sinusoidal endothelial denudation and focal hemorrhage into the portal connective tissue. Poor hepatic arterial flow can exacerbate these issues, leading to further complications such as ischemic cholangitis. The studies show that centrilobular hepatocyte ballooning and cholestasis are the most prominent and characteristic features of SFSS. SFSS typically affects centrilobular (zone 3) hepatocytes due to hyperperfusion and poor arterial flow.[267]

303. A 55-year-old man with cirrhosis due to chronic hepatitis C undergoes liver transplantation with a living donor graft. The graft volume is 42% of the standard liver volume, with a graft-to-recipient weight ratio of 0.81. Post-transplantation, he develops jaundice and ascites, raising concerns for small-for-size syndrome (SFSS). What is the most likely etiology of SFSS in this case?
a) Impaired regenerative capacity of mature hepatocytes due to chronic liver disease
b) Vascular shear stress and damage to hepatic sinusoids and parenchyma from excessive portal vein flow relative to graft size
c) Increased immunological rejection risk associated with a living donor graft
d) Pre-existing liver pathology causing inadequate blood flow to the transplanted graft
e) Downregulation of endothelin-1 causing reduced hepatic sinusoidal perfusion
**Answer: b**
The primary etiology of SFSS is vascular shear stress and damage to hepatic sinusoids and parenchyma due to excessive portal vein flow relative to the small graft size. This hyperperfusion, exacerbated by a graft-to-recipient weight ratio of 0.81 and low graft volume (42%), causes sinusoidal injury, leading to jaundice and ascites.

Overexpression, not downregulation, of endothelin-1 contributes to portal hypertension, worsening SFSS.[268]

304. A 58-year-old man (120 kg, BMI 38) with cirrhosis due to MASH undergoes liver transplantation with a 900 g graft. One week post-transplant, he develops small-for-size syndrome (SFSS), presenting with worsening jaundice and intractable ascites, unresponsive to maximal supportive therapy. Which treatment is most effective in addressing excessive portal vein flow in this patient?
a) Ligation of a portosystemic shunt to redirect portal flow
b) Splenic artery embolization to reduce splenic hyperemia
c) Continuation of maximal medical therapy awaiting liver hypertrophy
d) Delayed splenectomy to manage hypersplenism and portal hypertension
e) TIPS to lower portal vein pressure

**Answer: b**

Splenic artery embolization effectively reduces excessive portal vein flow by addressing splenic hyperemia, a key contributor to portal hypertension in SFSS. This targeted approach alleviates sinusoidal stress, improving jaundice and ascites, while avoiding the risks of other interventions.[266]

305. A 40-year-old female patient is scheduled to undergo minimally invasive donor hepatectomy (MIDH) to provide a portion of her liver for her brother in need of a transplant. Considering the current understanding of MIDH, which of the following statements is most accurate regarding this procedure?
a) MIDH is safer and more effective than open liver donation
b) The robotic approach has been shown to have inferior outcomes compared to the hand-assisted laparoscopic approach
c) Appropriate selection criteria and surgeon experience are crucial for minimizing complications and improving outcomes with MIDH
d) The learning curve is steep because retrieving a liver graft from a living donor is equivalent to a conventional hepatectomy
e) Data supporting the effectiveness of MIDH is widely accepted and donor safety has been fully validated

**Answer: c**

MIDH has the ability to improve donor safety and facilitate quicker recovery times. However, optimal outcomes depend on having skilled surgeons and appropriate selection of patients to minimize complications, blood loss, and hospital stay duration. Various techniques exist, including robotic-assisted methods, but proficiency is essential for managing the fragile liver tissue and maintaining the integrity of vascular structures during the surgery. Importantly, obtaining a liver graft from a living donor differs from a traditional hepatectomy, as the vascular connections of the removed section need to be carefully preserved. The validation of donor safety for this technique remains incomplete, and it is presently practiced in only a limited number of specialized centers due to its complexity. In discussions at the Second International Consensus Conference on laparoscopic liver resections, participants noted that while MIDH is not inferior to standard methods regarding donor safety, the procedure was still not advocated due to insufficient data on postoperative complications.[269]

306. A 50-year-old man with chronic liver failure due to hepatitis B cirrhosis is evaluated for living donor liver transplantation (LDLT). His condition requires a substantial graft volume to address his liver insufficiency. Two potential living donors are identified: his 25-year-old daughter, who has a right lobe volume that constitutes 75% of her total liver volume, and her uncle, who can donate the left lobe of his liver. What is the most appropriate recommendation for the transplant team?
a) Proceed with using the right lobe from the daughter, as she is a direct relative and ideally suited for donation
b) Proceed with using the left lobe combined with the caudate lobe from the daughter
c) Consider utilizing just the left lobe from the uncle, despite the potential for small-for-size graft syndrome
d) Evaluate combining the left lobes from both donors to increase overall graft volume while minimizing risk
e) Perform a dual graft LDLT using the right lobe from the uncle and the left lobe from the daughter to meet the size requirements
**Answer: d**
In this scenario, the daughter's right lobe is contraindicated for donation due to the disproportionate size (right lobe > 70% of total liver volume), which poses a significant risk to her as a donor. The uncle's left lobe alone may potentially result in small-for-size graft syndrome if he is the sole donor. Therefore, the appropriate course of action is to consider combining the left lobes from both donors if both demonstrate acceptable liver volumes to ensure sufficient graft size while maintaining donor safety. This option avoids the complications associated with using a disproportionate right lobe and effectively addresses the patient's need for a larger graft.[270]

307. A 38-year-old woman with autoimmune hepatitis and HCC is evaluated for living donor liver transplantation (LDLT). Her husband volunteers to donate his right lobe, but he is concerned about the potential risks associated with the donation procedure. What is the most critical information the transplant team should communicate to the potential donor and recipient?
a) The risk of HCC recurrence is slightly lower in LDLT recipients than in deceased donor liver transplant recipients

b) The overall frequency of severe complications in living donors is extremely low, reported to be between 0.2% and 0.5%
c) The overall frequency of severe complications in living donors is relatively low, reported to be between 2% and 5%
d) Right lobe donation consistently leads to a higher incidence of severe complications than left lobe donation
e) LDLT demonstrates higher graft and patient survival at 5 years in comparison to deceased donor liver transplant recipients

**Answer: b**

In this clinical scenario, it is essential for the transplant team to provide accurate information about the risks associated with living liver donation. While complications do occur in living donors (ranging from 15% to 30%), severe complications—defined as those requiring transplantation or resulting in death—are exceedingly rare, occurring in only about 0.2% to 0.5% of cases. This information can help alleviate the potential donor's fears and clarify that living donation is a relatively safe procedure when performed in experienced centers. The statement regarding the risk of HCC recurrence is misleading, HCC recurrence has been modeled to be slightly higher in LDLT recipients. There is the sense that some of the HCC patients are "fast-tracked" with LDLT, not allowing the biological character of the tumor to be recognized on the waiting list. There is no evidence that the overall morbidity differs between right and left lobe donors. Studies show comparable 5-year patient survival among LDLT and deceased donor liver transplant recipients (approximately 70%).[271]

308. A 45-year-old woman with end-stage liver disease secondary to autoimmune liver disease is being evaluated for living donor liver transplantation (LDLT). She is facing a critical situation, with her condition deteriorating rapidly. Her medical team discusses the option of dual graft LDLT, involving two potential living donors: her sister, who would donate her left lobe, and a family friend who is also willing to donate his left lobe as well. Considering the risks and benefits involved, what is the most ethically sound approach for the transplant team to convey to the potential living donors?
a) Assure the donors that the surgical risks are minimal and emphasize the life-saving potential of the transplant for the recipient
b) Clearly communicate the surgical risks involved for each donor, including potential complications and the low incidence of donor death
c) Encourage the donors to proceed with dual donation since it is likely to facilitate a better physiological outcome for the recipient
d) Given that the overall risk of living donation effectively doubles for dual donors, the ethical implications of dual graft LDLT may render this option unethical

e) Focus discussion largely on the emotional benefits of being a successful living donor

**Answer: b**

In the context of living donor liver transplantation, it is paramount to uphold the ethical principle of nonmaleficence, which emphasizes avoiding harm to donors. Therefore, the surgical risks associated with donating a liver must be explicitly communicated to potential donors. While the dual graft LDLT option may offer advantages for the recipient, it also places two individuals at risk for the same procedure. By informing the donors about the potential complications and the overall low incidence of severe issues (including donor death), the transplant team supports informed consent and respects the autonomy of each donor.[271]

309. A 38-year-old woman presents to a liver transplant clinic seeking to become a living donor for a patient she met through a social media platform aimed at connecting potential organ donors and recipients. She expresses a strong desire to help the patient, stating they had several discussions online and formed a close bond. However, the transplant team notices that her motivations seem unusually strong, and she is unaware of the medical risks involved in liver donation. Additionally, she has no known personal connection to the patient, raising concerns among the medical staff. Which of the following factors raises suspicion for potential organ trading in this clinical scenario?
a) The donor expresses overwhelming enthusiasm and commitment to the procedure despite lacking understanding of the medical risks involved
b) The donor frequently discusses her intention to donate on public forums, bringing attention to her persona
c) The transplant center maintains publicly accessible records detailing both successful outcomes and complications, including donor morbidity and mortality
d) The transplant team discovers that the donor has received gifts or financial incentives from the patient or associated parties.
e) The donor has made multiple previous attempts to donate her liver to her younger sister, who passed away from biliary atresia

**Answer: d**

The discovery that the donor has received gifts or financial incentives from the patient or associated parties raises significant suspicion for potential organ trading. This points toward a potential quid pro quo arrangement, which is illegal and unethical in the context of organ transplantation. While the other answer choices raise concerning aspects of the situation, none indicate the unethical implications of potential organ trading as clearly as the presence of incentives or gifts involved in the donation process.[272]

# 8. Complex Operative Scenarios

310. What is the most common arterial complication in liver transplantation?
a) Hepatic artery obliteration
b) Hepatic arterial thrombosis
c) Hepatic arterial pseudoaneurysm
d) Hepatic arterial rupture
e) Hepatic arterial embolism
**Answer: b**
The primary complication related to hepatic artery reconstruction is hepatic artery thrombosis, occurring in approximately 5% of adult and 7% of pediatric liver transplants. Hepatic artery thrombosis is linked to biliary complications and can adversely affect both patient and graft survival, often necessitating retransplantation.[273]

311. The main objectives of pretransplant imaging include all of the following:
a) To identify the arterial anatomy
b) To assess the adequacy of the inflow vessel
c) To identify the relationship of the optimal inflow vessel to other structures (varices, portal vein, and its tributaries)
d) To assess the quality of the infrarenal aorta for aortohepatic grafting, if necessary
e) To evaluate iliac artery vessels for potential use as a conduit
**Answer: e**
If the aortic conduit is used, donor iliac vessels are typically utilized, or third-party vessels may be used. If no other vessels are available, prosthetic material is employed. Recipient iliac vessels are never used as conduits due to the associated high morbidity.[274]

312. A 58-year-old female with end-stage liver disease is scheduled for liver transplantation. Preoperative CT reveals normal anatomy and portal hypertension. However, during the initial hepatectomy stage, the surgeon observes significant respiratory variation in the intensity of the pulse and thrill of the hepatic artery, noting that the pulse is stronger during deep inhalation than during exhalation. How should the surgeon modify the surgical technique in this case?
a) This indicates the presence of median arcuate ligament syndrome; the arterial reconstruction should be done utilizing an infrarenal aortic conduit
b) Surgical division of the median arcuate ligament may be necessary to alleviate compression on the celiac axis during arterial reconstruction

c) This indicates the presence of pulmonary embolism and associated right-sided heart failure; cardiopulmonary bypass should be implemented
d) The respiratory variation in the hepatic artery pulse is a normal variant, and no further action is needed
e) This indicates the presence of severe arterial plaque at the takeoff of the celiac trunk; the arterial reconstruction should be done utilizing an infrarenal aortic conduit
**Answer: b**
In this scenario, the significant respiratory variation in hepatic artery pulse intensity suggests the possibility of median arcuate ligament syndrome (MALS), which can compromise the celiac axis and arterial inflow during liver transplantation. As a result, the surgeon should anticipate the need for surgical division of the median arcuate ligament to relieve the compression on the celiac axis during arterial reconstruction. This intervention is crucial for improving arterial flow and minimizing the risk of hepatic arterial thrombosis. On CT or MRI, MALS is best identified in the sagittal view, where celiac compression is readily and often dramatically apparent.[275]

313. A 64-year-old male with end-stage liver disease secondary to MASH, diabetes, ESRD (dialysis-dependent), and mild coronary artery disease is being evaluated for liver transplantation. His preoperative CT scan reveals a replaced right hepatic artery and a relatively small main hepatic artery. Additionally, there is extensive calcification of the aorta at the origins of the celiac trunk, superior mesenteric artery (SMA), and the main aorta, which covers the majority of the vessel, including the supraceliac aorta. Given these findings, how should the transplant team proceed?
a) The patient is not a candidate for a liver transplant given the extent of arterial disease
b) The transplant team should plan for a liver transplant in conjunction with the replacement of the infrarenal aorta using a prosthetic graft, connecting donor iliac vessels as a conduit to the donor's main celiac trunk
c) The transplant team should plan for a liver transplant using a double aortic conduit from the external right iliac vessels using donor iliac arteries
d) The transplant team should plan for a liver transplant using a double aortic conduit from the external left iliac vessels using donor iliac arteries
e) The transplant team should plan for a liver transplant using an extended polytetrafluoroethylene as an inflow from the recipient's external right iliac artery
**Answer: a**
The extensive calcification of the aorta at the origins of the celiac trunk, SMA, and main aorta significantly impacts the surgical approach to liver transplantation. Because these vascular anomalies increase the risk of complications during aortohepatic grafting and may render the patient a high-risk candidate for the procedure, the patient is not a suitable surgical candidate. Even though aortic replacement and liver

transplant are technically feasible, it will not be clinically possible, especially on this older patient with multiple comorbidities.[276]

314. A 57-year-old female diagnosed with end-stage liver disease secondary to MASH, she is listed for liver transplant. The CT scan at the time of listing revealed a partial thrombus in the main portal vein. However, six months later, the patient was admitted to the hospital with peritonitis. A repeat CT scan indicated the progression of the portal vein thrombus (PVT), resulting in complete occlusion of the main portal vein down to the confluence of the splenic and superior mesenteric veins. At the time of her hospital admission, the patient received an offer for a liver transplant. What is the most appropriate course of action for the transplant team?
a) The patient is no longer a candidate for a liver transplant
b) Place the patient on hold, initiate anticoagulation therapy, and consult interventional radiology for thrombectomy
c) Accept the liver offer only on the condition that interventional radiology can perform thrombectomy prior to the transplant
d) Accept the liver offer and plan for a thromboendovenectomy at the time of the transplant
e) Accept the liver offer and plan for the construction of a venous conduit using the donor iliac vein as a conduit from the superior mesenteric vein to the donor's main portal vein
**Answer: d**
The optimal approach in this scenario is to accept the liver offer and plan for a thromboendovenectomy at the time of the transplant. Most instances of PVT can be effectively treated through thromboendovenectomy alone. If the thrombus is acute and pliable, it can often be removed using a Fogarty catheter. This catheter is carefully inserted into the proximal vein, the balloon is inflated, and the clot is then extracted. Extreme caution is necessary to avoid damaging the proximal vein behind the pancreas with the catheter, as this would be challenging to repair. For more chronic and well-formed thrombi, a spatula may be employed to gently dislodge the thrombus, similar to the technique used in an endarterectomy. The vein is carefully everted to reveal more proximal portions and extend the endovenectomy until the clot can be removed. Given that the thrombus extends to the confluence of the splenic and superior mesenteric veins, careful dissection of the portal vein will be necessary to establish control over the inflow. Although this presents a challenging yet feasible situation, the surgeon must ensure preparedness and strategic planning. Inexperienced surgeons should consider involving a senior colleague to assist with this complex segment of the operation. Additionally, the anesthetic team must be fully informed to anticipate significant blood loss during the procedure.[277]

315. A 62-year-old man with a history of alcohol-related cirrhosis presents to the emergency department with abdominal pain, ascites, and bilateral lower extremity swelling. An abdominal ultrasound reveals significant occlusion of the portal vein. Given the unique vascular characteristics of the portal venous system and the high compliance of the portal vein in healthy individuals, which of the following factors is most likely contributing to the development of portal vein thrombosis (PVT) in this patient?
a) Increased intra-abdominal pressure from ascites causing direct compression of the portal vein
b) Alcoholic cardiomyopathy leading to decreased overall blood flow and stasis in the portal system
c) The presence of valvular insufficiency in the splanchnic veins promoting retrograde flow
d) The low-pressure, slow-flow environment of the portal venous system altered due to increased hepatic sinusoidal resistance in cirrhosis
e) Systemic venous hypertension from heart failure influencing splanchnic circulation
**Answer: d**
In patients with cirrhosis, architectural distortion and increased resistance in the hepatic sinusoids alter portal venous hemodynamics, promoting the development of PVT. Normally, the portal venous system is characterized by low pressure, slow flow, and high volume, but these changes create a state that is particularly susceptible to thrombosis. The portal vein's lack of valves and pulsatile flow further distinguishes it from systemic venous circulation and contributes to this vulnerability.[278]

316. A 58-year-old woman with a history of hepatitis C-related cirrhosis presents for routine follow-up. An abdominal Doppler ultrasound reveals a portal vein diameter of 1.6 cm and a flow velocity of 12 cm/second. The patient is asymptomatic, with normal LFT and no signs of decompensation. Which of the following statements is most accurate regarding the patient's risk of developing portal vein thrombosis (PVT) in the upcoming year?
a) The patient has a low risk for PVT due to her asymptomatic status despite the reduced flow velocity
b) The patient is likely at high risk for developing PVT due to the portal vein flow velocity being below the established threshold (15 cm/second)
c) The presence of a widened portal vein diameter suggests a decreased risk of PVT
d) The patient's normal LFT and absence of ascites indicate a negligible risk of PVT
e) The asymptomatic nature of the patient indicates that portal flow velocity is not a reliable predictor for PVT development
**Answer: b**

Studies indicate that a portal vein flow velocity below 15 cm/second is an independent predictive factor for the occurrence of portal vein thrombosis in cirrhotic patients. In this case, the patient's flow velocity of 12 cm/second places her at high risk for developing PVT within the next year, despite her asymptomatic status and normal LFT. The increase in portal vein diameter and the "steal effect" related to porto-collateral circulation results in reduced portal blood flow, further contributing to this risk.[279]

317. A 65-year-old man with a history of alcohol-related cirrhosis presents to the clinic for ongoing management of portal hypertension and esophageal varices. He is currently taking a nonselective β-blocker (NSBB) for primary prevention of variceal bleeding. During the visit, he expresses concern about potential side effects, specifically the risk of developing portal vein thrombosis (PVT). Which of the following statements most accurately reflects current evidence regarding NSBB use in patients with cirrhosis and portal hypertension?
a) NSBBs should be avoided in all cirrhotic patients with portal hypertension due to an increased risk of PVT
b) Recent meta-analyses confirm that NSBB use significantly increases the risk of PVT in cirrhotic patients
c) The severity of portal hypertension and reduced portal vein flow velocity are more predictive of PVT than NSBB use
d) NSBBs are contraindicated in any patient with esophageal varices who has developed portal vein thrombosis
e) NSBBs effectively reduce portal hypertension but are strongly associated with a decline in portal blood flow velocity, increasing PVT risk

**Answer: c**

Although concerns have been raised about a possible link between NSBB use and the development of PVT, current evidence does not establish a causal relationship. Prospective studies suggest that the severity of portal hypertension and a portal vein flow velocity below 15 cm/s are the most significant risk factors for PVT. The heterogeneity and limitations of earlier studies, many of which were retrospective and did not adjust for confounders, weaken claims that NSBBs independently increase PVT risk. As such, NSBBs remain a cornerstone in the management of portal hypertension and variceal bleeding prevention in appropriately selected patients.[280]

318. A 57-year-old male with a history of alcoholic cirrhosis and severe main portal vein thrombosis, which has resulted in significant collateral circulation, undergoes a liver transplant. During the procedure, a thromboendovenectomy is performed successfully. However, after reperfusion of the allograft, the surgical team notes that portal blood flow remains suboptimal. The surgeon ligates a large portosystemic

shunt, but it only slightly improves portal flow. Which of the following factors is most likely contributing to the inadequate portal venous flow?
a) Insufficient inflow from the hepatic artery leading to overall decreased hepatic perfusion
b) The presence of an undetected splenorenal shunt siphoning blood from the portal circulation
c) Inadequate anticoagulation therapy prior to portal vein clamping, resulting in new thrombus formation
d) Distal mesenteric clots that have traveled to the liver, creating embolic phenomena
e) Problems with hepatic outflow causing liver congestion and decreased portal inflow

**Answer: b**

In this scenario, the ongoing suboptimal portal blood flow after successful thromboendovenectomy may be attributed to the presence of a splenorenal shunt. Such shunts can develop in patients with significant portal hypertension and often divert blood away from the portal system into systemic circulation, thereby compromising the effective portal venous flow to the transplanted liver. Although portosystemic shunts can be ligated to improve portal flow, undetected splenorenal shunts may continue to siphon blood from the portal system. This vascular alteration can be a common complication in patients with cirrhosis and must be carefully evaluated and identified on CT images preoperatively as part of surgical planning.[277]

319. A 54-year-old male with end-stage liver disease due to hepatitis C is listed for a combined liver-kidney transplant (CLKT). The patient receives an organ offer from a young DBD donor; however, preoperative testing reveals a positive T-cell crossmatch (XM) against the donor. Which of the following statements best reflects the current understanding of the implications of a positive XM in CLKT?
a) A positive XM in CLKT patients guarantees the success of the renal allograft due to the liver's immunoprotective effects
b) Recent studies have shown that sensitized recipients with a positive XM may have compromised kidney graft and patient survival despite liver transplantation
c) The development of immunosuppressive therapies has completely mitigated the risks associated with positive XM in liver and kidney transplants but not in heart transplants
d) Historical data indicates that kidney allografts from CLKT procedures are more successful than those from isolated kidney transplants, regardless of XM status
e) Positive XM results should lead to automated exclusion from transplantation in all organ types due to guaranteed poor outcomes.

**Answer: b**

Recent analyses indicate that sensitized recipients of CLKT with positive XM face significant risks, including reduced graft and patient survival. Unlike earlier beliefs that the liver allograft provides protective immunity to the kidney, current data suggest that the presence of preformed or de novo donor-specific antibodies can lead to adverse outcomes in the kidney graft, challenging the previously held assumptions about the liver's protective role. Therefore, while the liver may be less susceptible to hyperacute rejection, the implications of a positive XM in terms of kidney allograft success must be considered carefully.[281]

320. A 62-year-old man with end-stage liver disease and renal failure is scheduled for a combined liver-kidney transplant. The liver transplant is successfully completed; however, following reperfusion of the liver allograft, the patient becomes hemodynamically unstable, requiring high doses of two vasopressors while remaining coagulopathic and hypothermic. The kidney allograft awaits implantation on ice. What should the surgical team do next?
a) Proceed immediately with kidney implantation to restore renal perfusion while addressing abdominal hemostasis and bile duct reconstruction
b) Achieve hemostasis by controlling major surgical bleeding, pack the abdomen with temporary skin closure, and delay the kidney transplant until the patient is hemodynamically stable
c) Achieve hemostasis by controlling major surgical bleeding, pack the abdomen with temporary skin closure, and proceed with the kidney transplant
d) Achieve hemostasis by controlling major surgical bleeding, pack the abdomen with temporary skin closure, and cancel the kidney transplant, reallocating the kidney to another recipient
e) Initiate intraoperative dialysis while addressing hemostasis and bile duct reconstruction, then proceed with the kidney transplant
**Answer: b**
The patient's hemodynamic instability following liver reperfusion demands immediate stabilization before proceeding with the kidney transplant. Controlling significant surgical bleeding to achieve hemostasis is paramount, given the heightened risk of complications from coagulopathy post-liver reperfusion and arterial reconstruction. A damage control strategy is optimal: control bleeding, pack the abdomen with temporary closure, and transfer the patient to the ICU for resuscitation and warming. If hemodynamic stability is restored within 24 hours, the patient may proceed with kidney transplantation. This approach prioritizes patient safety, minimizing risks associated with simultaneous transplantation in a compromised state and ensuring a stable environment for subsequent procedures.[282]

321. A 64-year-old man with a history of alcohol-related liver cirrhosis and hepatorenal syndrome underwent successful liver transplantation. Four months later,

despite stable liver function, he remains dependent on hemodialysis due to persistent renal failure. Which of the following statements is most accurate?
a) Continue hemodialysis while monitoring renal function for potential spontaneous recovery
b) Renal failure contributes to approximately 10% of mortality in patients surviving beyond five years post-liver transplant
c) Enroll the patient in the Kidney Allocation for Liver Transplant program to facilitate placement on the kidney transplant waitlist
d) Kidney transplantation after liver transplant is less invasive, but survival is lower compared to liver transplant recipients without renal failure
e) Given the nephrotoxicity of tacrolimus, initiate withdrawal of immunosuppressive therapy to promote renal recovery

**Answer: c**

The patient's persistent renal failure following liver transplantation, likely due to hepatorenal syndrome and possibly exacerbated by calcineurin inhibitor nephrotoxicity, necessitates a strategic approach. With stable liver function but ongoing dependence on hemodialysis, enrolling in the Kidney Allocation for Liver Transplant (KALT) program is the most appropriate course. KALT facilitates access to kidney transplantation for patients with ESRD post-liver transplant, preserving liver function while improving overall health outcomes. Renal failure significantly impacts long-term survival, contributing to nearly 40% of deaths in patients surviving beyond five years post-liver transplant, either as a primary (9%) or secondary (30%) cause. KALT offers a lower-morbidity procedure, increased kidney availability (when not allocated for combined liver-kidney transplantation), and survival rates comparable to those of liver transplant recipients without renal impairment. While kidney transplantation may be less invasive, the survival outcomes for patients who receive a kidney transplant after liver transplant through programs like KALT can be comparable to those of liver transplant recipients without renal failure, especially when managed appropriately.[283]

322. The most common causes of early graft loss (within 7 to 30 days after primary transplant) requiring retransplantation are hepatic arterial thrombosis and primary nonfunction (PNF). PNF has been reported to serve as an indication for retransplantation in up to 30% of cases. The cause is often multifactorial and includes both donor and recipient factors. Significant donor factors include all of the following, except:
a) Degree of steatosis in the donor allograft
b) Increased cold ischemic time (>12 hours)
c) Reduced-size allograft
d) Older donor age (>50 years old)

e) Female donor gender
**Answer: e**
Even though females generally have smaller livers and reduced-size allografts are associated with PNF, the female gender by itself is not associated with PNF. Key recipient risk factors encompass deteriorating medical conditions, renal insufficiency, and the need for retransplantation. Moreover, extended warm ischemic time has been identified as a crucial perioperative risk factor for PNF. The interplay of these factors can lead to cumulative effects, resulting in notably poor outcomes.[284]

323. A 58-year-old man with a MELD score of 12, listed for liver transplantation due to HCC, is advised to consider a marginal donor liver if one becomes available. Which statement about marginal liver transplantation is most accurate?
a) Marginal livers should be prioritized for critically ill patients at higher risk of death while awaiting a standard donor liver
b) Accepting a marginal liver typically yields a worse prognosis than remaining on the waitlist for a standard donor liver
c) The use of marginal livers has significantly increased the incidence of primary nonfunction among transplant recipients
d) Recipients of marginal donor livers generally face longer wait times for retransplantation compared to those receiving standard donor livers
e) Marginal livers are preferentially allocated to fulminant liver failure patients to minimize organ discard
**Answer: c**
For this patient, a marginal liver transplant presents both opportunity and risk. Marginal livers, increasingly utilized to expand the donor pool, are associated with a higher incidence of primary nonfunction, particularly as their use has grown among healthier recipients or those with underreported risks. While marginal grafts may benefit non-critically ill patients, such as those with HCC at risk of tumor progression beyond transplant criteria or those whose MELD score underestimates mortality risk, their elevated risk of graft failure discourages use in high-risk candidates. By attempting transplantation with marginal livers, the organ pool is expanded, as failing grafts would otherwise be discarded, though this comes with an increased likelihood of retransplantation.[285]

324. A 47-year-old female patient with a history of liver cirrhosis secondary to hepatitis C virus infection receives a liver transplant. Unfortunately, she develops recurrent episodes of rejection and requires retransplantation after six months. Preoperatively, she is found to need mechanical ventilation and has a serum creatinine level of 2.5 mg/dL. During the procedure, she requires multiple units of blood

products. All of the following are significant independent risk factors predictive of poor survival after her retransplantation, except:
a) Age older than 40 years
b) Renal insufficiency
c) Requirement for mechanical ventilation
d) Use of intraoperative blood products
e) Preoperative ICU status

**Answer: a**

In this context, age older than 40 years is not an independent risk factor predictive of poor survival after retransplantation. Previous studies have identified age greater than 50 years as a significant risk factor. Other factors listed, such as renal insufficiency, mechanical ventilation requirement, the use of intraoperative blood products, and preoperative ICU status, are all associated with worse outcomes.[286]

325. What is the normal resistive index (RI) in the hepatic artery following early liver transplantation, and how is it calculated?
a) 1.0 to 1.2, calculated as the peak systolic velocity minus the end diastolic velocity, divided by the peak systolic velocity
b) 0.7 to 0.9, calculated as the peak systolic velocity minus the end diastolic velocity, divided by the peak systolic velocity
c) 0.5 to 0.7, calculated as the peak systolic velocity minus the end diastolic velocity, divided by the peak systolic velocity
d) 0.7 to 0.9, calculates as the peak systolic velocity divided by the end diastolic velocity
e) 0.5 to 0.7, calculated as the peak systolic velocity minus the end diastolic velocity, divided by the end diastolic velocity

**Answer: b**

The RI is calculated as the difference between the peak systolic (PS) velocity and the end diastolic (ED) velocity, divided by the peak systolic velocity (RI = [PS − ED] / PS). The normal RI in the hepatic artery early after liver transplantation is typically between 0.7 and 0.9. A low RI, along with increased flow velocities, may indicate hepatic artery stenosis.[287]

326. A 24-year-old woman with a BMI of 35 underwent emergent liver transplantation for fulminant hepatic failure due to acetaminophen overdose following a suicide attempt. The procedure was complicated by prolonged portal vein clamping, causing bowel edema. Moderate tension was noted during fascial closure. Postoperatively, in the ICU, her pressor requirements increased, peak airway pressure rose to 35 mmHg, and urinary output significantly decreased. How should she be managed?
a) Suspect increased intra-abdominal pressure; obtain an urgent CT scan

b) Suspect increased intra-abdominal pressure; perform an urgent laparotomy
c) Suspect increased intra-abdominal pressure; measure bladder pressure to confirm
d) Suspect primary nonfunction of the liver; relist for transplantation
e) Suspect intra-abdominal bleeding; transfuse red blood cells and obtain an urgent CT angiogram

**Answer: b**

The patient's symptoms—rising pressor needs, elevated peak airway pressure, and reduced urinary output—suggest abdominal compartment syndrome, a surgical emergency following liver transplantation. Contributing factors include prolonged portal vein clamping causing bowel edema and tension during fascial closure. Urgent laparotomy is required to relieve intra-abdominal pressure, as delays for diagnostic measures like bladder pressure measurement or imaging could worsen outcomes.[288]

327. A 34-year-old man with fulminant hepatic failure due to acute liver decompensation from Wilson's disease presents with worsening hemodynamic instability, refractory metabolic acidosis, elevated lactate levels, and an increasing base deficit. He is intubated, on hemodialysis, and listed for liver transplantation. A CT scan confirms a patent hepatic artery and portal vein but reveals extensive liver necrosis. A suitable liver donor has been identified, with transplantation feasible within 24 hours. The patient's wife requests all possible measures to save his life. What is the most appropriate immediate management step to stabilize his condition and optimize his transplant candidacy?
a) Accept the liver offer and perform an emergent total hepatectomy to remove the necrotic liver
b) Decline the liver offer and focus on medical stabilization with vasopressors and bicarbonate infusion
c) Accept the liver offer but delay hepatectomy until the transplant, monitoring metabolic status
d) Decline the liver offer and initiate molecular adsorbent recirculating system therapy to manage acidosis
e) Accept the liver offer and pursue veno-venous extracorporeal membrane oxygenation to support hemodynamics.

**Answer: a**

The patient's critical condition, driven by extensive liver necrosis, necessitates immediate action to address the source of refractory metabolic acidosis and systemic toxicity. Accepting the liver offer and performing an emergent total hepatectomy removes the necrotic liver, potentially stabilizing hemodynamics and metabolic status, thus optimizing the patient for the imminent transplantation.[289]

328. A 20-year-old man with end-stage liver disease due to biliary atresia, diagnosed shortly after birth, presents for liver transplantation evaluation. He underwent a Kasai procedure at 1 month of age but has progressed to transplant candidacy. He has situs inversus, with his heart on the right side and visceral organs laterally inverted. His medical history includes recurrent respiratory infections but no known cardiac dysfunction. Imaging reveals significant portal vein anomalies. Which statement regarding his management and surgical considerations is most accurate?
a) Due to high mortality from vascular anomalies in situs inversus, the patient's transplant candidacy is limited, and surgical options are restricted
b) Donor selection should prioritize a graft matching the native liver's dimensions to ensure optimal spatial fit and compatibility
c) A combined heart-liver transplant evaluation is warranted, as situs inversus increases the risk of cardiac anomalies, potentially improving outcomes with co-transplantation
d) Orthotopic allograft positioning is essential for success, but suprahepatic venous outflow location may compromise outcomes
e) Portal vein reconstruction, guided by the size and location of the native portal vein, is a critical consideration in heterotaxy patients undergoing liver transplantation.
**Answer: e**
Liver transplantation in patients with situs inversus, as pioneered by Lilly and Starzl in 1974, is now feasible with careful surgical planning. The primary challenge in heterotaxy, such as situs inversus, lies in portal vein reconstruction due to vascular anomalies that can impair graft perfusion. Meticulous evaluation of the native portal vein's size and location is essential to guide effective reconstruction, often requiring vascular conduits. Donor selection should favor smaller or segmental grafts to enhance placement flexibility, not grafts matching the native liver's size. Orthotopic positioning is often achievable, and suprahepatic venous outflow location does not typically compromise outcomes. Situs inversus does not inherently limit candidacy or correlate with high mortality, and while cardiac evaluation is necessary, combined heart-liver transplantation is unwarranted without cardiac dysfunction.[290]

329. An 18-year-old male presents to the emergency department after an intentional overdose of acetaminophen in a suicide attempt. Following comprehensive treatment for acute liver failure, he has been stabilized but is now exhibiting signs of worsening hepatic encephalopathy and toxic liver syndrome. The patient is listed for a liver transplant as status 1A. Given his youth and a documented history of poor medical compliance, the transplant team is considering an auxiliary liver transplant (ALT) instead of a whole liver transplant. All of the following are considered contraindications for an auxiliary liver transplant, except:
a) Presence of significant hepatic encephalopathy, grade III or IV

b) Significant hemodynamic instability necessitating continuous high dose IV vasopressor support
c) Radiological evidence of significant necrosis throughout the majority of the native liver corresponding with toxic liver syndrome
d) Elevated intracranial pressure requiring monitoring and intervention
e) Previous history of non-compliance with medical instructions related to his care

**Answer: e**

ALT presents more technical challenges than a whole liver transplant, and careful consideration must be given to the patient's condition at the time of surgery. Patients experiencing hemodynamic instability or elevated intracranial pressure may not withstand the surgical procedure, making a whole liver transplantation a more suitable option. Those with hyperacute liver failure may experience toxic liver syndrome due to liver necrosis, and they can sometimes improve temporarily with hepatectomy or portocaval shunt. As a result, it may be necessary to remove most of the native liver to mitigate the systemic effects of the insults. Leaving a significant volume of necrotic liver in place can lead to ongoing issues such as cerebral edema and further hemodynamic instability after transplantation, which have frequently resulted in neurological injury. To minimize the risks of poor compliance and also reduce the long-term risks of immunosuppression associated with liver transplant, an ALT may be considered as an alternative.[291]

330. A 5-year-old boy with propionic acidemia is evaluated for auxiliary partial liver transplantation (APLT) from a living donor to manage his metabolic disorder. The transplantation team is planning an orthotopic approach, resecting a portion of the native liver to accommodate the graft. Which statement regarding the surgical considerations for this procedure is most accurate?
a) A heterotopic approach avoids resection of the native liver, simplifying the procedure and preserving native liver function
b) An orthotopic approach ensures lower venous outflow pressure in the graft, improving perfusion compared to a heterotopic graft
c) A heterotopic approach allows for easier accommodation of larger grafts without requiring native liver resection
d) An orthotopic approach increases venous outflow pressure when the patient is upright, risking graft congestion
e) A heterotopic approach provides better anatomical alignment for the graft, minimizing vascular complications

**Answer: b**

APLT for propionic acidemia involves placing a partial liver graft to supplement metabolic function while retaining the native liver. In the orthotopic approach, a segment of the native liver is resected to create space for the graft, minimizing compression of major venous vessels and ensuring optimal graft perfusion. This approach maintains lower venous outflow pressure (typically a 2 mm Hg gradient between liver sinusoids and hepatic veins), enhancing perfusion dynamics compared to heterotopic grafts, which are placed below the native liver and experience higher outflow pressure. Heterotopic APLT does not simplify the procedure and may complicate vascular connections, risking compression.[292]

331. A 22-year-old female with a history of acute liver failure secondary to intentional acetaminophen overdose underwent auxiliary partial orthotopic liver transplantation (ALT). Postoperatively, her recovery shows delayed normalization of coagulation parameters, and her serum transaminases remain elevated beyond expected levels. Despite her stable clinical condition and a modest increase in serum bilirubin, the transplant team becomes concerned about the possibility of acute rejection. Which of the following statements best describes a potential challenge in managing this patient's postoperative recovery?
a) Coagulopathy typically resolves more rapidly following ALT compared to whole-liver transplantation
b) The serum transaminase levels in ALT usually demonstrate a more rapid downward trajectory than in whole-liver transplantation
c) Mild unconjugated hyperbilirubinemia should not warrant further investigation unless accompanied by marked transaminase elevation
d) The diagnosis of acute rejection may be more difficult in ALT due to less pronounced transaminase elevation compared to whole-liver transplantation
e) The postoperative recovery of liver function after ALT is similar to recovery following whole-liver transplantation
**Answer: d**
In the context of ALT, the postoperative recovery trajectory for liver function may present unique challenges. Specifically, serum transaminases may not decrease as expected because of the involvement of the injured native liver, making it difficult to identify acute rejection. Compared to whole-liver transplantation, where transaminase levels provide clearer guidance on graft function, ALT patients may display only modest elevations in these enzymes. This complicates the diagnosis of acute rejection, and a liver biopsy may be needed for confirmation, particularly in patients with mild unconjugated hyperbilirubinemia, necessitating further investigation to exclude rejection in such scenarios.[293]

## 9. Medical Care of Transplant Recipents

332. A 28-year-old man with alcohol-related liver cirrhosis undergoes successful liver transplantation. Despite significant intraoperative coagulopathy, the procedure is otherwise uncomplicated. To manage hypovolemia and support recovery, he receives multiple blood products, including PRBC, platelets, FFP, cryoprecipitate, and albumin. Which blood product carries the highest risk of bacterial contamination?
a) PRBC
b) Platelets
c) FFP
d) Cryoprecipitate
e) Albumin
**Answer: b**
Platelets carry the highest risk of bacterial contamination among the listed products, with an estimated incidence of 1 in 1,000 to 1 in 2,500 units. This risk stems from skin flora introduced during collection and the room-temperature storage conditions that facilitate bacterial growth. Critically ill patients, such as transplant recipients in the ICU, are particularly susceptible to complications like infection or sepsis due to their immunocompromised state. In contrast, PRBC, FFP, and cryoprecipitate are stored at lower temperatures, and albumin undergoes rigorous sterilization, significantly reducing their contamination risk.[294]

333. A 62-year-old female is one day post-liver transplantation after a prolonged history of MASH. Her vital signs show a stable blood pressure and a heart rate, but laboratory tests indicate a drop in her hemoglobin level to 7.8 g/dL from 9.6 g/dL. What is the most appropriate management strategy to optimize splanchnic perfusion to the liver allograft in this patient?
a) Administer IV fluids aggressively to achieve normovolemia
b) Initiate PRBC transfusions to correct the hemoglobin drop
c) Start aggressive diuresis to prevent fluid overload in the setting of postoperative swelling
d) Administer vasodilators to improve systemic circulation and reduce splanchnic vasoconstriction
e) Monitor the patient closely and continue current management without transfusion of products
**Answer: b**
In the immediate post-liver transplantation period, maintaining adequate splanchnic perfusion is crucial for the health of the graft. The splanchnic vasculature is more

sensitive to decreases in blood volume compared to the systemic circulation. A relatively small drop in intravascular volume can lead to compromised perfusion of the liver. Although a normal person can tolerate a 25% to 30% decrease in blood volume without a change in systemic blood pressure or heart rate, splanchnic perfusion becomes compromised after only a 10% to 15% reduction in intravascular volume. In this scenario, although the patient's blood pressure is stable, the drop in hemoglobin suggests potential blood loss, which can inhibit adequate perfusion to the liver allograft. Administering PRBC transfusions will help restore hemoglobin levels, correct intravascular volume, and thus optimize splanchnic perfusion, supporting the functioning of the new liver.[295]

334. A 42-year-old woman, one day post-liver transplant for autoimmune hepatitis, is intubated in the ICU. She tolerated surgery well but is hypotensive (systolic BP 85 mmHg, MAP 60 mmHg) with elevated cardiac output and low systemic vascular resistance (SVR, 400 dynes-sec/cm$^5$). She has reduced urinary output, hemoglobin of 8.3 g/dL (previously 8.5 g/dL), mildly elevated creatinine, and serosanguineous drain output. What is the most appropriate next step in management?
a) Start vasopressors to maintain MAP above 65–70 mmHg
b) Transfuse 1 unit of PRBC and monitor hemoglobin every 4 hours
c) Administer two 500 mL boluses of 5% albumin, followed by 1.5 times maintenance IV fluids
d) Obtain a cardiac echocardiogram and initiate dobutamine for inotropic support
e) Restrict fluids and prepare for hemodialysis
Answer: a
Post-liver transplant, this patient exhibits a hyperdynamic state with hypotension, elevated cardiac output, and low SVR due to vasodilation. Her MAP of 60 mmHg compromises organ perfusion, particularly to the kidneys, contributing to reduced urinary output and rising creatinine. Initiating vasopressors, such as norepinephrine or vasopressin, is the priority to restore MAP above 65–70 mmHg, ensuring adequate perfusion to the graft and vital organs. While her hemoglobin is slightly low, transfusion is not urgent, as bleeding appears minimal. Fluid boluses risk graft congestion, and her hypotension is primarily vasogenic, not hypovolemic. Inotropic support is unnecessary with elevated cardiac output, and hemodialysis is premature without clear renal failure.[296]

335. A 64-year-old woman, one day post-liver transplant for MASH, is intubated in the ICU. She tolerated surgery well despite intraoperative bradycardia during reperfusion. She is now hypotensive with reduced cardiac output (CO) and elevated systemic vascular resistance (SVR, 1500 dynes-sec/cm$^5$). Fluid resuscitation has not improved her hemodynamics. She has decreased urinary output, hemoglobin of 8.4

g/dL (previously 8.7 g/dL), and increasing creatinine. What is the most appropriate next step in her management?
a) Initiate norepinephrine to improve blood pressure
b) Transfuse PRBC to restore intravascular volume
c) Start vasopressin with maintenance IV fluids and monitor closely
d) Obtain a cardiac echocardiogram and initiate dobutamine for inotropic support
e) Restrict fluids and prepare for hemodialysis

**Answer: d**

This patient's hypotension, coupled with low cardiac output and high SVR (1500 dynes-sec/cm$^5$), suggests cardiac dysfunction rather than hypovolemia, especially since fluid resuscitation was ineffective. Her intraoperative bradycardia raises concern for potential cardiac issues. Obtaining a cardiac echocardiogram is critical to evaluate for underlying dysfunction, and initiating inotropic support with dobutamine can enhance cardiac contractility and perfusion if confirmed.[296]

336. A liver transplant recipient is evaluated in the ICU for allograft function using clinical and laboratory parameters. Which of the following findings suggests potential allograft dysfunction?
a) Rising ALT and AST levels
b) Improving mentation and wakefulness
c) Increased insulin requirement
d) Fever
e) Persistent hypoglycemia

**Answer: e**

A functioning liver allograft typically demonstrates specific postoperative trends. ALT and AST levels often rise, peaking within 1–2 days before declining, reflecting transient ischemia-reperfusion injury. Improving mentation and normothermia indicate metabolic and synthetic recovery. Increased insulin requirements are common due to high-dose steroids and transient hyperglycemia. However, persistent hypoglycemia, resistant to treatment, suggests impaired glycogenolysis and gluconeogenesis, indicating potential allograft dysfunction and warranting urgent evaluation.[297]

337. A 61-year-old female with a history of MASH underwent a successful liver transplant. On the 9th postoperative day, she developed a fever of 39.8°C, and her serum transaminase levels rose dramatically, with AST exceeding 7000 U/L. An emergent ultrasound did not reveal hepatic arterial flow. What is the next step in management?
a) Immediately initiate high-dose corticosteroids for suspected acute graft rejection
b) Begin broad-spectrum IV antibiotics and consult for urgent retransplantation

c) Obtain an immediate CT angiogram to assess the hepatic artery
d) Immediately initiate anticoagulation therapy and repeat liver ultrasound in 6 hours
e) Immediately initiate anticoagulation and consult for urgent retransplantation
**Answer: c**
Hepatic artery thrombosis and stenosis can lead to significant increases in transaminase levels, such as AST exceeding 5000 U/L. While doppler ultrasound evaluates arterial flow, if it fails to identify hepatic arterial flow and the resistance index falls below 0.5, further investigation is crucial. An immediate CT angiogram or surgical exploration is necessary to confirm the status of the hepatic artery, as delays can result in irreversible ischemic damage to the liver and biliary tree. If thrombosis is confirmed and the graft is not salvageable, the patient may need to be urgently listed for retransplantation.[298]

338. A 62-year-old female with a history of MASH underwent a successful liver transplant and is currently recovering in the ICU. The patient tolerated transplant well, but the medical team struggles to wean her off the ventilator. After 48 hours, her respiratory parameters are as follows: respiratory rate of 22 breaths/min, tidal volume of 4 mL/kg, PaO2 at 85 mm Hg, minute ventilation of 8.8 L/min, maximal inspiratory force of -30 cm H2O, and satisfactory cough and gag reflex. Which of the following factors is most likely contributing to her inability to be extubated?
a) High respiratory rate exceeding 20 breaths/min
b) Insufficient tidal volume less than 5 mL/kg
c) PaO2 below 90 mm Hg
d) Minute ventilation less than 10 L/min
e) Maximal inspiratory force of -30 cm H2O,
**Answer: b**
Weaning from the ventilator in liver transplant recipients should parallel the protocols used in the general ICU patient. Parameters for successful ventilator weaning include respiratory rate less than 30 breaths/min; tidal volume greater than 5 mL/kg; PaO2 greater than 70 mm Hg; minute ventilation less than 10 L/min; fractional inspired oxygen concentration of less than 0.4; maximal inspiratory force of greater than −25 cm H2O; frequency/tidal volume ratio less than 100 breaths/min/L; satisfactory cough and gag reflex; and return of muscle tone.[299]

339. A 55-year-old man, post-liver transplant, is admitted to the ICU following a procedure complicated by significant blood loss and reperfusion syndrome. The liver allograft is functioning well, but he develops ARDS. He is mechanically ventilated using a low tidal volume strategy (6 mL/kg), higher respiratory rates, and PEEP set at 14 cm H2O. Which statement best reflects the impact of high PEEP in this clinical scenario?

a) PEEP above 10 cm H2O significantly reduces splanchnic perfusion and hepatic blood flow
b) PEEP below 10 cm H2O is required to preserve hepatic blood flow in liver transplant recipients
c) PEEP up to 15 cm H2O does not adversely affect hepatic vein outflow or portal blood flow in the allograft
d) High PEEP increases intra-abdominal pressure, risking hepatic venous congestion in the allograft
e) PEEP above 12 cm H2O impairs portal vein inflow, necessitating lower PEEP settings

**Answer: c**

In liver transplant recipients with ARDS, ventilatory strategies like low tidal volume and high PEEP (up to 15 cm H2O) are used to manage hypoxemia. Evidence suggests that PEEP levels up to 15 cm H2O do not significantly impair hepatic vein outflow or portal blood flow in the liver allograft, making it safe for use in this context.[300]

340. A 60-year-old male patient with a history of cirrhosis and pulmonary hypertension (PH) undergoes orthotopic liver transplantation. Post-operatively, he experiences worsening of his PH, characterized by elevated pulmonary arterial pressures and signs of hypoxemia. What is the most appropriate initial treatment strategy?
a) Continue mechanical ventilation but increase tidal volumes to improve oxygenation
b) Initiate IV epoprostenol and adjust according to vital signs
c) Transfuse PRBC in order to increase the oxygen-carrying capacity of the blood
d) Continue mechanical ventilation and initiate oral sildenafil
e) Employ high PEEP strategies to enhance lung recruitment and improve oxygenation

**Answer: b**

In this scenario, the patient is experiencing worsening of the PH following liver transplantation. The initial management of PH requires maintaining oxygen saturation above 90% while correcting contributing factors. IV epoprostenol is an effective pulmonary vasodilator and has been shown to reduce mortality. Epoprostenol is started at 2 ng/kg/min and increased by 2 ng/kg/min until the blood pressure falls significantly or the heart rate increases. The intravascular volume should be reduced using IV loop diuretics or dialysis, decreasing the central venous pressure to 0 to 5 mm Hg, because significant fluid overload can cause a rapid regression that can lead to patient death. Mechanical ventilation can both compromise venous return from the allograft and increase pulmonary vascular resistance through overdistension of alveoli. Ventilator strategies include using low lung volumes (6 mL/kg), lower plateau airway pressure, and reduced PEEP to prevent alveolar overdistension.[301]

341. A 55-year-old female patient with end-stage liver disease secondary to alcohol abuse undergoes orthotopic liver transplantation. Post-operatively, she experiences atrial fibrillation with a rapid ventricular response. The patient's heart rate ranges from 130 to 140 beats per minute, with a blood pressure of 86/48 mmHg, but she maintains her mentation. What is the most appropriate initial treatment strategy?
a) Administer metoprolol 5 mg IV intermittent doses for rate control
b) Initiate an IV esmolol infusion with rapid titration
c) Begin IV amiodarone with a loading dose of 150 mg IV, followed by a maintenance infusion, and convert to the oral form
d) Administer desynchronized electrical cardioversion
e) Start diuretics immediately to manage volume overload while avoiding any antiarrhythmic medications due to hepatotoxicity concerns

**Answer: c**

With a functioning liver allograft, conversion is best accomplished with IV amiodarone (150 mg IV loading dose followed by 1 mg/min IV for 6 hours and 0.5 mg/min IV for 18 hours). Despite debatable concerns of hepatotoxicity associated with amiodarone use, there are only rare case reports of possible hepatotoxicity with IV amiodarone, and only one report of possible hepatotoxicity in a liver transplant allograft.[302]

342. A 42-year-old male with chronic liver disease, awaiting liver transplant, presents to the emergency department with diffuse muscle weakness, cramps, and altered mental status. He has a history of significant ascites and edema, managed with spironolactone 50 mg daily and furosemide 100 mg daily. His edema improved, but he developed abdominal pain and has been unable to tolerate oral intake for 3 days, though he remained compliant with his medications. On exam, he has sinus tachycardia, blood pressure of 92/68 mmHg, and appears dehydrated. Labs are significant for serum sodium of 155 mmol/L. His weight is 70 kg. What is the patient's total body water deficit?
a) 2.2 L
b) 4.5 L
c) 6 L
d) 9 L
e) 12 L

**Answer: b**

This patient has acute hypernatremia (Na 155 mmol/L) due to free water loss from excessive diuresis (furosemide and spironolactone) and inadequate intake for less than 48 hours. His symptoms—muscle weakness, cramps, and altered mental status—are

consistent with hypernatremia, and dehydration is evident from tachycardia and hypotension. The formula for free water deficit is:
Water Deficit = TBW × [(Na_current / Na_normal) - 1].
TBW = 0.6 × 70 kg = 42 L.
Na_current = 155 mmol/L, Na_normal = 140 mmol/L.
Water Deficit = 42 × [(155 / 140) - 1] = 42 × 0.107 ≈ 4.5 L.[303]

343. A 53-year-old Hispanic female, listed for liver transplant, presents to the emergency department with generalized weakness. She has significant ascites managed with spironolactone, furosemide, and occasional paracentesis. She couldn't refill her furosemide prescription and instead doubled her spironolactone dose for the past weeks. Blood work shows K 5.9 mmol/L. Which medication can eliminate potassium from the body?
a) Calcium gluconate
b) Insulin
c) Nebulized albuterol
d) IV metoprolol
e) Furosemide
**Answer: e**
This patient has hyperkalemia (K 5.9 mmol/L) from doubling spironolactone, a potassium-sparing diuretic, while stopping furosemide. Calcium gluconate stabilizes cardiac membranes but doesn't remove potassium. Insulin (with dextrose) and nebulized albuterol shift potassium into cells, lowering serum levels by ~1 mmol/L within 2 hours, but don't eliminate it. Furosemide, a loop diuretic, removes potassium via urine.[304]

344. A 38-year-old female, 7 days post-liver transplant for autoimmune hepatitis, is in the ICU with persistent anemia (Hb 7.8 g/dL), thrombocytopenia (platelets 18,000/μL), and elevated serum creatinine (2.8 mg/dL, baseline 1.0 mg/dL). She is on tacrolimus, a prednisone taper, and mycophenolate mofetil (MMF). Initial workup shows schistocytes on peripheral smear, attributed to intraoperative transfusions. Her AST and ALT have normalized, but LDH is persistently elevated and haptoglobin is <1 mg/dL. Which is the most appropriate next step in management?
a) Continue tacrolimus and MMF at current dose but repeat stress-dose steroids
b) Discontinue tacrolimus and initiate plasmapheresis
c) Administer eculizumab 900 mg IV immediately
d) Transfuse 2 units of platelets and continue to monitor
e) Consider splenic artery embolization or splenectomy
**Answer: b**

This patient has hemolytic uremic syndrome (HUS), likely triggered by tacrolimus, a known cause in posttransplant patients. The triad of anemia, thrombocytopenia, and elevated creatinine, plus high LDH and low haptoglobin, confirms HUS despite schistocytes being nonspecific here. Standard treatment is discontinuing the calcineurin inhibitor (CNI) and starting plasmapheresis until LDH and haptoglobin normalize. Eculizumab is a first-line option for atypical HUS, but its use in CNI-associated HUS is supported only by case reports, not yet standard. Platelet transfusion is unnecessary and may worsen microangiopathy. Splenic intervention is irrelevant to HUS.[305]

345. A 55-year-old male, 4 days post-liver transplant for hepatitis C cirrhosis, is in the ICU on tacrolimus, prednisone, and mycophenolate mofetil. His tacrolimus dose was increased yesterday due to subtherapeutic levels. Today, he develops acute confusion, slurred speech, and a generalized tonic-clonic seizure. His blood pressure is 160/95 mmHg, and tacrolimus level is 18 ng/mL. Brain MRI reveals T2 hyperintensities in the subcortical white matter of the occipital and parietal lobes. What is the most appropriate next step in management?
a) Administer IV lorazepam 2 mg and aspirin for ischemic stroke
b) Switch tacrolimus to cyclosporine and repeat head CT in 12 hours
c) Reduce tacrolimus dose and start IV levetiracetam
d) Administer IV lorazepam 2 mg, discontinue tacrolimus, initiate antihypertensive therapy, and perform EEG
e) Order EEG, administer IV lorazepam 2 mg, and give aspirin for ischemic stroke
**Answer: d**
This patient has posterior reversible encephalopathy syndrome (PRES), likely due to tacrolimus neurotoxicity, common in early post-transplant patients with elevated calcineurin inhibitor levels and compromised blood-brain barriers. Acute confusion, slurred speech, seizures, and MRI findings of T2 hyperintensities in the occipital and parietal subcortical white matter confirm PRES, not ischemic stroke. Management involves discontinuing tacrolimus to eliminate the neurotoxic trigger, administering IV lorazepam to control seizures, initiating antihypertensive therapy to reduce vasogenic edema, and performing an EEG to assess seizure activity.[306]

346. A 62-year-old female, 10 days post-liver transplant for MASH, develops two witnessed generalized tonic-clonic seizures. The first seizure resolved spontaneously after 3 minutes, but the second, occurring 2 hours later, persists for 6 minutes. After controlling the active seizure with IV lorazepam 4 mg, what is the most appropriate antiepileptic drug?
a) Phenytoin 15 mg/kg IV loading dose, then 100 mg orally three times daily for 3 months

b) Valproic acid 20 mg/kg IV loading dose, then 500 mg orally twice daily for 3 months
c) Levetiracetam 2 g IV loading dose over 60 minutes, then 1 g orally twice daily for 3 months
d) Carbamazepine 200 mg IV loading dose, then 200 mg orally twice daily for 3 months
e) Lorazepam 2 mg IV every 5 minutes as needed, then 1 mg orally as needed for 12 months

**Answer: c**

This post-liver transplant patient has seizures, with the second episode exceeding 5 minutes, suggesting evolving status epilepticus. After lorazepam controls the active seizure, an antiepileptic is needed for acute IV initiation and long-term oral use. Levetiracetam is ideal in transplant recipients due to its broad efficacy, minimal hepatic metabolism, and lack of interaction with immunosuppressants like tacrolimus, with seamless IV-to-oral transition. Phenytoin and carbamazepine induce cytochrome P-450, reducing immunosuppressant levels. Valproic acid is hepatically metabolized and hepatotoxic, risking graft injury. Lorazepam is for acute control, not suitable for long-term oral therapy.[307]

347. A 58-year-old male, 8 days post-liver transplant for alcohol-related cirrhosis, presents with lethargy and mild confusion. His history includes severe hepatic encephalopathy before transplant. The transplant used an extended criteria donor, with delayed graft function but slowly improving LFT. Blood work shows creatinine 3.5 mg/dL (baseline 0.9 mg/dL), BUN 98 mg/dL, and ammonia 28 μmol/L. What is the most likely cause of his persistent encephalopathy?
a) Recurrent hepatic encephalopathy from delayed graft function
b) Uremic encephalopathy from acute kidney injury
c) Unrecognized stroke due to coagulopathy before transplant
d) Undiagnosed dementia obscured by pre-transplant hepatic encephalopathy
e) Tacrolimus-induced posterior reversible encephalopathy syndrome (PRES)

**Answer: b**

This patient, 8 days post-liver transplant with improving graft function and pre-transplant hepatic encephalopathy, presents with lethargy and mild confusion. Uremic encephalopathy from acute kidney injury (creatinine 3.5 mg/dL, BUN 98 mg/dL) is the most likely cause. Uremic encephalopathy, associated with renal failure, causes symptoms ranging from mild confusion to coma, likely due to neurotransmitter imbalances, toxins, and blood-brain barrier injury. Recurrent hepatic encephalopathy is unlikely with normalizing liver function and near-normal ammonia (28 μmol/L). Stroke is improbable without focal neurologic signs or coagulopathy evidence. Dementia is chronic and unlikely to present acutely post-transplant. Tacrolimus-induced PRES typically involves seizures and characteristic MRI findings, absent here.[308]

348. A 22-month-old male underwent liver transplantation for biliary atresia. The procedure was uneventful, with intraoperative transfusions of 340 mL PRBCs and 220 mL FFP. In the pediatric ICU, initial blood work at 2:00 PM shows a prothrombin time (PT) of 14 seconds and INR of 2.1. Repeat blood work 12 hours later reveals PT 22 seconds, INR 2.4, AST 360 U/L, ALT 255 U/L, and total bilirubin 4.8 mg/dL. What is the most likely cause of the prolonged PT and INR 12 hours post-transplant?
a) Inadequate intraoperative clotting factor replacement
b) Delayed graft function impairing clotting factor synthesis
c) Dilutional coagulopathy from excessive PRBCs transfusion
d) Ongoing bleeding consuming coagulation factors
e) Reduced potency of transfused FFP due to expiration
**Answer: b**
The prolonged PT and INR 12 hours post-liver transplant, accompanied by elevated bilirubin, suggest delayed graft function impairing synthesis of clotting factors, particularly factor VII, which has a short half-life of 4–6 hours. Intraoperative FFP, administered over 12 hours ago, would no longer significantly contribute to factor VII levels. The initial PT and INR reflect intraoperative support, but the worsening coagulopathy indicates inadequate graft production of clotting factors.[309]

349. A 3-year-old female, 12 hours post-liver transplant for biliary atresia, is in the pediatric ICU. Intraoperative transfusions included 250 cc of PRBCs and 150 cc of FFP. Her initial postoperative hematocrit is 24%, platelet count is 25,000/mm3, and INR 2.1. The abdominal drain output increases to 50 cc/hour of mostly serous fluid in the next 4 hours, with a drain hematocrit of 3%. She remains hemodynamically stable with no overt bleeding. What is the most appropriate next step in management?
a) Transfuse 100 cc of PRBCs to raise hematocrit to 30%
b) Transfuse 10 cc/kg of platelets to increase platelet count above 30,000/mm3
c) Administer 50 cc of FFP to bring INR below 2
d) Proceed to surgical reexploration for suspected intra-abdominal bleeding
e) Continue observation and regular hemoglobin check
**Answer: e**
This 3-year-old, 12 hours post-liver transplant, has a hematocrit of 24%, within the target range of 20-30% to ensure oxygen delivery while minimizing hepatic artery thrombosis risk. The drain output of 50 cc/hour is mostly serous (hematocrit 3%), indicating no significant bleeding, and her stability supports this. Platelet count (25,000/mm3) exceeds 20,000/mm3, so transfusion isn't warranted without active bleeding. In an effort to decrease the incidence of hepatic artery thrombosis,

postoperative care should include no correction of coagulopathy in the absence of clinical bleeding and an INR of less than 2.5, FFP administration should be avoided.[310]

350. A 35-year-old male, 3 weeks post-liver transplant for hepatitis C cirrhosis, presents with new-onset, unrelenting, throbbing, unilateral headaches worsening over 5 days. He is on tacrolimus (level 12 ng/mL), prednisone, and mycophenolate mofetil. He denies fever, confusion, seizures, or neck stiffness, and his blood pressure is 130/85 mmHg. Blood work shows a white blood cell (WBC) count of $6.5 \times 10^9$/L. Acetaminophen provides no relief. What is the most appropriate next step in management?
a) Perform lumbar puncture and consult neurology
b) Reduce tacrolimus dose and monitor levels closely
c) Administer sumatriptan 50 mg orally as needed
d) Order head CT to rule out cerebrovascular event
e) Switch tacrolimus to cyclosporine

**Answer: b**

This patient's throbbing, unilateral headaches, 3 weeks post-liver transplant, suggest tacrolimus neurotoxicity, a common side effect even at therapeutic levels (12 ng/mL). Reducing the tacrolimus dose is the most appropriate initial step to alleviate symptoms while maintaining graft protection. The normal WBC count and absence of fever, neck stiffness, or confusion make meningitis unlikely, deferring the need for lumbar puncture. If headaches persist despite dose reduction, a head CT is warranted, followed by lumbar puncture and neurology consultation if imaging is negative.[311]

351. A 28-year-old female, 9 months post-liver transplant for fulminant hepatic failure secondary to mushroom toxicity, presents to the clinic for preconception counseling. She is on tacrolimus (level 8 ng/mL), prednisone 5 mg daily, and mycophenolate mofetil 750 mg twice per day. Her graft function is stable, with AST 25 U/L, ALT 30 U/L, and bilirubin 0.8 mg/dL. She has had no rejection episodes, and her blood pressure is 120/78 mmHg. What is the most appropriate recommendation regarding the timing of pregnancy?
a) Proceed with pregnancy planning immediately
b) Wait until at least 12 months post-transplant
c) Wait until at least 24 months post-transplant
d) Delay pregnancy until tacrolimus is discontinued for 6 weeks
e) Advise against pregnancy after solid organ transplant

**Answer: c**

This 28-year-old liver transplant recipient has stable graft function at 9 months, but guidelines recommend waiting 1-2 years post-transplant for pregnancy to ensure graft stability and minimize risks of rejection or complications. Studies suggest 24 months is optimal, especially with mycophenolate mofetil, which requires discontinuation 6 weeks prior due to teratogenicity, but timing alone doesn't address this here.[312]

352. A 21-month-old female undergoes liver transplantation for fulminant liver failure secondary to adenovirus. The donor is a 13-month-old pediatric patient who died from a brain injury. Of note, the donor had multiple traumas consistent with abuse and was severely malnourished. All of the following can be signs of primary nonfunction except:
a) Liver with poor color and firm texture at the time of reperfusion
b) Persistent hemodynamic instability
c) Persistent coagulopathy
d) Serum bilirubin rise after surgery
e) Failure to recover neurological function
**Answer: d**
This 21-month-old post-liver transplant patient is at risk for primary nonfunction, a rare but serious complication. Signs include poor liver color and firmness at reperfusion, hemodynamic instability, persistent coagulopathy, and failure to regain neurological function, all reflecting immediate graft failure. Serum bilirubin rise, however, is not a reliable indicator of primary nonfunction, as it can increase post-surgery due to volume shifts, hemolysis, or other issues like bile leak or sepsis, even with a functioning graft.[313]

353. A 4-year-old male, 8 days post-liver transplant for biliary atresia, presents with fever, lethargy, and jaundice. He is on tacrolimus (level 10 ng/mL), prednisone, and mycophenolate mofetil. Labs show ALT 150 U/L, AST 180 U/L, ALP 400 U/L, GGT 350 U/L, bilirubin 6.2 mg/dL, and WBC $14.5 \times 10^9$/L, all elevated after initial normalization. Liver ultrasound reveals heterogeneous echotexture, periportal edema, and patent hepatic artery. What is the most appropriate next step in management?
a) Order MRCP to assess biliary tree
b) Administer IV methylprednisolone 10 mg/kg daily for 3 days
c) Start broad-spectrum antibiotics and obtain blood cultures
d) Perform liver biopsy to diagnose acute rejection
e) Increase tacrolimus dose to target level 12–15 ng/mL
**Answer: c**
Ultrasound findings of heterogeneous echotexture and periportal edema are nonspecific but consistent with infection or inflammation. Starting broad-spectrum antibiotics and obtaining blood cultures is the most appropriate initial step to address potential sepsis. Given the elevated liver enzymes and bilirubin, a liver biopsy should

follow promptly to evaluate for acute rejection or other graft dysfunction once infection is stabilized, as these conditions may coexist.[314]

354. A 6-year-old female, 18 months post-liver transplant for biliary atresia, presents for routine follow-up. She was initially on tacrolimus, mycophenolate mofetil (MMF), and prednisone. Per protocol, prednisone was tapered off by 6 months, MMF discontinued by 12 months, and she is now on tacrolimus monotherapy (trough level 5 ng/mL). Labs show ALT 35 U/L, AST 40 U/L, and bilirubin 0.9 mg/dL. Her mother reports a recent upper respiratory infection treated with antibiotics. What is the most appropriate adjustment to her immunosuppression regimen at this visit?
a) Increase tacrolimus dose to target a trough level of 8-10 ng/mL
b) Restart MMF at half-dose to prevent late rejection
c) Restart prednisone 5 mg daily to prevent late rejection
d) Discontinue tacrolimus and start cyclosporine to preserve kidney function
e) Maintain current tacrolimus monotherapy and monitor levels
**Answer: e**
This 6-year-old, 18 months post-liver transplant, is on tacrolimus monotherapy, appropriate for long-term management after prednisone and MMF were tapered off per protocol. Normal ALT, AST, and bilirubin suggest stable graft function, and the resolved upper respiratory infection doesn't indicate rejection or need for adjustment. Pediatric protocols favor tacrolimus monotherapy after 12 months, with trough levels lowered over time. Higher tacrolimus troughs (8-10 ng/mL) are for early post-transplant, not now.[315]

355. A 16-year-old male, 5 years post-liver transplant for Wilson's disease, presents for follow-up as he prepares to transition to adult care. He is on tacrolimus monotherapy (trough level 2.7 ng/mL), with a history of inconsistent adherence reported by his parents. Blood work show ALT 80 U/L, AST 95 U/L, and bilirubin 1.8 mg/dL, up from previously normal values. He admits to missing doses due to school stress and reluctance to move to adult care. What is the most appropriate next step to address his nonadherence and graft dysfunction?
a) Increase tacrolimus dose to target a trough level of 8-10 ng/mL
b) Refer to a health care transition coordinator to facilitate the transition process, achieve self-management skills and promote independence in health care management
c) Delay transition till patient reaches 18 years of age
d) Add mycophenolate mofetil to enhance immunosuppression
e) Obtain liver biopsy to assess for acute rejection
**Answer: b**

Valeria Ripa, MD and Fady M. Kaldas, MD

This 16-year-old, 5 years post-liver transplant, exhibits graft dysfunction (elevated ALT, AST, bilirubin) and nonadherence, common in adolescents (17-53% prevalence), driven by school stress and transition reluctance. His tacrolimus level (2.7 ng/mL) is subtherapeutic due to missed doses. Referral to a health care transition coordinator addresses psychosocial barriers, enhances self-management, and supports adherence during this high-risk period, rather than delaying transition or escalating immunosuppression prematurely.[316]

356. A 42-year-old male, severely malnourished due to chronic liver disease, undergoes liver transplantation for alcohol-induced liver cirrhosis. Pre-transplant, he had a protein-poor diet and muscle wasting. Postoperatively, on day 3, he develops oliguria (urine output 0.4 mL/kg/hour) despite aggressive fluid resuscitation with normal saline. Labs show serum creatinine 0.7 mg/dL (baseline 0.5 mg/dL), estimated GFR 95 mL/min/1.73 m² (via Cockcroft-Gault), ALT 120 U/L, AST 150 U/L, and bilirubin 3.8 mg/dL. What is the most appropriate next step?
a) Rely on current estimated GFR as sufficient evidence of normal renal function
b) Patient most likely has urinary retention, initiate tamsulosin therapy
c) Obtain renal ultrasound to evaluate for post-renal obstruction
d) Perform cystatin C-based GFR estimation
e) GFR is the accurate estimate of kidney function, patient most likely developed retention, place a Foley catheter
**Answer: d**
This 42-year-old, malnourished post-liver transplant patient develops oliguria on day 3, suggesting possible acute kidney injury, but serum creatinine (0.7 mg/dL) and estimated GFR (95 mL/min/1.73 m²) via Cockcroft-Gault appear reassuring. In malnutrition and liver disease, low muscle mass, poor protein intake, and elevated bilirubin lower creatinine production, falsely elevating GFR estimates. Cystatin C-based GFR estimation is more accurate here, as it's less influenced by these factors. Flomax assumes retention without evidence; bladder ultrasound is preferred first. Foley placement monitors output, not function; bladder ultrasound should precede it.[317]

357. A 68-year-old male with a history of liver cirrhosis secondary to MASH underwent a successful liver transplant. His postoperative course was complicated by acute kidney injury requiring inpatient dialysis for one week, with subsequent recovery of kidney function. He presents for his first follow-up clinic visit reporting resolution of leg swelling and normal urine output. His current medications include furosemide 40 mg daily, tacrolimus 2.5 mg BID (trough level 10.8 ng/mL today), mycophenolate mofetil (MMF) 500 mg BID, and a prednisone taper. LFT are within normal limits, but his serum creatinine has increased to 2.4 mg/dL (from 1.7 mg/dL at hospital

discharge), and his potassium is 4.9 mEq/L. What is the most appropriate next step in management?
a) Obtain urinalysis and kidney ultrasound
b) Discontinue furosemide and decrease tacrolimus dose to target a trough of 6–8 ng/mL
c) Continue current medications, encourage free water intake, and schedule repeat blood work in one week
d) Switch tacrolimus to cyclosporine and initiate Lokelma to lower potassium
e) Discontinue tacrolimus, increase mycophenolate mofetil to 1000 mg BID, and continue prednisone taper

**Answer: b**

The rising creatinine (2.4 mg/dL) and mild hyperkalemia (4.9 mEq/L) suggest tacrolimus nephrotoxicity, exacerbated by a trough of 10.8 ng/mL. Reducing the tacrolimus dose to a 6–8 ng/mL trough minimizes renal toxicity in this older patient, who has a lower rejection risk. With resolved edema and normal urine output, furosemide is unnecessary and can be discontinued.[318]

358. A 55-year-old female with end-stage liver disease due to alcohol-related cirrhosis undergoes liver transplantation. Post-reperfusion, she develops persistent hypotension requiring increased norepinephrine, a base excess worsening from -8 to -15 mEq/L, and a core temperature drop to 34°C despite warming. Profuse coagulopathic bleeding prompts packing and temporary abdominal closure. In the ICU, 6 hours post-reperfusion, labs show INR 4.2 (unresponsive to FFP), AST 6700 U/L, ALT 4500 U/L, and lactate 8 mmol/L. What is the most appropriate next step in management?
a) Administer high-dose corticosteroids and monitor for 24 hours
b) Initiate bicarbonate drip and maximize supportive care
c) Urgently list for retransplantation and initiate CRRT
d) Perform urgent transplant hepatectomy and list for retransplantation
e) Transition to comfort care due to poor prognosis

**Answer: c**

This patient exhibits primary nonfunction (PNF) post-liver transplant, evidenced by hemodynamic instability, severe acidosis, hypothermia, refractory coagulopathy, and markedly elevated transaminases. Urgent listing for retransplantation is the most appropriate next step. PNF requires rapid retransplantation to replace the nonfunctional graft, as supportive measures alone are insufficient.[319]

359. A 55-year-old Asian male with cirrhosis due to hepatitis B undergoes deceased donor liver transplantation. The donor, a 56-year-old male, sustained a reversible cardiac arrest lasting 20 minutes before hospital arrival. Donor laboratory values

showed a peak AST of 1200 IU/L and ALT of 900 IU/L, which normalized by the time of brain death declaration, with a peak INR of 1.7 and a final INR of 1.2. What is the primary risk associated with using this donor liver?
a) Increased incidence of primary nonfunction in the recipient
b) Elevated 12-month mortality risk for the recipient
c) Higher peak liver transaminases in the recipient post-transplant
d) Prolonged ICU and hospital stay for the recipient
e) Greater likelihood of acute cellular rejection due to increased inflammation after reperfusion in the recipient

**Answer: c**

Studies show that brief and reversible cardiac arrest in organ donors does not affect overall allograft performance or patient survival. Donors with reversible cardiac arrest are associated with higher peak liver transaminases in the recipient post-transplant. There is no indication for transplant hepatectomy at this stage, as the patient's instability can still be managed with supportive care while awaiting a new graft. Hepatectomy is a rare, extreme measure reserved for cases where the graft itself drives uncontrollable systemic deterioration, which is not yet evident here.[320]

360. A 67-year-old male underwent a liver transplant for MASH complicated by HCC. Prior to the transplant, he received transarterial chemoembolization (TACE) and radiofrequency ablation of the tumor. The hepatectomy was complicated by adhesions and a stricture at the hilar plate, which was also short. The donor liver was a small graft weighing 900 grams with type 1 arterial anatomy. The transplant was performed using the bicaval technique. The biliary reconstruction was performed under some tension. On postoperative day 7, the patient developed an anastomotic bile leak. What is the most likely cause of the complication and how should the complication be managed?
a) Technical error of anastomosis performed under tension; convert choledocholedocostomy to choledocojejunostomy
b) Technical error of anastomosis performed under tension; perform ERCP with uncovered self-expandable metal stent
c) Technical error of anastomosis performed under tension; perform ERCP with partially covered self-expandable metal stent
d) Adhesions from previous TACE and radiofrequency ablation causing thinning of the bile duct wall; perform ERCP with fully covered self-expandable metal stent
e) Stricture at the hilar plate; perform ERCP and balloon dilation of the stricture followed by placement of fully covered self-expandable metal stent

**Answer: a**

The anastomotic bile leak likely resulted from a technical error due to the biliary reconstruction being performed under tension, which can impair healing. Converting the choledocholedocostomy to a choledocojejunostomy is the best approach as it relieves tension and promotes healing. Stent placement is not effective for this issue. The complication could be prevented by preserving as much length as possible of the recipient bile duct and ensuring adequate blood supply.[321]

361. A 45-year-old male patient with a history of HCC underwent orthotopic liver transplant. During the procedure, the donor liver was implanted, and the transected distal end of the cystic duct remnant was incorporated into the suture line of the biliary anastomosis to facilitate drainage. Six months post-transplant, the patient presents with right upper quadrant pain, fever, and elevated liver enzymes. Imaging reveals a dilated, fluid-filled structure adjacent to the biliary anastomosis. Which of the following best explains the underlying pathophysiology of this complication?
a) Hepatic artery pseudoaneurysm causing compression of the common bile duct
b) Delayed stricturing of the biliary anastomosis obstructing drainage from the cystic duct remnant
c) Bacterial overgrowth within the cystic duct remnant leading to inflammatory occlusion
d) Ischemic necrosis of the cystic duct remnant causing secondary fluid accumulation
e) Malignant transformation of the cystic duct epithelium resulting in obstructive mucin production
**Answer: b**
The development of a cystic duct remnant mucocele following liver transplantation is an uncommon complication, often linked to impaired drainage of the cystic duct. In this case, the distal end of the transected cystic duct was incorporated into the biliary anastomosis to ensure drainage, a standard surgical technique. However, delayed anastomotic stricturing can occur post-transplant due to fibrosis, inflammation, or technical factors, obstructing the outflow from the cystic duct remnant. This obstruction leads to the accumulation of mucus produced by the cystic duct epithelium, forming a mucocele.[322]

362. A 44-year-old woman with intrahepatic cholangiocarcinoma underwent chemoirradiation, followed by liver transplantation. During the procedure, a choledochocholedochostomy was performed, a donor bile duct noted to be longer than optimal. Six weeks post-transplant, she develops jaundice, pruritus, and elevated bilirubin levels. Tumor markers remain normal. MRCP reveals a tortuous, sharply angulated bile duct with proximal dilatation and narrowing at the angulation point. What is the most likely mechanism contributing to this biliary pathology?
a) Excessive donor bile duct length causing kinking and obstruction
b) Acute rejection leading to cholestatic liver injury
c) Ischemic bile duct injury from inadequate arterial supply

d) Allergic reaction to suture material causing fibrotic narrowing
e) Cholangiocarcinoma recurrence causing biliary obstruction
**Answer: a**
The MRCP findings of a tortuous, sharply angulated bile duct with proximal dilatation and distal narrowing indicate a mechanical obstruction due to an excessively long donor bile duct, resulting in kinking and impaired bile flow. The rapid onset at six weeks, normal tumor markers, and specific imaging findings make cholangiocarcinoma recurrence unlikely, as it typically presents later with distinct radiologic features. Ischemic injury from inadequate arterial supply usually causes diffuse biliary strictures or necrosis, not localized kinking.[321]

363. A 58-year-old man with liver cirrhosis secondary to alcohol abuse undergoes liver transplantation. The donor is a 67-year-old individual who suffered a fatal stroke, and the cold ischemia time (CIT) is 7 hours and 20 minutes. Which of the following is the correct statement regarding elderly liver allografts and biliary complications?
a) The short CIT mitigated the risk of biliary complications typically associated with older grafts
b) The donor's advanced age inherently increases the likelihood of biliary strictures
c) The donor's advanced age is associated with an increased risk arterial but not biliary complications
d) The use of ursodiol prevents biliary inflammation and stricture formation
e) The elderly donor liver has a larger bile duct size, reducing the risk of anastomotic strictures
**Answer: a**
Elderly donor livers ($\geq 65$ years) are traditionally associated with a higher risk of biliary complications, such as strictures and leakage, due to increased susceptibility to ischemic injury. However, a short CIT minimizes this risk by reducing the duration of ischemia, thereby preserving biliary epithelial integrity and preventing complications like non-anastomotic or anastomotic strictures.[323]

364. A 45-year-old woman with primary sclerosing cholangitis undergoes liver transplantation from a donor weighing 48 kg. She has a history of prior upper abdominal surgery. On postoperative day 18, she develops fever, elevated liver enzymes, and imaging suggestive of hepatic artery thrombosis (HAT), confirmed by angiography. Based on the available data, what is the most significant risk factor contributing to the development of early HAT in this patient?
a) Low donor weight
b) Recipient age above 40 years
c) History of upper abdominal surgery
d) Single arterial anastomosis during surgery

e) Primary sclerosing cholangitis
**Answer: a**
The most significant risk factor for early HAT in this patient is the low donor weight. Studies identify low donor weight as an independent risk factor for early HAT, defined as occurring within 21 days post-transplant, alongside prior HAT and multiple arterial anastomoses. The low weight likely contributes to smaller vessel caliber, increasing thrombosis risk.[324]

365. A 55-year-old man undergoes liver transplantation for cirrhosis secondary to MASH. His postoperative course is complicated by a bile leak requiring reoperation on day 7, with delayed biliary anastomosis. On day 12, he experiences hypotension and a hemoglobin drop from 10 g/dL to 7 g/dL. Cultures from an intraabdominal drain grow Escherichia coli. On day 18, he develops sudden massive gastrointestinal bleeding and is diagnosed with a hepatic artery pseudoaneurysm. What is the correct statement regarding hepatic artery pseudoaneurysm following liver transplant?
a) It is related to intraabdominal infection and managed with antibiotics
b) It has a low incidence with a high mortality rate of 25%
c) It is typically asymptomatic and diagnosed incidentally
d) Abdominal ultrasound is a fast and accurate imaging modality
e) Bile leak and intraabdominal infection increase the risk of its development
**Answer: e**
Hepatic artery pseudoaneurysm, a rare post-transplant complication (0.3-2.6% incidence) with a mortality rate approaching 75%, is linked to bile leaks and intraabdominal infections. These factors, present here with a bile leak and intraabdominal infection, weaken the arterial wall, increasing pseudoaneurysm risk.[325]

366. A 67-year-old woman with cirrhosis due to alcoholic liver disease undergoes liver transplantation from a 64-year-old donor. The total cold ischemia time is 6 hours and 25 minutes. The procedure involves a standard arterial anastomosis between the donor celiac trunk and the recipient common hepatic artery. Notably, both donor and recipient exhibit atheromatous disease in the aorta, celiac trunk, and hepatic arteries. On postoperative day 10, she develops elevated liver enzymes, and imaging confirms hepatic artery thrombosis (HAT). Based on the available data, what is the most significant factor contributing to the development of HAT in this patient?
a) Presence of atherosclerosis in the donor hepatic artery
b) Donor age above 60 years
c) Presence of atherosclerosis in the recipient vessels
d) Recipient age above 65 years
e) Prolonged cold ischemia time

**Answer: a**
The most significant factor contributing to HAT in this patient is atherosclerosis in the donor hepatic artery. Studies show that donor hepatic artery atherosclerosis is a strong, independent risk factor for HAT, likely due to plaque-related clot formation. Recipient hepatic artery atherosclerosis showed no significant effect.[326]

367. Trimethoprim-sulfamethoxazole (Bactrim) is commonly utilized after liver transplantation for Pneumocystis jirovecii pneumonia (PJP) prophylaxis. Based on current guidelines, in which of the following scenarios is atovaquone not indicated as a replacement for Bactrim post-liver transplant?
a) Neutropenia
b) Hyperkalemia
c) Pregnancy
d) Known hypersensitivity to trimethoprim, sulfamethoxazole, or a past sulfa allergy
e) Stable chronic kidney disease with no adverse effects

**Answer: e**
Bactrim is commonly used post-liver transplant for PJP prophylaxis but has contraindications necessitating alternatives like atovaquone. Atovaquone is indicated for neutropenia, as Bactrim can exacerbate bone marrow suppression; hyperkalemia, as trimethoprim can increase potassium levels; pregnancy, due to teratogenic risks; and known hypersensitivity or sulfa allergy, due to potential severe reactions.[327]

368. Which statement best identifies the highest-risk group and the peak timing for CMV infection in the context of liver transplantation?
a) CMV-seronegative recipients with CMV-seropositive donors; peak incidence at 5 weeks post-transplant
b) CMV-seronegative recipients with CMV-seronegative donors; peak incidence at 8 weeks post-transplant
c) CMV-seropositive recipients with CMV-seronegative donors; peak incidence at 2 weeks post-transplant
d) CMV-seropositive recipients with CMV-seropositive donors; peak incidence at 5 weeks post-transplant
e) CMV-seronegative recipients with CMV-seropositive donors; peak incidence at 7 days post-transplant

**Answer: a**
CMV-seronegative recipients receiving a liver from a CMV-seropositive donor (D+/R-) face the highest risk of primary CMV infection and symptomatic disease, as the donor liver transmits the virus, amplified by blood transfusions. Without prophylaxis, CMV infections typically occur between 3 and 8 weeks post-transplant, peaking at 5 weeks when immunosuppression is most intense.[327]

369. A 50-year-old woman undergoes liver transplantation for autoimmune liver disease. Pre-transplant, she is CMV-seronegative, and her donor is also CMV-seronegative (D-/R-). Post-transplant, she is started on valganciclovir for CMV prophylaxis per protocol, alongside tacrolimus and prednisone. On postoperative day 14, laboratory results reveal neutropenia with an absolute neutrophil count (ANC) of 600/mm³, she remains afebrile with no signs of infection. What is the most appropriate management step?
a) Continue valganciclovir and treat neutropenia with filgrastim
b) Switch valganciclovir to acyclovir and recheck CMV titer in 2 weeks
c) Hold valganciclovir and monitor CMV every 3 months
d) Increase valganciclovir dose to prevent CMV and hold prednisone
e) Hold valganciclovir and monitor CMV titer weekly
**Answer: e**
This patient is at low risk for CMV infection post-liver transplant, as neither donor nor recipient harbors latent virus. Valganciclovir, used for CMV prophylaxis, commonly causes neutropenia, as seen here (ANC < 800/mm³). In low-risk patients with this side effect, the best step is to hold valganciclovir to allow neutrophil recovery, and monitor CMV titer weekly to ensure no unexpected infection emerges.[328]

370. A 55-year-old man undergoes liver transplantation for cirrhosis due to alcohol abuse. He is CMV-seropositive, and his donor is CMV-seronegative (D-/R+). Post-transplant, he receives valganciclovir prophylaxis, tacrolimus, and mycophenolate mofetil (MMF) immunosuppression. On postoperative day 28, routine monitoring shows a serum CMV PCR increase from 200 copies/mL to 700 copies/mL over one week. His creatinine clearance is 45 mL/min, and he has no symptoms of CMV disease. What is the most appropriate next step in management?
a) Increase valganciclovir dose from 450 mg BID to 900 mg BID until one negative CMV PCR
b) Start IV ganciclovir 5 mg/kg BID for 2 weeks
c) Continue current therapy and monitor CMV PCR weekly
d) Add acyclovir 400 mg BID until one negative CMV PCR
e) Hold MMF and start IV ganciclovir 5 mg/kg BID for 2 weeks
**Answer: a**
This patient's rising CMV viremia (200 to 700 copies/mL over one week) indicates early CMV replication, warranting preemptive therapy despite the absence of symptoms. Guidelines recommend increasing valganciclovir to 900 mg twice daily (adjusted for creatinine clearance of 45 mL/min) until one negative CMV PCR

confirms viral clearance. This approach is effective (~85% efficacy) and appropriate for asymptomatic viremia.[327]

371. A 60-year-old male who underwent liver transplantation 2 weeks ago is being discharged home from the hospital. He resides in a rural area of southern Nevada. His immunosuppressive regimen includes tacrolimus, a steroid taper, and mycophenolate mofetil. Pretransplant serology showed no evidence of prior coccidioidomycosis exposure. What is the most appropriate management strategy for his antifungal prophylaxis at this time?
a) Continue fluconazole prophylaxis for 6 months posttransplant
b) Continue fluconazole prophylaxis as long as he resides in an endemic area, with regular monitoring for symptoms and serology
c) Continue fluconazole prophylaxis indefinitely
d) Continue fluconazole prophylaxis for 42 days posttransplant
e) Switch fluconazole to voriconazole prophylaxis to broaden antifungal coverage for 12 months

**Answer: b**

This asymptomatic liver transplant recipient resides in southern Nevada, an endemic region for Coccidioides species, which cause coccidioidomycosis. The provided data indicate that de novo coccidioidomycosis developed in 3% of liver transplant recipients posttransplant, with 66% of cases occurring within the first year, and recommend universal antifungal prophylaxis for 6-12 months in endemic areas. However, given the fact that this patient had no pretransplant exposure (negative serology), continuing prophylaxis is critical while he remains in the endemic area.[329]

372. A 45-year-old female underwent liver transplantation one year ago for primary sclerosing cholangitis complicated by ulcerative colitis. Her past medical history includes a subtotal colectomy with ileostomy 5 years prior to transplant. She is currently on tacrolimus and a low-dose prednisone. She presents for an elective ileostomy reversal. During surgery, multiple adhesions are encountered, leading to an aborted procedure, and inadvertent enterotomies and a gastrotomy are made, which are repaired intraoperatively. How should the patient be managed following this procedure?
a) Initiate fluconazole prophylaxis only if she develops signs of infection
b) Start fluconazole prophylaxis immediately and continue for at least 6 months
c) Administer a single dose of fluconazole intraoperatively, then discontinue antifungal therapy
d) In addition to 24-hour antibiotic coverage, start fluconazole therapy immediately in the operating room and continue for 1 to 2 weeks postoperatively
e) Continue antibiotic coverage for 24 hours following the surgery

**Answer: d**
This immunosuppressed liver transplant recipient faces an elevated fungal infection risk due to intraoperative gastrotomy. These breaches in mucosal integrity, combined with her ongoing immunosuppression, heighten the risk of fungal translocation, particularly Candida, common in posttransplant patients. Immediate fluconazole therapy in the operating room, alongside 24-hour antibiotic coverage for bacterial risk, is appropriate to prevent early postoperative infections.[330]

373. A 62-year-old male underwent liver transplantation 3 years ago for cryptogenic cirrhosis. He has been maintained on single-agent tacrolimus with stable graft function until 2 weeks ago, when he developed severe T cell-mediated rejection confirmed by biopsy. He was treated with antithymocyte globulin (ATG) and high-dose corticosteroids. How should his medication be managed to prevent secondary infections?
a) Initiate trimethoprim-sulfamethoxazole, fluconazole, and valganciclovir prophylaxis
b) Start valganciclovir and atovaquone prophylaxis for 6 months
c) Administer fluconazole prophylaxis for 1 month, with no other changes
d) Begin valganciclovir prophylaxis only if CMV PCR becomes positive
e) Continue current immunosuppression without additional prophylaxis

**Answer: a**
This liver transplant recipient received ATG for severe rejection, intensifying immunosuppression and raising the risk of opportunistic infections. Valganciclovir prevents CMV, trimethoprim-sulfamethoxazole covers PJP, and fluconazole targets fungal prophylaxis, all critical post-ATG.[331]

374. A 58-year-old male underwent liver transplantation 6 months ago for alcoholic cirrhosis. He has been stable on tacrolimus and low-dose prednisone but experienced early rejection 3 months posttransplant, treated with a short course of high-dose corticosteroids. He now presents with a 10-day history of fever, productive cough, and dyspnea. Chest imaging reveals multiple bilateral nodules and a cavitary lesion in the right upper lobe. Sputum culture confirms Nocardia asteroides. He has no neurological symptoms, and his absolute neutrophil count is normal. What is the most appropriate management?
a) Start trimethoprim-sulfamethoxazole monotherapy
b) Initiate ceftriaxone and azithromycin
c) Begin levofloxacin monotherapy
d) Start amoxicillin-clavulanate and doxycycline
e) Administer meropenem and vancomycin

**Answer: a**

This liver transplant recipient with Nocardia asteroides pneumonia requires targeted antibiotic therapy. The data indicate Nocardia infections occur in 3.7% of liver transplant patients, often presenting as pneumonia, with risk factors including early rejection and enhanced immunosuppression—both present here. Trimethoprim-sulfamethoxazole is the first-line treatment for Nocardia due to its efficacy against most species and ability to cover potential dissemination (e.g., brain, skin), despite no current extrapulmonary symptoms.[332]

375. A 55-year-old female underwent liver transplantation 8 weeks ago for hepatitis C-related cirrhosis. She is on tacrolimus, mycophenolate mofetil, and prednisone. She presents with a 5-day history of nonproductive cough, myalgia, confusion, and watery diarrhea. Vital signs show a temperature of 39.2°C, pulse of 70 bpm, and blood pressure of 110/70 mmHg. Laboratory results reveal sodium of 128 mEq/L, AST of 150 U/L, and ALT of 180 U/L. Chest X-ray demonstrates a left lower lobe consolidation with a small pleural effusion. She is staying with her sister in an old house with an outdated water system prone to contamination. What is the most likely pathogen?
a) Pneumocystis jirovecii
b) Nocardia asteroides
c) Legionella pneumophila
d) Streptococcus pneumoniae
e) Aspergillus fumigatus
**Answer: c**
This liver transplant recipient shows classic Legionella pneumonia signs: nonproductive cough, temperature-pulse dissociation, elevated liver enzymes, diarrhea, hyponatremia, myalgia, confusion, and consolidation with effusion on X-ray. The clue of an old house with an outdated water system suggests contamination, a typical Legionella source, thriving in stagnant or warm water.[333]

376. A 60-year-old male, 14 months post-liver transplantation for MASH, has been stable on tacrolimus and low-dose prednisone without recent rejection episodes. He presents with a 3-day history of fever, headache, and confusion. Vital signs show a temperature of 38.8°C, heart rate of 90 bpm, and normal blood pressure. Neurological examination reveals neck stiffness and disorientation. Labs show a white blood cell count of $10.5 \times 10^3/\mu L$ with a left shift. CSF culture confirms Listeria monocytogenes. What behavior most likely contributed to his Listeria infection?
a) Consuming pasteurized cheese
b) Consuming smoked salmon
c) Handling raw poultry without gloves
d) Eating well-done steaks

e) Swimming in a local lake
**Answer: b**
Smoked salmon, often consumed without further cooking, is a common vehicle for Listeria, unlike pasteurized cheese, which is heat-treated to eliminate pathogens. Handling raw poultry is more associated with Salmonella or Campylobacter, not Listeria. Well-done steaks, thoroughly cooked, pose minimal risk. Swimming in a lake is unlikely to cause Listeria infection, which is primarily foodborne.[334]

377. A 52-year-old male underwent liver transplantation 2 years ago for MASH. He has been maintained on tacrolimus and mycophenolate mofetil with stable graft function. He presents for routine follow-up, asymptomatic, with recent labs showing mildly elevated AST (60 U/L) and ALT (80 U/L). His BMI is 32 kg/m², and he has poorly controlled type 2 diabetes mellitus. A protocol ultrasound reveals moderate hepatic steatosis (>30% parenchymal involvement), without masses or ascites. Which statement is most accurate regarding his condition?
a) Recurrent MASH occurs in less than 10% of liver transplant recipients
b) Liver biopsy remains the gold standard for diagnosing recurrent MASH after liver transplantation
c) Pre-transplant hyperlipidemia is a strong predictor of increased risk for post-transplant NAFLD (non-alcoholic fatty liver disease)
d) Recurrent MASH post-liver transplantation progresses to fibrosis more rapidly than pre-transplant MASH
e) Post-transplant MASH is associated with a significantly elevated risk of graft loss at 10 years
**Answer: b**
Studies indicate a 100% recurrence rate of NAFLD within 5 years in protocol biopsies. Liver biopsy remains the gold standard for confirming MASH recurrence. Pre-transplant hyperlipidemia is not associated with an increased risk of post-transplant NAFLD, despite its known association with NAFLD. Despite recurrent steatosis and inflammation after liver transplantation, the risk of progression to advanced fibrosis (≥F3 stage) or cirrhosis is overall low. Post-liver transplantation MASH, whether recurrent or de novo, is not associated with decreased survival or graft loss across retrospective studies with up to 15 years of follow-up data.[335]

378. A 38-year-old female, who underwent liver transplantation 3 years ago for autoimmune hepatitis (AIH), presents with fatigue and jaundice. She has been maintained on tacrolimus and mycophenolate mofetil, with steroids tapered 18 months ago due to stable graft function. Labs show AST 120 U/L, ALT 150 U/L, and IgG 2000 mg/dL. Liver biopsy confirms recurrent AIH with moderate inflammation and interface hepatitis. Which statement is true?

a) Premature withdrawal of corticosteroids caused recurrence of AIH
b) The rate of AIH recurrence is high, close to 70% within the first 3 years
c) Risk factors for recurrence include high preoperative aminotransferase and IgG levels
d) Episodes of late rejection (>6 months after transplant) are not associated with recurrence rate
e) Although AIH is more common in females, recurrence is more common in males

**Answer: c**

Risk factors for AIH recurrence post-transplant include high preoperative aminotransferase and IgG levels. The median time to recurrence is 2 years, with 12% recurrence at 1 year and 36% recurrence at 5 years. Premature steroid withdrawal typically does not directly cause recurrence, and recurrence rates are not higher in males. Late rejection is often linked with recurrence.[336]

379. Which of the following statements is accurate regarding the recurrence of primary biliary cholangitis (PBC) after liver transplantation?
a) The median time to recurrence is approximately 12 months
b) Most patients with recurrence require retransplantation
c) Recurrence rates are significantly higher in female recipients
d) Recurrence is associated with older recipient and donor age
e) Recurrence typically leads to rapid graft dysfunction

**Answer: d**

Recurrence of PBC after liver transplantation is more strongly associated with older recipient and donor age. The median time to recurrence is approximately 3–5 years. Most patients with recurrent PBC do not require retransplantation, as the disease typically progresses slowly and is manageable with medical therapy, such as ursodeoxycholic acid. Although PBC predominantly affects females, sex is not a significant risk factor for recurrence post-transplant.[337]

380. A 34-year-old man with a history of ulcerative colitis and primary sclerosing cholangitis (PSC) underwent liver transplantation 5 years ago. He now presents with progressive fatigue, pruritus, and elevated cholestatic liver enzymes. MRCP reveals multifocal stricturing and beading of the intrahepatic bile ducts. A liver biopsy shows periductal fibrosis and ductopenia. What is the correct statement regarding PSC recurrence after liver transplant?
a) Patients with ulcerative colitis and active disease have a higher risk of recurrence
b) High-dose maintenance steroids decrease the risk of recurrence
c) Ursodeoxycholic acid therapy delays the onset of recurrence
d) PSC recurrence is universal
e) Recurrence of the disease is usually asymptomatic and clinically insignificant

**Answer: a**
Recurrent PSC occurs in a subset of patients after transplant, with an estimated risk from 7% to 47%. Active ulcerative colitis is associated with a higher risk of recurrence, while colectomy may reduce this risk. No immunosuppressive regimen, including steroids, has been proven to prevent recurrence. Ursodeoxycholic acid is commonly used but has not been shown to delay recurrence. Unfortunately, patients with recurrence can progress to graft failure.[338]

381. A 62-year-old woman with a history of cirrhosis due to alcoholic liver disease underwent liver transplantation six months ago. Before transplantation, she experienced two documented episodes of overt hepatic encephalopathy (OHE), one requiring hospitalization. Post-transplant, her liver function has normalized, and she no longer shows overt neurological symptoms. However, neuropsychological testing reveals mild, persistent memory deficits, with near-normal attention and psychomotor speed. Which of the following best explains her persistent cognitive impairment following liver transplantation?
a) Complete reversibility of cognitive deficits is expected, and her memory issues are unrelated to prior hepatic encephalopathy
b) Hepatic encephalopathy before transplantation is correlated with persistent cognitive deficits after liver transplantation
c) The effects of hepatic encephalopathy on the brain in the post-transplant period usually completely resolve in younger patients (less than 50 years old)
d) Her memory deficits are a normal part of post-transplant recovery and will resolve within a year
e) Persistent cognitive deficits are uncommon after transplantation and suggest a new, unrelated neurological condition
**Answer: b**
Studies show that pre-transplant OHE is linked to persistent cognitive deficits post-transplantation, particularly in memory, due to potentially irreversible brain damage. Studies on neuropsychiatric outcomes in patients transplanted for alcoholic liver disease reveal overall improvement in the neurocognitive profiles of this population. However, this group appears to be at increased risk for persistent cognitive impairment after liver transplantation particularly in the domain of memory.[339]

382. A 38-year-old man with Wilson's disease presents with progressive neurological symptoms, including dysarthria, tremor, ataxia, and bradykinesia, alongside evidence of liver cirrhosis. His liver disease is well compensated, but his neurological symptoms have worsened despite optimal medical therapy. Which of the following best describes the role of liver transplantation in managing severe neurological symptoms in Wilson's disease?

a) Liver transplantation is contraindicated due to the severity of neurological symptoms and lack of guaranteed improvement
b) Neurological symptoms reliably resolve within 6 to 12 months post-transplant, making transplantation the preferred treatment
c) Transplantation may lead to slow, partial neurological recovery, supporting its use in severe cases
d) Neurological improvement post-transplant is unlikely, and outcomes are worse than in patients without neurological symptoms
e) Transplantation is only indicated for decompensated cirrhosis, with no impact on neurological manifestations

**Answer: c**

Liver transplantation for Wilson's disease is well-established for decompensated cirrhosis but remains controversial for severe neurological symptoms. Emerging evidence suggests that even patients with significant pre-transplant neurological manifestations can experience slow, partial recovery post-transplant, often requiring adjunctive therapies like amantadine and multidisciplinary care.[340]

383. A 57-year-old man with a 10-year history of cirrhosis due to MASH, complicated by esophageal varices and portal hypertension, presents with progressive difficulty walking, resting tremor, and slowed movements over the past year. He has no history of overt hepatic encephalopathy. Neurological examination reveals parkinsonism with bradykinesia, rigidity, and a shuffling gait, alongside mild cognitive impairment. T1-weighted MRI shows symmetric hyperintensities in the bilateral globus pallidus and putamina. What is the most likely diagnosis?
a) Wilson's disease
b) Parkinson's disease
c) Hepatic encephalopathy
d) Acquired hepatocerebral degeneration
e) Stroke

**Answer: d**

Acquired hepatocerebral degeneration is characterized by parkinsonism and cognitive impairment in advanced cirrhosis, often linked to manganese accumulation. The patient's symptoms—bradykinesia, rigidity, and tremor—along with T1-weighted MRI hyperintensities in the globus pallidus and putamina, align with the diagnosis.[341]

384. A 34-year-old woman underwent liver transplantation 4 months ago due to acute liver failure from an acetaminophen overdose. Her post-transplant course was uneventful except for persistent depression, for which she was started on venlafaxine 150 mg daily. She was discharged home with stable liver function and good adherence

to her immunosuppressive regimen. She was slowly tapered off steroids, diuretics, and opioids over 4 months period. Her mood normalized, and she stopped venlafaxine abruptly 2 days ago. She now presents with nausea, dizziness, irritability, electric-shock-like sensations in her limbs, and difficulty sleeping. Physical examination and labs, including LFT, are normal. Which of the following best explains her symptoms?
a) Adrenal insufficiency due to prolonged steroid use
b) Opioid withdrawal
c) Discontinuation syndrome from abrupt cessation of venlafaxine
d) Acute delirium due to fluid overload after diuretic withdrawal
e) Adverse reaction to immunosuppressive therapy mimicking neurological symptoms
**Answer: c**
Abrupt cessation of venlafaxine, a serotonin-norepinephrine reuptake inhibitor with a short half-life, causes discontinuation syndrome, characterized by nausea, dizziness, irritability, electric-shock sensations, and insomnia—matching her symptoms.[342]

385. A 58-year-old man underwent liver transplantation 5 days ago for cirrhosis secondary to alcohol use. His postoperative course has been stable, with normalizing liver function tests, but he has not slept well since surgery. On day 5, he becomes agitated, disoriented, and has visual hallucinations, suggesting delirium. His vital signs are normal, and there is no evidence of infection or graft dysfunction. Which of the following is the most appropriate next step to manage his delirium in the context of his insomnia?
a) Initiate zolpidem 10 mg at bedtime to improve sleep and reduce delirium
b) Administer lorazepam 1 mg IV as needed to sedate and calm the patient
c) Implement nonpharmacological sleep hygiene measures and melatonin (1-2 mg)
d) Increase nighttime monitoring to identify delirium triggers
e) Prescribe eszopiclone 3 mg nightly to restore sleep and address hallucinations
**Answer: c**
Post-liver transplant delirium is often worsened by insomnia, prevalent in hospitals. Nonpharmacological sleep hygiene (e.g., reducing noise, minimizing nighttime disruptions, promoting daytime activity) is the preferred initial strategy, combined with melatonin (1-2 mg), which enhances sleep quality safely. Benzodiazepines and non-benzodiazepine hypnotics like zolpidem or eszopiclone may aggravate delirium.[343]

386. A 28-year-old man underwent liver transplantation 10 days ago for acute liver decompensation due to excessive alcohol intake. His postoperative course was initially stable; however, on day 10, he develops confusion, unsteady gait, and difficulty

moving his eyes upward. Neurological exam reveals ataxia, vertical gaze palsy, and delirium. Laboratory results show normal electrolytes and no infection, but MRI reveals symmetric T2 hyperintensities in the mamillary bodies and dorsomedial thalami. Which of the following is the most appropriate initial management for his condition?
a) Administer lorazepam 2 mg IV to manage delirium and potential alcohol withdrawal
b) Initiate IV thiamine 500 mg daily for 3 days, followed by oral supplementation
c) Start lactulose therapy to treat possible hepatic encephalopathy overlap
d) Switch tacrolimus to cyclosporine for possible tacrolimus toxicity
e) Provide IV fluids with dextrose to correct nutritional deficits and improve mentation

**Answer: b**

Wernicke encephalopathy, likely from thiamine deficiency in this alcoholic post-transplant patient, presents with delirium, ataxia, and gaze palsy, confirmed by symmetric T2 MRI hyperintensities. Immediate IV thiamine (500 mg daily) is the standard treatment to reverse symptoms and prevent progression.[344]

387. A 63-year-old man underwent liver transplantation 18 months ago for cirrhosis due to hepatitis B. He has been maintained on tacrolimus and mycophenolate mofetil for immunosuppression. Over the past 6 weeks, he reports progressive difficulty with speech, right arm weakness, and intermittent confusion. Neurological exam reveals expressive aphasia and right-sided hemiparesis. Brain MRI shows multifocal, asymmetric subcortical white matter lesions without enhancement. CSF analysis detects JC virus. Which of the following is the most appropriate next step in managing his condition?
a) Initiate high-dose IV acyclovir to target JC virus replication
b) Reduce tacrolimus dosage and monitor for graft rejection
c) Initiate IV ganciclovir 900 mg BID to target JC virus replication
d) Obtain brain biopsy for definitive diagnosis
e) Continue observation, as the disease is usually self-limiting

**Answer: b**

Progressive multifocal leukoencephalopathy (PML), indicated by JC virus DNA in CSF and MRI findings, results from immunosuppression in this transplant patient. Reducing tacrolimus to bolster immunity is the primary management step, despite limited efficacy, while monitoring graft function. The prognosis is grim: PML is fatal in 84% of posttransplant cases, with death occurring within 1 year in roughly half of patients.[345]

# 10. Transplant Pathology and Immunology

388. A transplant surgery fellow is performing liver retrieval surgery at a small community hospital. Upon inspection, the liver appears fatty, prompting the fellow to perform a core needle biopsy. Which of the following is the most appropriate way to handle the fresh liver biopsy specimen?
a) Place the specimen in a container with physiologic saline to maintain hydration
b) Wrap the specimen in dry gauze to prevent contamination during transport
c) Place the specimen on nonabsorbent material such as Telfa and put it in a plastic specimen container
d) Allow the specimen to air dry briefly to stabilize it before transport
e) Store the specimen in a sterile plastic container with an absorbent pad to soak up excess fluid

**Answer: c**

To preserve a fresh liver biopsy for accurate histological assessment, placing it on nonabsorbent material like Telfa in a plastic container prevents fat loss and artifacts. Storing the sample in "physiologic" saline, letting it air dry, or placing it on an absorbent material must be strictly avoided. Both air drying and saline storage can make hepatocytes look shrunken or necrotic, exaggerating ischemic damage. Absorbent materials remove fat from the tissue, falsely reducing the apparent degree of steatosis.[346]

389. A 55-year-old man underwent liver transplantation 2 hours ago for alcohol-induced cirrhosis. The donor liver, retrieved from a 40-year-old with a history of obesity, showed 25% macrovesicular steatosis on pre-transplant assessment. A postreperfusion needle biopsy is performed 1 hour after revascularization. The pathology report describes scattered microvesicular steatosis, mild hepatocellular swelling, and focal areas of large lipid droplets in the sinusoids with associated neutrophilia and fibrin deposition. There is no evidence of coagulative necrosis or subcapsular neutrophilia. Which of the following best characterizes the observed injury?
a) Severe preservation-reperfusion injury due to prolonged warm ischemia
b) Mild preservation-reperfusion injury exacerbated by donor macrovesicular steatosis
c) Surgical hepatitis from manipulation, unrelated to reperfusion
d) Late ischemic insult despite lack of necrosis

e) Resolving reperfusion injury with macrophage-mediated fat clearance
**Answer: b**
Postreperfusion biopsies within hours of revascularization assess preservation-reperfusion injury. This biopsy shows microvesicular steatosis and hepatocellular swelling (mild injury) plus lipid droplets, neutrophilia, and fibrin in sinusoids, consistent with donor macrovesicular steatosis (>20%) amplifying reperfusion damage. Severe injury requires necrosis. Surgical hepatitis involves perivenular neutrophilia without lipid findings; late ischemia fits biopsies days later with apoptosis. Resolution occurs weeks later with macrophages, not hours.[347]

390. The diagnosis of chronic rejection, based on biliary epithelial cell senescence, bile duct loss, or perivenular fibrosis, requires exclusion of non–rejection-related causes of ductal injury, such as obstructive cholangiopathy, hepatic artery stricturing or thrombosis, cholangitic drug-induced liver injury, and CMV infection. Which of the following features is least suggestive of obstructive cholangiopathy?
a) Bile duct loss in some portal tracts with ductular reaction in others
b) Neutrophil clusters within hepatic lobules
c) Copper or copper-associated protein deposition in periportal hepatocytes
d) Bile duct changes with central perivenulitis and/or fibrosis
e) Hepatocanalicular cholestasis disproportionate to ductopenia (<50% of portal tracts)
**Answer: d**
Bile duct changes combined with central perivenulitis and/or fibrosis are characteristic of chronic rejection, not obstructive cholangiopathy. Obstructive cholangiopathy typically presents with features like bile duct loss with ductular reaction, neutrophil clusters in lobules, copper deposition in periportal hepatocytes, and hepatocanalicular cholestasis out of proportion to ductopenia, reflecting biliary obstruction and cholestatic injury.[348]

391. A 47-year-old male undergoes liver transplantation due to fulminant hepatic failure. Pre-transplant testing reveals high donor-specific antibody (DSA) levels (MFI >10,000). On postoperative day 4, he develops rising liver enzymes and coagulopathy. A liver biopsy shows marked microvascular endothelial cell hypertrophy, eosinophilic and neutrophilic microvasculitis, diffuse C4d staining in the portal microvasculature, and scattered blastic lymphocytes in the portal tracts. Additionally, there is portal edema, focal necrosis, and prominent sinusoidal congestion. What is the most likely diagnosis?
a) Preservation-reperfusion injury
b) Obstructive cholangiopathy
c) Acute antibody-mediated rejection (AMR)

d) Acute cellular rejection (ACR) alone
e) Viral hepatitis
**Answer: c**
The biopsy findings align with acute AMR, favored in the presence of high DSA levels (MFI >10,000). Portal edema, necrosis, and congestion further support this diagnosis. Preservation-reperfusion injury lacks C4d staining and microvasculitis, while obstructive cholangiopathy shows ductular reaction and cholestasis, not seen here. ACR alone does not account for microvascular changes or C4d deposition. Viral hepatitis is unlikely given the timing and specific findings.[349]

392. A 39-year-old female, 6 months post-liver transplantation for autoimmune hepatitis, presents with fatigue and elevated liver enzymes. A liver biopsy is performed. The pathologist identifies an unusual finding and must determine if it aligns with acute cellular rejection (ACR). Which of the following is not a typical sign of acute cellular rejection?
a) Lymphocytic cholangitis
b) Portal and peribiliary granulomas
c) Subendothelial inflammation of portal and/or terminal hepatic venules
d) Predominantly mononuclear but mixed portal inflammation
e) Greater than 50% of the ducts or terminal hepatic veins are damaged
**Answer: b**
ACR, also known as referred to as "T-cell mediated" rejection, is characterized histopathologically by predominantly mononuclear but mixed portal inflammation containing blastic or activated lymphocytes, neutrophils, and eosinophils; subendothelial inflammation of portal and/or terminal hepatic venules; and bile duct inflammation and damage. The diagnosis is strengthened if greater than 50% of the ducts or terminal hepatic veins are damaged. Portal and/or peribiliary granulomas are not a feature of either acute or chronic rejection. If portal-based granulomas are encountered, a non–rejection-related cause of duct injury, such as primary biliary cirrhosis, mycobacterial or fungal infection or sarcoidosis.[350]

393. A 55-year-old female, 5 years post-liver transplantation for primary biliary cholangitis (PBC), presents with pruritus and elevated liver enzymes (ALT 60 U/L, AST 50 U/L, ALP 380 U/L, bilirubin 3 mg/dL). A liver biopsy is performed. The histopathology report notes portal inflammation and lymphocytic cholangitis. Which of the following statements is correct regarding PBC versus rejection?
a) PBC-associated inflammation is patchy and preferentially involves medium-sized bile ducts (>40 to 50 μm in diameter)
b) Rejection-associated inflammation is patchy and preferentially involves medium-sized bile ducts (>40 to 50 μm in diameter)

c) PBC-associated inflammation involves most portal tracts and targets small bile ducts (<20 μm in diameter)
d) Rejection-associated inflammation is patchy and targets small bile ducts (<20 μm in diameter)
e) PBC-associated inflammation is uniform across portal tracts and involves medium-sized bile ducts (>40 to 50 μm in diameter)
Answer: a
In rejection, portal inflammation and lymphocytic cholangitis typically involve the majority of portal tracts and target small bile ducts (<20 μm in diameter). In contrast, PBC-associated inflammation is patchy and preferentially affects medium-sized bile ducts (>40 to 50 μm in diameter).[350]

394. Which mechanism is least likely to explain the liver allograft's resistance to rejection compared to other transplanted organs?
a) Secretion of soluble MHC class I molecules by hepatocytes
b) Clonal exhaustion due to the liver's large antigenic mass
c) Clonal deletion of recipient T cells via interaction with donor hepatocytes
d) Hematopoietic chimerism driven by donor stem cells and tolerogenic dendritic cells
e) Alloantigen presentation in an active inflammatory state
Answer: e
The liver allograft's relative resistance to rejection, compared to other organs, is attributed to unique tolerogenic mechanisms. Secretion of soluble MHC class I molecules suppresses recipient immune responses. The liver's large antigenic mass induces clonal exhaustion of recipient T cells. Interaction between recipient leukocytes and donor hepatocytes promotes clonal deletion, reducing alloreactivity. Hematopoietic chimerism, facilitated by donor stem cells and tolerogenic dendritic cells, fosters immune tolerance. However, alloantigen presentation in an active inflammatory state is least likely to contribute, as inflammation typically enhances immune activation and rejection, counteracting the liver's tolerogenic environment.[351]

395. A 28-year-old male, 3 years post-liver transplantation for alcohol-related cirrhosis, has normal liver function and enrolls in an immunosuppression (IS) weaning trial. A preweaning biopsy showed minimal portal inflammation and no fibrosis. After gradual IS reduction, a repeat biopsy reveals increased portal mononuclear infiltration, interface hepatitis resembling low-grade chronic hepatitis, and subtle perivenular fibrosis, with no significant bile duct damage or C4d deposits. Liver enzymes remain normal and donor-specific antibodies (DSA) are absent. What is the most appropriate next step?
a) Discontinue immunosuppression completely

b) Resume full immunosuppression immediately
c) Continue gradual weaning with close monitoring
d) Perform immediate antiviral therapy for suspected CMV infection
e) Initiate treatment with lymphocyte-depleting antibodies
**Answer: b**
The repeat biopsy findings indicate potential immunological damage consistent with latent rejection during IS weaning. These changes, even without bile duct damage, C4d deposits, or elevated enzymes, warrant concern per follow-up biopsy criteria, suggesting early rejection. Resuming full immunosuppression is appropriate to halt progression.[352]

396. A 35-year-old female, 4 years post-liver transplantation for autoimmune hepatitis (AIH), presents with fatigue and elevated liver enzymes. A liver biopsy reveals moderate portal inflammation with significant lymphocytic infiltrates, prominent interface hepatitis, and lobular necroinflammatory activity. However, there is also notable atrophy and loss of interlobular bile ducts in 50% of portal tracts. Autoantibody titers (ANA and anti-smooth muscle) are elevated, and immunosuppression has been stable. What is the most likely diagnosis?
a) Chronic cellular rejection
b) Recurrent AIH
c) Overlap of recurrent AIH and chronic rejection
d) Acute cellular rejection
e) Chronic antibodies mediated rejection
**Answer: c**
The biopsy shows significant lymphocytic infiltrates, interface hepatitis, and lobular activity, strongly favoring recurrent AIH over chronic rejection, which is typically paucicellular with bile duct atrophy and loss. However, the presence of significant bile duct atrophy and loss (50% of portal tracts) complicates the diagnosis, as this is characteristic of chronic rejection. The combination suggests an overlap of recurrent AIH and chronic rejection.[353]

397. A 42-year-old male, 5 years post-liver transplantation for primary sclerosing cholangitis (PSC), presents with pruritus and elevated liver enzymes. The transplant team debates the likelihood of recurrent PSC versus other causes. A liver biopsy is performed. What is the most typical histological presentation of recurrent PSC?
a) Interlobular and septal bile ducts with concentric "onion skin" fibrosis
b) A mixed portal infiltrate with eosinophils
c) Atrophy and loss of interlobular bile ducts with minimal or no portal inflammation
d) Diffuse microvascular C4d deposits
e) Intranuclear inclusions and owl's eye cells

**Answer: a**
Recurrent PSC typically shows concentric "onion skin" fibrosis around interlobular and septal bile ducts. A mixed portal infiltrate with eosinophils favors acute rejection. Chronic rejection is a paucicellular process that results in atrophy and loss of interlobular bile ducts with minimal portal fibrosis. Diffuse C4d deposits indicate antibody-mediated rejection. Intranuclear inclusions and owl's eye cells are classic for CMV infection.[353]

398. A 52-year-old male, 3 years post-liver transplantation for MASH presents with elevated liver enzymes and a history of recent alcohol use. A liver biopsy reveals macrovesicular steatosis in acinar zone III, ballooning degeneration of hepatocytes, mild lobular mononuclear inflammation, and early sinusoidal fibrosis. The pathologist notes eosinophilic cytoplasmic inclusions in ballooned hepatocytes and uses ubiquitin staining to confirm their identity. Which of the following best describes these inclusions?
a) Lipid droplets indicative of severe steatosis
b) Ropey Mallory-Denk bodies typical of steatohepatitis
c) Intranuclear inclusions and owl's eye cells suggestive of CMV hepatitis
d) Hyaline deposits associated with chronic rejection
e) Granular iron aggregates suggestive of Pappenheimer bodies
**Answer: b**
Mallory-Denk bodies are eosinophilic, rope-like structures found in the cytoplasm of hepatocytes showing ballooning degeneration. They may vary from conspicuous and distinct to faint and hard to discern. Ubiquitin immunohistochemistry can aid in their detection when identification is uncertain. While these bodies are often more noticeable in alcoholic liver disease than in MASH, this difference isn't consistently dependable for differentiation.[354]

399. A 55-year-old male, 10 years post-liver transplantation, presents for a routine follow-up. He has been on long-term immunosuppression with tacrolimus and mycophenolate. Given his transplant history, he is at increased risk of which type of malignancy compared to the general population?
a) Squamous cell carcinoma
b) Basal cell carcinoma
c) Melanoma
d) Non-hodgkin lymphoma
e) Kaposi sarcoma
**Answer: a**
The most common malignancy after solid organ transplantation is non-melanoma skin cancer, with squamous cell carcinoma, being the predominant type. The risk of

squamous cell carcinoma is significantly elevated (65- to 250-fold) in transplant recipients due to chronic immunosuppression, which impairs immune surveillance, and is often associated with ultraviolet light exposure.[355]

400. A 52-year-old male underwent liver transplantation for cirrhosis secondary to chronic hepatitis B virus infection. Six months post-transplant, while maintained on tacrolimus and mycophenolate mofetil immunosuppression, the patient presents with pyrexia, generalized lymphadenopathy, and multiple violaceous cutaneous lesions on the lower extremities. Histopathological examination of a biopsied lesion reveals spindle cell proliferation with vascular slits, and PCR confirms escalating HHV8 viremia. Which of the following represents the most probable diagnosis?
a) Post-transplant lymphoproliferative disorder
b) Graft versus host disease
c) Kaposi sarcoma
d) Primary effusion lymphoma
e) Multicentric Castleman disease
**Answer: c**
The presentation of violaceous cutaneous lesions, histopathological findings of spindle cells and vascular slits, rising HHV8 viremia in an immunosuppressed patient strongly support a diagnosis of Kaposi sarcoma. Multicentric Castleman disease presents with lymphadenopathy and systemic symptoms but lacks the characteristic cutaneous pathology observed here.[356]

401. The risk for developing lung cancer after liver transplantation is closely linked to which of the following?
a) Extended duration of immunosuppressive therapy
b) Combined history of heavy smoking and alcoholic liver disease
c) Administration of induction immunosuppression during transplantation
d) Reactivation of latent EBV
e) Oncogenic effects mediated by calcineurin inhibitors
**Answer: b**
The heightened risk of lung cancer post-liver transplantation is predominantly associated with his extensive smoking history and alcoholic liver disease. Research from a multicenter U.S. registry indicates that patients with alcoholic liver disease face a 5-year lung cancer risk of 2% and a 10-year risk of 4.8%, significantly higher than the 0.15% and 1.3% observed in nonalcoholic recipients.[357]

402. A 60-year-old male who underwent liver transplantation 5 years ago for alcoholic cirrhosis presents with fatigue, weight loss, and diffuse lymphadenopathy. He is EBV-positive and received an EBV-negative organ. He has been maintained on tacrolimus

and mycophenolate mofetil. Imaging reveals multiple enlarged lymph nodes in the neck, chest, and abdomen, and a biopsy confirms post-transplant lymphoproliferative disorder (PTLD). Which of the following interventions or characteristics is most likely to improve this patient's survival outcome?
a) Discontinue tacrolimus
b) High-dose steroid therapy
c) Switching from tacrolimus to sirolimus
d) Extended interval (>2 years) between transplantation and PTLD diagnosis
e) EBV-positive status in the recipient

**Answer: c**

Data from a single large-volume center showed excellent short- and long-term survival in patients after liver transplantation and PTLD who were EBV-negative, had early-stage disease, and achieved complete response. Switching from a calcineurin inhibitor (e.g., tacrolimus) to sirolimus at PTLD diagnosis improved survival compared to reducing or stopping immunosuppression alone, leveraging sirolimus's antiproliferative effects.[358]

403. A 58-year-old male with a history of hepatitis C underwent liver transplantation 18 months ago for HCC. Pre-transplant imaging revealed a single 6.3 cm tumor in the right lobe, AFP level of 96,000 ng/mL. Pathology of the explanted liver confirmed a poorly differentiated HCC with vascular invasion. He now presents with fatigue and abdominal pain. Imaging shows multiple hepatic nodules, and a biopsy confirms HCC recurrence. Which of the following is least associated with increased risk of tumor recurrence?
a) Tumor diameter exceeding 5 cm
b) Vascular invasion
c) Poor histological differentiation
d) Elevated pre-transplant AFP
e) Hepatitis C as the underlying etiology

**Answer: e**

The most prominent factors linked to posttransplant recurrence of HCC include pretransplant AFP levels, tumor size and number, poor histological differentiation, vascular invasion, and the immunosuppressive regimen.[359]

404. A 52-year-old male with unresectable perihilar cholangiocarcinoma underwent neoadjuvant chemoradiotherapy followed by liver transplantation 18 months ago. The explanted liver revealed a 3.2 cm moderately differentiated tumor with evidence of residual viable tumor cells despite treatment. He has been maintained on sirolimus for immunosuppression. Recent imaging shows a 1.5 cm lesion in the transplanted

liver, and biopsy confirms cholangiocarcinoma recurrence. Which of the following factors most significantly contributed to this patient's recurrence?
a) Use of sirolimus as immunosuppressive therapy
b) Presence of residual tumor on explant pathology
c) Moderately differentiated tumor histology
d) Tumor size of 3.2 cm at transplantation
e) Extended interval (>12 months) between transplantation and cholangiocarcinoma recurrence

**Answer: b**

Recurrence of cholangiocarcinoma after liver transplantation occurs in 19% of recipients and carries a high mortality rate. The primary predictor of posttransplant recurrence is residual tumor on explant pathology, indicating incomplete tumor control despite neoadjuvant therapy.[360]

405. The appearance of which cell in the portal tracts predicts transplant liver rejection even before biochemical evidence is present?
a) Neutrophils
b) CD4 cells
c) CD8 cells
d) Eosinophils
e) Macrophages

**Answer: b**

CD4+ lymphocytes in the portal tracts are an early predictor of liver transplant rejection, appearing before biochemical changes like elevated ALP. CD8+ cells predominate later during active rejection, targeting bile ducts, while CD4+ cells initiate and amplify the immune response.[361]

406. Type 2 CD4+ helper T cells secrete IL-5, which is detected in rejecting liver allografts and attracts eosinophils to the portal triads, exacerbating inflammation and tissue injury. The presence of IL-5 mRNA in these allografts underscores the role of eosinophils in liver graft rejection. Studies have investigated whether peripheral blood eosinophil counts can predict acute cellular rejection and monitor treatment response. Which of the following statement is the most accurate?
a) Elevated peripheral blood eosinophil counts are associated with steroid treatment rather than liver rejection
b) Elevated peripheral blood eosinophil counts have a positive predictive value for acute cellular rejection
c) Only eosinophil infiltration in liver tissue, not peripheral blood eosinophil levels, is associated with rejection

d) Due to increased eosinophil migration to the liver during a rejection episode, peripheral blood eosinophil levels are decreased
e) Increased peripheral blood eosinophilia is associated with eosinophil migration from the liver and resolution of rejection

**Answer: b**

An elevated peripheral blood eosinophil count has a positive predictive value for acute cellular rejection of the liver, while a normal count typically rules out moderate or severe rejection. Additionally, a decrease in peripheral eosinophilia may indicate histological improvement following treatment for rejection.[362]

407. Which of the following is the incorrect statement about liver Kupffer cells?
a) Located in the liver sinusoids
b) Able to remove immune complexes and activated complement
c) Restore liver tissue integrity following injury
d) Also known as liver-resident dendritic population
e) Contribute to liver disease progression

**Answer: d**

Kupffer cells are liver-resident macrophages located in the sinusoids. Kupffer cells help to restore tissue integrity following injury, able to remove immune complexes and activated complement but can also contribute to liver disease progression.[363]

408. Which cell type is the most abundant non-parenchymal population in the liver, efficiently scavenging and presenting hepatocyte-derived antigens on MHC class I or II molecules, constitutively expressing CD40, and upregulating CD80 and CD86 during inflammation?
a) Hepatic stellate cells
b) Kupffer cells
c) Dendritic cells
d) Liver sinusoidal endothelial cells
e) Liver-resident T cells

**Answer: d**

Liver sinusoidal endothelial cells are the most prevalent non-parenchymal cells in the liver. They act as efficient scavengers, processing and presenting hepatocyte-derived antigens on MHC class I or II molecules. These cells constitutively express CD40, with CD80 and CD86 expression induced during inflammatory conditions.[363]

409. A 45-year-old male underwent liver transplantation 10 years ago for alcoholic liver disease. He has been stable on tacrolimus-based immunosuppression with no rejection episodes. His transplant team considers withdrawing immunosuppression. Recent tests show normal liver function, low lymphocyte proliferation index, and

reduced circulating regulatory T cell levels. Which of the following factors is least likely to support this decision?
a) Young age at the time of transplantation
b) Male gender
c) Extended duration since transplantation
d) Low lymphocyte proliferation index
e) Reduced circulating concentrations of regulatory T cells

**Answer: e**

Factors favoring successful immunosuppression withdrawal in liver transplantation include younger age at transplant, male gender, and a prolonged post-transplant period, and reduced lymphocyte proliferation index, suggesting immune adaptation. However, low circulating levels of regulatory T cells have been associated with acute rejection.[364]

410. A 55-year-old male undergoes a successful liver transplantation from a deceased donor. Immunosuppressive therapy with tacrolimus, steroids, and mycophenolate mofetil is initiated. On post-transplant day 14, flow cytometry detects a small population of donor-derived leukocytes in the recipient's peripheral blood. Repeat flow cytometry is performed on day 90. Based on current understanding of donor leukocyte dynamics post-transplantation, what is it most likely to show?
a) No detectable donor leukocytes due to immune elimination by the recipient's immune system
b) Persistent donor leukocytes integrated as tissue-resident cells in the recipient's circulation
c) Low levels of donor leukocytes persisting as part of long-term microchimerism
d) Increased donor leukocytes due to migration and proliferation in the recipient's periphery
e) Reduced but detectable donor leukocytes due to ongoing apoptosis from insufficient growth factors

**Answer: a**

Based on historical data and recent insights into donor leukocyte dynamics post-solid organ transplantation, donor-derived leukocytes typically migrate into the recipient's circulation shortly after transplantation but are cleared within 30 to 60 days, as detected by flow cytometry. By day 90, in the absence of graft-versus-host disease or other complications, these cells are most likely to be undetectable due to immune elimination by the recipient's immune system. Recent data has explored microchimerism, where low levels of donor cells may persist long-term in some recipients and contribute to immune tolerance. However, this is less common, often tissue-specific, and typically below the detection threshold of standard flow cytometry by day 90 in most cases.[365]

411. A 50-year-old male with cirrhosis due to hepatitis C is evaluated for liver transplantation at a U.S. transplant center. Due to a shortage of deceased donor organs, his 42-year-old sister offers to be a living donor. Blood typing reveals the patient is type A and the donor is type B. Based on current global practices and strategies for ABO-incompatible living donor liver transplantation (ABO-I LDLT), what is the most accurate statement regarding the management of this case?
a) ABO-I LDLT is routinely performed in the U.S. across adult and pediatric populations using standard immunosuppression, rendering it a feasible option
b) ABO-I LDLT is infrequently performed in the U.S. but prevalent in Japan, where induction therapy precedes standard immunosuppression
c) ABO-I LDLT is broadly adopted in the U.S. and Japan, utilizing pre-transplant plasmapheresis as the primary desensitization strategy
d) ABO-I LDLT is universally avoided due to elevated risks of acute antibody-mediated rejection and graft failure
e) ABO-I LDLT is universally avoided due to decreased 5-year rates of patient and graft survival
**Answer: b**
Since 2014, Japan has developed and refined methods to prevent antibody-mediated rejection for ABO -I LDLD, a practice that has spread primarily to Asia, where LDLT predominates due to limited brain-dead donor availability. The optimal approach for safety and effectiveness involves a pre-transplant desensitization regimen of rituximab, plasmapheresis, tacrolimus, and mycophenolate mofetil, followed by conventional immunosuppression.[366]

412. A 62-year-old female with cirrhosis due to MASH undergoes deceased donor liver transplantation. Pre-transplant testing reveals preformed donor-specific anti-HLA antibodies (DSA) with a median fluorescence intensity (MFI) of 11,000 by Luminex assay. At 1 month post-transplant, repeat testing shows persistent DSA with an MFI of 6,500. What is the most likely implication of her persistent DSA?
a) Elevated risk of chronic rejection due to persistent high-MFI DSA
b) Negligible impact on long-term graft survival
c) Imminent risk of acute antibody-mediated rejection necessitating urgent intervention
d) Non-significant finding, as DSA typically resolves by 12 months, warranting repeat testing at 6 months
e) Indication of immunological tolerance, obviating further DSA surveillance
**Answer: a**
Persistent high-MFI DSA (>5,000) post-liver transplantation is associated with a heightened risk of chronic rejection.[367]

413. A 62-year-old male with decompensated liver disease due to autoimmune hepatitis underwent liver transplantation from a 24-year-old DBD male donor. He has a 9-year history of diabetes mellitus and prior steroid-treated sarcoidosis. By postoperative day 35, he presents with fever, rash, mucocutaneous ulcers, leukopenia (260 cells/mm$^3$), and thrombocytopenia (80,000 cells/mm$^3$). Short tandem repeat analysis confirms >50% donor-derived lymphocytes in his marrow, diagnosing graft-versus-host disease (GVHD). Which of the following is least likely to have contributed to the development of GVHD in this patient?
a) Recipient age exceeding 60 years
b) Younger donor age relative to recipient
c) Pre-existing glucose intolerance
d) Donor-recipient age disparity greater than 20 years
e) Autoimmune disease in donor

**Answer: e**

Known GVHD risk factors in liver transplantation include recipient age >60, younger donor age, glucose intolerance, and donor-recipient age difference >20 years, all present here and tied to increased donor lymphocyte reactivity.[368]

414. All of the following statements accurately describe graft-versus-host disease (GVHD) in liver transplant recipients, except:
a) It can manifest in both humoral and cellular forms
b) It typically presents between 1 and 8 weeks post-transplantation
c) The most common clinical features include fever, skin rash, diarrhea, and pancytopenia
d) The most common clinical presentation is acutely worsening liver graft function
e) Diarrhea is the most frequent gastrointestinal manifestation

**Answer: d**

GVHD in liver transplantation arises from donor lymphocytes attacking host tissues, typically presenting 1–8 weeks post-transplant with fever, rash, diarrhea, and pancytopenia, while sparing the liver graft, which remains functional.[368]

415. A 67-year-old man with cirrhosis from alcoholic liver disease undergoes liver transplantation. On postoperative day 8, he develops a fever and a maculopapular rash on his trunk, with peripheral blood analysis showing 25% donor T-cell chimerism. By postoperative day 14, the rash spreads to his extremities, and he experiences diarrhea and leukopenia, with donor T-cell chimerism remaining at 22%. Based on the current understanding of graft-versus-host disease (GVHD) in liver transplantation, what is the most appropriate interpretation of these findings?
a) Persistent donor T-cell chimerism above 20% strongly supports a GVHD diagnosis

b) The observed chimerism levels indicate typical donor lymphoid engraftment
c) Chimerism below 30% rules out GVHD as a likely cause
d) Elevated chimerism is a transient post-transplant event unrelated to GVHD
e) Chimerism suggests donor-specific tolerance, with symptoms likely due to infection

**Answer: a**

In liver transplantation, donor T-cell chimerism typically peaks within the first week and falls below 1% by 4 weeks. Persistent chimerism exceeding 20% beyond this period, combined with symptoms such as fever, rash, diarrhea, and leukopenia, strongly suggests GVHD caused by donor lymphocyte-mediated injury to the host.[369]

416. Based on current understanding of graft-versus-host disease in liver transplantation, what is the most common cause of mortality?
a) Fulminant liver failure
b) Sepsis secondary to infectious complications
c) Gastrointestinal hemorrhage from mucosal ulceration
d) Multiorgan failure from cytokine storm
e) Cardiac arrhythmia leading to cardiac arrest

**Answer: b**

Most patient die of end-organ failure caused by causing fulminant sepsis due to Enterobacteriaceae, Vancomycin resistant enterococci, invasive aspergillosis, or disseminated candida.[368]

## 11. Immunosuppression

417. Following a solid organ transplant, T-cell activation occurs through a process known as the three-signal hypothesis. Which of the following represents the second signal in this process?
a) Interaction of the T-cell receptor with MHC molecules
b) Binding of CD28 on the T cell to CD80/CD86 on the APC
c) Release of IL-2 and its binding to the IL-2 receptor on T cells
d) Activation of nuclear factor of activated T cells and cytokine transcription
e) Transition of the T cell from the G0 to G1 phase, leading to proliferation and differentiation

**Answer: b**
Signal 1: Interaction of the T-cell receptor (TCR-CD3) with MHC molecules on the APC.
Signal 2: Binding of CD28 on the T cell to CD80/CD86 on the APC, providing co-stimulation.
Signal 3: Release of IL-2 and its binding to the IL-2 receptor, promoting T-cell proliferation and differentiation.[370]

418. All current immunosuppressive medications target one of the three essential signaling pathways involved in immune system activation. Which of the following agents is not a signal 1 blocker?
a) Cyclosporine
b) Tacrolimus
c) Sirolimus
d) Rabbit-derived antithymocyte globulin (rATG)

**Answer: c**
Signal 1 is the first step in the three-signal hypothesis of T-cell activation, it involves the interaction between the T-cell receptor (TCR) on the surface of a T cell and MHC molecule presenting an antigen on an APC. This interaction is stabilized by the CD3 complex on the T cell, which helps transmit the activation signal intracellularly. Signal 1 blockers include calcineurin inhibitors (e.g., cyclosporine and tacrolimus) and anti-CD3 monoclonal antibodies (e.g., OKT3 and rATG), which inhibit the T-cell receptor complex. Sirolimus primarily acts as a Signal 2 blocker by inhibiting mTOR, affecting T-cell proliferation and differentiation.[371]

419. Which of the following agents works by blocking immune stimulation signal 2 by binding to the costimulatory molecule CD28, thereby preventing its interaction with CD80/CD86?
a) Belatacept
b) Simulect
c) Campath
d) Rituximab
e) Azathioprine
**Answer: a**
Belatacept is the only agent that competes with CD28 for binding to its ligands, CD80 and CD86, thus inhibiting the necessary costimulatory signal required for T-cell activation and proliferation.[371]

420. All of the following agents are considered signal 3 immune activation blockers, except for:
a) Basiliximab
b) Sirolimus
c) Everolimus
d) Tacrolimus
**Answer: d**
Signal 3 blockers include anti-CD25 antibodies, such as basiliximab, which competitively bind to the IL-2 receptor (IL-2R), as well as mTOR inhibitors like sirolimus and everolimus, which prevent further downstream signal transduction if the IL-2R is activated. Tacrolimus is a calcineurin inhibitor that acts primarily as a signal 1 blocker.[371]

421. Which of the following statements best describes the mechanism of action of calcineurin inhibitor in preventing T-cell activation?
a) It blocks the binding of IL-2 to its receptor on T cells
b) It inhibits the phosphorylation and activation of nuclear factor of activated T cells (NFAT)
c) It decreases intracellular calcium levels, thus preventing T-cell receptor signaling
d) It promotes the upregulation of co-stimulatory molecules on the APC
e) It promotes the phosphorylation of NFAT, thus inhibiting its activity
**Answer: b**
Calcineurin inhibitor acts by inhibiting the activity of calcineurin, preventing the phosphorylation and activation of NFAT. This action stops NFAT from translocating to the nucleus, which in turn inhibits the transcription of IL-2 and other cytokines necessary for T-cell activation and proliferation.[372]

422. This drug was isolated from the fungus Tolypocladium inflatum, which was first identified in soil samples obtained in 1969. It works by inhibiting signal 1 immune activation.
a) Tacrolimus
b) Cyclosporine
c) Sirolimus
d) Everolimus
e) Mycophenolate mofetil
**Answer: b**
In 1972, cyclosporine's immunosuppressive properties were identified, and by 1978 it was shown to prevent rejection in kidney transplants at Cambridge and in liver transplants by the Denver/Pittsburgh group, significantly improving allograft survival and advancing the field of transplantation.[373,374]

423. A 38-year-old man underwent liver transplantation for alcohol-induced cirrhosis. His postoperative course was complicated by seizures, prompting a change in his immunosuppressive regimen from tacrolimus and prednisone to cyclosporine (150 mg BID, target serum levels 150–200 ng/mL) and prednisone, with levetiracetam (500 mg BID) added for seizure control. Four weeks post-discharge, he switched from levetiracetam to phenytoin for ongoing seizures. He now presents with elevated LFT (ALT 120 U/L, AST 100 U/L, ALP 300 U/L) and bilirubin (3.5 mg/dL), with a cyclosporine level of 75 ng/mL. Which recent medication change most likely caused these findings?
a) Switching from levetiracetam to phenytoin
b) Starting erythromycin for skin cellulitis
c) Increased grapefruit juice consumption
d) Starting verapamil for hypertension
e) Starting sertraline for depression
**Answer: a**
Cyclosporine is metabolized by the cytochrome P450 3A4 (CYP3A4) enzyme system. Drugs that induce CYP3A4, such as phenytoin, accelerate cyclosporine metabolism, reducing its serum levels and increasing the risk of graft rejection. Conversely, CYP3A4 inhibitors like erythromycin, verapamil, and grapefruit juice increase cyclosporine levels. Sertraline has minimal impact on CYP3A4. Switching from levetiracetam to phenytoin likely caused the decreased cyclosporine level, contributing to elevated LFT and bilirubin due to possible graft rejection.[375,376]

424. A 41-year-old woman underwent a liver transplant for primary sclerosing cholangitis with Roux-en-Y biliary reconstruction. Her postoperative course was uneventful, and she was discharged on a triple immunosuppressive regimen:

cyclosporine 175 mg twice daily (serum level 200 ng/mL), a prednisone taper, and mycophenolate mofetil 1000 mg twice daily. Three weeks post-discharge, she presents with jaundice and elevated LFT, bilirubin and GGT. Liver MRI reveals stent migration and biliary obstruction, while the liver biopsy indicates biliary obstruction with features of transplant rejection. What is the most likely cause of the transplant rejection?
a) Biliary obstruction triggering inflammation and immune upregulation
b) Subtherapeutic cyclosporine levels due to impaired absorption
c) Chronic rejection from prolonged biliary obstruction
d) Infection-induced immune-mediated response
e) Undiagnosed underlying autoimmune hepatitis

**Answer: b**

Cyclosporine absorption depends on bile for emulsification and uptake in the gut. Biliary obstruction, as seen with stent migration, impairs bile flow, reducing cyclosporine absorption and leading to subtherapeutic levels, which can precipitate transplant rejection. Tacrolimus, unlike cyclosporine, does not rely on bile for absorption and is unaffected by biliary obstruction.[375,376]

425. Which of the following is not a side effect of cyclosporine?
a) Nephrotoxicity
b) Neurotoxicity
c) Weight loss
d) Gingival hyperplasia
e) Hirsutism

**Answer: c**

Cyclosporine is associated with side effects including nephrotoxicity, neurotoxicity, gingival hyperplasia, hirsutism, hypertension, hyperlipidemia, hyperkalemia, and weight gain.[311]

426. Tacrolimus, a potent immunosuppressive agent (100 times more potent than cyclosporine), suppresses T-cell activation through a specific binding mechanism. Which statement best describes its mechanism of action?
a) Inhibits CD28 interaction with CD80/CD86 on antigen-presenting cells, blocking Signal 2
b) Binds to FK506-binding protein (FKBP-12), inhibiting calcineurin and preventing nuclear factor of activated T cells (NFAT) activation
c) Directly blocks IL-2 transcription by inhibiting the IL-2 receptor on T cells
d) Increases intracellular calcium, enhancing T-cell proliferation
e) Promotes regulatory T-cell activation, increasing immune tolerance

**Answer: b**

Tacrolimus binds to FK506-binding protein (FKBP-12), forming a complex that inhibits calcineurin. This prevents the activation of NFAT, reducing transcription of cytokines like IL-2 and IFN-γ, thereby suppressing T-cell proliferation and promoting immunosuppression.[377]

427. What is the half-life of tacrolimus?
a) 6 hours
b) 12 hours
c) 18 hours
d) 24 hours
e) 36 hours
**Answer: b**
The half-life of tacrolimus is approximately 12 hours.[378]

428. What is the pathogenesis of the chronic form of tacrolimus-induced nephrotoxicity?
a) Afferent arterial vasoconstriction, leading to activation of the renin-angiotensin system
b) Efferent arterial vasoconstriction, leading to activation of the renin-angiotensin system
c) Downregulation of TGF-β, which promotes fibrosis
d) Hyaline thickening in the efferent arterioles, along with downregulation of TGF-β, interstitial fibrosis, tubular atrophy, and glomerulosclerosis
e) Hyaline thickening in the afferent arterioles, along with interstitial fibrosis, tubular atrophy, and glomerulosclerosis
**Answer: e**
The chronic form of tacrolimus-induced nephrotoxicity is characterized by hyaline thickening in the afferent arterioles, interstitial fibrosis, tubular atrophy, and glomerulosclerosis. Upregulation of TGF-β is a key etiological factor that promotes fibrosis in this condition. The acute form of nephrotoxicity is linked to endothelin and other vasoconstrictors that cause afferent arterial vasoconstriction, as well as an activation of the renin-angiotensin system.[379,380]

429. What is the most common manifestation of tacrolimus-induced neurotoxicity?
a) Tremor
b) Headache
c) Confusion
d) Agitation
e) Seizure
**Answer: b**

The most common manifestation of tacrolimus-induced neurotoxicity is headache. Neurotoxicity occurs more frequently with tacrolimus compared to cyclosporine. Symptoms can often be improved with a dose reduction.[381,382]

430. A 52-year-old male underwent a liver transplant due to MASH. His postoperative course was uncomplicated, and he was discharged home on tacrolimus 2 mg BID, with steady trough levels between 8 and 9 ng/mL, mycophenolate mofetil 1000 mg BID, and a prednisone taper. On postoperative day 42, fluconazole was discontinued. What is the expected adjustment to the current immunosuppressive regimen?
a) Increase the tacrolimus dose to 3 mg BID
b) Decrease the tacrolimus dose to 1.5 mg BID
c) Decrease mycophenolate mofetil to 500 mg BID
d) Discontinue prednisone
e) No changes to the current regimen
**Answer: a**
Fluconazole is an azole antifungal that inhibits the cytochrome P450 3A4 enzyme system, which metabolizes tacrolimus. Discontinuing fluconazole may result in an increase in tacrolimus metabolism, potentially leading to lower serum levels. Therefore, it may be necessary to increase the tacrolimus dose to maintain therapeutic levels after fluconazole is discontinued.[375,376]

431. mTOR inhibitors, a class of immunosuppressive agents, target the mTOR signaling pathway, which regulates the p70S6 kinase gene. This gene controls the translation of cell cycle-regulating proteins, such as cyclin E and cyclin-dependent kinases (CDKs), critical for cell cycle progression. Which cell cycle phase transition is primarily facilitated by this mechanism?
a) G0 to G1 phase
b) G1 to S phase
c) S to G2 phase
d) G2 to M phase
e) G1 to M phase
**Answer: b**
mTOR inhibitors block the mTOR pathway, which regulates p70S6 kinase and the translation of proteins like cyclin E and CDKs. These proteins drive the transition from the G1 to S phase of the cell cycle. By inhibiting mTOR, these agents prevent G1 to S phase progression, suppressing lymphocyte proliferation and activation, key to their immunosuppressive effect.[383]

432. Sirolimus, an immunosuppressive agent, binds to FKBP-12 to inhibit a key signaling pathway. Which statement best describes how sirolimus suppresses T- and B-cell proliferation and activation?
a) Sirolimus-FKBP-12 complex inhibits calcineurin, blocking nuclear factor of activated T cells (NFAT) activation and Signal 1 of T-cell activation
b) Sirolimus-FKBP-12 complex inhibits mTOR, blocking IL-2 and IL-15 induction, thus preventing T- and B-cell proliferation by halting cell cycle progression from G1 to S phase
c) Sirolimus increases IL-2 and IL-15 production, suppressing T-cell proliferation and immune response
d) Sirolimus-FKBP-12 complex inhibits p70S6 kinase, disrupting Signal 2 of T-cell activation and reducing T-cell proliferation
e) Sirolimus blocks IL-2 binding to its receptor, directly inhibiting T-cell activation and proliferation
**Answer: b**
Sirolimus binds to FKBP-12, forming a complex that inhibits the mTOR pathway. This blocks the induction of IL-2 and IL-15, critical cytokines for T- and B-cell proliferation, by preventing cell cycle progression from G1 to S phase (Signal 3 of T-cell activation). Unlike tacrolimus, sirolimus does not affect calcineurin. This mechanism also inhibits B-cell immunoglobulin synthesis, antibody-dependent cellular cytotoxicity, natural killer cells, and lymphocyte-activated killer cells.[383]

433. What is the half-life of sirolimus?
a) 12 hours
b) 24 hours
c) 36 hours
d) 48 hours
e) 63 hours
**Answer: e**
Sirolimus has a half-life of 63 hours; however, because it has a shorter effective half-life, the drug reaches steady state in 7 days.[384]

434. Which of the following is not a commonly reported side effect of sirolimus?
a) Hyperlipidemia
b) Cytopenia
c) Impaired wound healing
d) Pneumonitis
e) Renal tubular dysfunction
**Answer: e**

Although mTOR inhibitors, including sirolimus, are not associated with renal tubular dysfunction, they are linked to a higher incidence of proteinuria. Other commonly reported side effects include hyperlipidemia, cytopenia, impaired wound healing, and pneumonitis.[385]

435. Which mechanism best explains how everolimus impairs wound healing?
a) Enhances fibroblast migration via overactivation of the α-1β-3 integrin pathway, disrupting normal tissue repair
b) Reduces type 1 collagen mRNA synthesis, critical for tissue tensile strength
c) Promotes excessive fibroblast apoptosis through downregulation of profibrotic growth factors
d) Inhibits TGF-β signaling, reducing fibroblast differentiation and collagen deposition
e) Upregulates PDGF receptor expression, leading to dysregulated fibroblast proliferation
**Answer: b**
Everolimus, an mTOR inhibitor, impairs wound healing by reducing type 1 collagen mRNA synthesis, which is essential for collagen production and wound strength. Additionally, mTOR inhibition decreases fibroblast proliferation and suppresses profibrotic growth factors, contributing to poor healing. For elective surgeries, switching from mTOR inhibitors to calcineurin inhibitors 2 weeks before and continuing for 4 weeks after surgery is recommended to optimize healing.[386–388]

436. Everolimus has the same mechanism of action as sirolimus but a different half-life. What is the half-life of everolimus?
a) 12 hours
b) 24 hours
c) 30 hours
d) 40 hours
e) 68 hours
**Answer: c**
Everolimus has a shorter half-life of approximately 30 hour.[389]

437. The mechanism of action of mycophenolic acid involves blocking de novo purine synthesis by inhibiting type 2 inosine monophosphate dehydrogenase (IMPDH), which is the rate-limiting enzyme in the production of which molecule?
a) Guanosine monophosphate
b) Adenosine monophosphate
c) Adenosine diphosphate
d) ATP

e) Inosine monophosphate
**Answer: a**
Mycophenolic acid inhibits de novo purine synthesis by blocking the activity of type 2 IMPDH, the rate-limiting enzyme in the production of guanosine monophosphate. This reduction in guanosine monophosphate decreases DNA synthesis and limits cellular replication, particularly in B and T lymphocytes, which lack hypoxanthine-guanine phosphoribosyltransferase, a critical enzyme in the purine salvage pathway, thus causing the cell cycle to remain in the S phase.[390]

438. What is the half-life of mycophenolate mofetil?
a) 6 hours
b) 10 hours
c) 17 hours
d) 20 hours
e) 24 hours
**Answer: c**
Mycophenolate mofetil is rapidly hydrolyzed in the stomach to mycophenolic acid with a bioavailability of 94%, but its absorption is reduced by food, necessitating administration before meals; it has a half-life of 17 hours and is converted to the inactive mycophenolate glucuronide in the liver before being excreted in urine.[391,392]

439. Which of the following is the most commonly reported side effect associated with the use of mycophenolate mofetil?
a) Nausea and diarrhea
b) Neutropenia
c) Hyperlipidemia
d) Hypertension
e) Headache and peripheral neuropathy
**Answer: a**
Gastrointestinal disturbances, particularly nausea, diarrhea, and abdominal pain, are the most common side effect of mycophenolate mofetil use.[393]

440. Given the associated risks, which of the following is an absolute contraindication to the use of mycophenolate mofetil?
a) Pregnancy
b) Active hepatitis C
c) Active cutaneous malignancy
d) Active smoking
e) Active alcohol intake

**Answer: a**
The use of mycophenolate mofetil during pregnancy is associated with an increased risk of first-trimester pregnancy loss and congenital malformations and is therefore contraindicated in pregnant women. The Food and Drug Administration recommends that women of childbearing potential prescribed mycophenolate mofetil receive contraceptive counseling and use effective contraception to prevent these adverse outcomes.[394]

441. What is the standard premedication regimen recommended prior to the administration of rabbit antithymocyte globulin (rATG) to prevent cytokine release syndrome?
a) Diphenhydramine, antipyretics (typically acetaminophen), and corticosteroids
b) Famotidine, antipyretics (typically acetaminophen), and corticosteroids
c) Diphenhydramine, famotidine, and corticosteroids
d) Antipyretics (typically acetaminophen) and corticosteroids
e) Diphenhydramine and corticosteroids
**Answer: a**
The standard premedication regimen involves administering an antihistamine (such as diphenhydramine), antipyretics (typically acetaminophen), and corticosteroids approximately one hour prior to the infusion of rATG to mitigate the risk of cytokine release syndrome.[395]

442. A 22-year-old female underwent a multivisceral transplant (liver/intestine/pancreas) and is receiving an immunosuppressive regimen consisting of rabbit antithymocyte globulin (rATG) induction (three doses), a steroid taper, mycophenolate mofetil, and tacrolimus. She initially recovered well; however, on postoperative day 8, she began to experience high fevers, persistent polyarthralgias, jaw pain, and an erythematous morbilliform rash, accompanied by worsening renal function. An infectious workup was negative, but high levels of rabbit IgG antibodies were present. What is the most appropriate treatment?
a) Rituximab and dialysis
b) High-dose steroids with plasmapheresis
c) High-dose steroids and eculizumab
d) Hold tacrolimus and MMF but maintain an increased steroid dose
e) Supportive therapy and observation
**Answer: b**
High-dose steroids combined with plasmapheresis is the most effective treatment in this scenario, as the symptoms and high levels of rabbit IgG antibodies suggest a severe immune reaction to the rATG induction, which can lead to a condition resembling acute serum sickness or other antibody-mediated reactions. Eculizumab

is a monoclonal antibody that inhibits complement activation and is used for conditions such as atypical hemolytic uremic syndrome or paroxysmal nocturnal hemoglobinuria.[395]

443. A 45-year-old man received alemtuzumab as an experimental therapy for recurrent liver allograft rejection unresponsive to high-dose steroids. Alemtuzumab depletes specific lymphocyte populations. Which statement best describes its mechanism of action?
a) Inhibits T-cell proliferation by blocking the IL-2 receptor
b) Binds to CD28 on T cells, preventing interaction with CD80/CD86 on APC, blocking Signal 2
c) Disrupts the JAK-STAT pathway, reducing lymphokine expression and T-cell activation
d) Induces apoptosis of CD52-expressing lymphocytes via complement-dependent cytotoxicity and antibody-dependent cellular cytotoxicity
e) Selectively activates regulatory T cells, suppressing the immune response against the transplant
**Answer: d**
Alemtuzumab, a humanized monoclonal antibody, targets the CD52 antigen on T and B lymphocytes, triggering their depletion through complement-dependent cytotoxicity and antibody-dependent cellular cytotoxicity. This reduces the lymphocyte population, suppressing the immune response in conditions like allograft rejection.[396]

444. Rituximab is a chimeric monoclonal antibody directed against which protein?
a) CD 2
b) CD 3
c) CD 19
d) CD 20
e) CD 21
**Answer: d**
CD 20 is a protein that is widely expressed on B cells during early differentiation but is not expressed on differentiated plasma cells. Of note, the half-life of rituximab gets longer after each administration because the B cells that would otherwise have been targets for rituximab have been depleted by earlier infusions.[397]

445. Basiliximab is a chimeric monoclonal antibody directed against which protein?
a) IFN-γ
b) CD20
c) IL-2R

d) TNF-α
e) CD4
**Answer:** c
Basiliximab (Simulect) is a chimeric monoclonal antibody that consists of both mouse and human components. It is specifically directed against the alpha chain of the IL-2R, also known as CD25, which is prominently expressed on the surface of activated T cells.[398]

446. What is the half-life of basiliximab?
a) 6 hours
b) 24 hours
c) 48 hours
d) 72 hours
e) 168 hours
**Answer:** e
Basiliximab has a half-life of 7 days, and the effects on the IL-2R persist for up to 3 to 4 weeks.[399]

447. Belatacept, a modified CTLA4-Ig fusion protein, binds to CD80/CD86 on antigen-presenting cells, blocking CD28-mediated T-cell costimulation. Due to its association with post-transplant lymphoproliferative disorder (PTLD), in which patient group should belatacept be avoided?
a) EBV-seronegative patients
b) EBV-seropositive patients
c) CMV IgG-seropositive patients
d) CMV IgG-seronegative patients
e) Hepatitis B core antibody-positive patients
**Answer:** a
Belatacept increases the risk of PTLD, particularly in EBV-seronegative patients, who are more susceptible to EBV-related complications. Its use is also contraindicated in patients receiving lymphocyte-depleting therapies due to heightened PTLD risk.[400]

448. A 6-year-old girl, who underwent liver transplantation at age 2 for biliary atresia, was exposed to a classmate with varicella (chickenpox). She received one dose of the varicella vaccine at 14 months and is currently on tacrolimus monotherapy with normal LFT and no symptoms. What is the recommended course of action following this exposure?
a) Administer varicella vaccine
b) Initiate IV acyclovir at 20 mg/kg
c) Initiate IV acyclovir at 20 mg/kg with steroids

d) Administer intramuscular varicella-zoster immune globulin (VZIG) immediately
e) Observe in an inpatient setting

**Answer: d**

In immunocompromised patients, such as this liver transplant recipient, exposure to varicella requires prompt administration of VZIG to provide passive immunity and reduce the risk of varicella infection. VZIG should be given intramuscularly at a dose of one vial per 10 kg of body weight within 96 hours of exposure.[401]

449. A 46-year-old female with a history of autoimmune hepatitis underwent liver transplantation four years ago. Since the transplant, she has experienced multiple episodes of rejection, the most recent of which occurred 8 months ago and was managed with high-dose corticosteroids. She is currently stable, with normalized LFT, and is maintained on immunosuppressive therapy including prednisone 5 mg daily, tacrolimus, and mycophenolate mofetil. She is planning to travel to Ethiopia to visit her family and seeks medical advice regarding the yellow fever vaccine. Which of the following is the most appropriate recommendation regarding yellow fever vaccination for this patient?
a) The yellow fever vaccine is safe and can be administered given the patient's stable liver function
b) The yellow fever vaccine should be administered since high-dose steroids were last used over six months ago
c) The yellow fever vaccine should be avoided, but an inactivated alternative can be considered for protection
d) The yellow fever vaccine is contraindicated due to the patient's immunosuppressed state; she should instead take strict mosquito bite precautions and may be eligible for a medical waiver for travel
e) The yellow fever vaccine may be administered with close monitoring for adverse effects during the initial 72 hours.

**Answer: d**

Live attenuated vaccines, such as the yellow fever vaccine, are contraindicated in immunocompromised individuals due to the increased risk of vaccine-associated complications. In this case, alternative protective strategies should be recommended, including rigorous mosquito avoidance measures and considering a waiver for travel if vaccination is required by entry regulations.[402]

450. A 6-year-old male patient who underwent liver transplantation 1 year ago for biliary atresia presents for a routine follow-up visit in October. He is currently being treated with prednisone 5 mg daily and tacrolimus. The patient is doing well overall and has resumed attending school. Which of the following vaccinations should be avoided at this time due to his immunocompromised status?

a) COVID-19 vaccine
b) Influenza vaccine
c) MMR vaccine (measles, mumps, rubella)
d) Hepatitis A vaccine
e) DTaP vaccine (diphtheria, tetanus, and pertussis)
Answer: c
The MMR vaccine is a live attenuated vaccine and is generally contraindicated in patients who are significantly immunocompromised, such as those on long-term immunosuppressive therapy following organ transplantation. Other vaccines (COVID-19, influenza, hepatitis A, and DTaP) are recommended and safe for immunocompromised patients.[402]

451. Which of the following is not a side effect of corticosteroid therapy?
a) Increased weight
b) Increased growth
c) Increased blood pressure
d) Increased blood glucose
e) Increased cholesterol
Answer: b
Corticosteroids, such as prednisone, are commonly used as part of immunosuppressive therapy following organ transplantation. Increased growth is not a typical side effect of corticosteroid therapy. In fact, long-term use is associated with growth inhibition in children due to its effects on bone metabolism and suppression of the hypothalamic-pituitary-adrenal axis. Additionally, corticosteroids can interfere with nocturnal growth hormone secretion.[403,404]

452. A 3-year-old girl with hepatoblastoma underwent a living donor liver transplant from her HLA-compatible mother. She previously received chemotherapy, with tumor shrinkage from 12 cm to 9 cm, and her last session was 3 months ago. Post-transplant labs show persistent cytopenia, with a total white blood cell (WBC) count of $0.69 \times 10^9/L$ and an absolute neutrophil count (ANC) of $0.16 \times 10^9/L$. What is the most appropriate immunosuppressive strategy?
a) Reduce immunosuppression to a single agent due to good HLA match in a living donor graft
b) Increase immunosuppression regardless of HLA status, given the high rejection rate in the pediatric population
c) Use standard triple therapy: steroids, mycophenolate mofetil, and tacrolimus
d) Withhold mycophenolate mofetil and reduce tacrolimus due to neutropenia
e) Omit steroid induction due to prior chemotherapy
Answer: d

Living donor grafts with good HLA compatibility do not guarantee a lower rejection rate in pediatric cases. Given this patient's significant neutropenia, reducing immunosuppression is prudent. Mycophenolate mofetil should be held, and tacrolimus levels lowered to reduce infection risk while maintaining some level of graft protection.[405]

453. A 34-year-old male who underwent a liver transplant due to alcohol-induced liver disease had an uncomplicated hospital course and was discharged home on postoperative day 10. During his discharge consultation, the patient inquired about the earliest manifestations of acute rejection of the transplanted liver that he should monitor. What should he be aware of as the earliest signs?
a) Asymptomatic biochemical changes, with subtle increases first observed in bilirubin, ALP, and GGT
b) Fatigue, fever, malaise, and abdominal pain, followed by a rise in AST and ALT
c) Fatigue, fever, malaise, jaundice, and elevated nonspecific inflammatory markers (IL-2, TNF-α) along with increased white blood cell
d) Simultaneous increases in AST, ALT, bilirubin, ALP, and GGT levels, associated with a gradual onset of abdominal pain and fatigue
e) Jaundice, anorexia, fever, and nonspecific increases in inflammatory markers with normal LFT and bilirubin
**Answer: a**
In the context of acute rejection of a transplanted liver, the earliest manifestations are frequently biochemical changes that occur before any clinical symptoms develop. These asymptomatic changes typically include subtle increases in laboratory values such as bilirubin, ALP, and GGT. These alterations indicate cholestatic inflammation that initially affects the biliary epithelium and subsequently the hepatocytes.[406]

454. A 38-year-old female underwent a liver transplant due to cryptogenic liver cirrhosis. The patient is negative for Hepatitis C (HCV), positive for EBV, and negative for CMV. The liver graft is negative for HCV, positive for EBV, and negative for CMV. The patient tolerated the surgery well and was discharged home with normalized laboratory results. During her outpatient clinic visit, the patient reports experiencing fatigue, and her blood work shows elevated levels of AST, ALT, bilirubin, and ALP. The tacrolimus trough level is 13 ng/mL; additionally, she is taking prednisone and mycophenolate mofetil. A liver ultrasound is normal, and the hepatic vessels are patent. A transjugular liver biopsy reveals a mixed cellular infiltrate predominantly consisting of lymphocytes localized to the portal tracts and central vein areas. What is the most appropriate course of action?
a) Increase tacrolimus dose and repeat blood work in one week

b) Admit the patient for inpatient care and initiate IV steroid boluses with close monitoring of liver function
c) Admit the patient for inpatient care and initiate plasmapheresis followed by rituximab
d) Admit the patient for inpatient care and initiate IV steroid boluses plus thymoglobulin
e) Admit the patient for inpatient care, lower the tacrolimus dose, hold steroids, and start ganciclovir therapy

**Answer: b**

In this case, the patient is exhibiting signs suggestive of acute rejection, which is indicated by the abnormal LFT and findings from the liver biopsy. The most appropriate management for acute rejection post-transplant, particularly if it is suspected to be cellular rejection rather than infection or other causes, is to administer high-dose IV steroids.[407]

455. A 44-year-old female patient with a history of autoimmune hepatitis underwent a successful liver transplant two years ago. Even though the transplant was successful, the patient has ongoing chronic rejection that is unresponsive to increased immunotherapy and steroid boluses. She is currently being admitted to the hospital with food intolerance, worsening jaundice, pruritus, and significantly abnormal LFT. A transjugular liver biopsy showed progressive ductopenia, characterized by a significant loss of small bile ducts. What is the most appropriate management strategy for this patient?
a) Increase the patient's tacrolimus dosage and initiate high-dose corticosteroids therapy
b) Initiate treatment with anti-thymocyte globulin to deplete T-cells and reduce cellular-mediated rejection
c) Perform biliary stent placement to relieve any potential obstruction and provide biliary drainage
d) Start a course of IV immunoglobulin therapy to modulate the immune response
e) Evaluate for retransplantation due to the poor prognosis associated with ongoing chronic rejection and ductopenia

**Answer: e**

In cases of chronic rejection characterized by progressive ductopenia and histological findings suggestive of "vanishing bile duct syndrome," the prognosis can be quite poor. In this scenario, the ongoing cellular-mediated injury to the bile ducts indicates that typical augmentations to immunosuppression may not be sufficient to reverse the damage, and increasing immunosuppression, given the potential for bacterial infection or even sepsis, is not appropriate. Retransplantation is often considered the most appropriate management strategy for patients experiencing severe chronic rejection.[408]

456. A 53-year-old female patient underwent a liver transplant for MASH. Initially, the patient recovered well; however, on postoperative day 12, she began to exhibit worsening transaminitis and increased bilirubin levels. The CT scan did not reveal any abnormalities with the liver graft. A liver biopsy showed endothelial cell hypertrophy, portal capillary dilation, microvasculitis characterized by the presence of monocytes, eosinophils, and neutrophils, and portal/peri-portal edema. Notably, the liver biopsy was positive for high intensity C4d staining in the graft, and circulating donor-specific antibody levels were elevated. What is the most appropriate management strategy for this patient?
a) Initiate high-dose corticosteroids
b) Start plasmapheresis followed by IV immunoglobulin
c) Administer rituximab
d) Administer eculizumab
e) Combination therapy with plasmapheresis, rituximab, and high-dose corticosteroids
**Answer: e**
In cases of antibody-mediated liver rejection, a multi-faceted treatment approach is often required, especially when there is evidence of severe endothelial cell injury and indications of ongoing humoral rejection. The combination therapy of plasmapheresis, rituximab, and high-dose corticosteroids targets the removal of circulating donor-specific antibodies, depletes B-cells to reduce further antibody production, and provides immediate anti-inflammatory effects.[409]

457. A 67-year-old male patient underwent a liver transplant for HCC measuring 6.2 cm, with underlying liver cirrhosis secondary to Hepatitis C. The patient received previous antiviral therapy, which resulted in viral clearance. The patient had an uneventful recovery and is currently 4 weeks post-transplant. The explant pathology showed a viable 6.2 cm HCC, but no other lesions. What is the most beneficial immunosuppressive regimen for this patient?
a) A combination of everolimus, low-dose tacrolimus, and a prednisone taper
b) A combination of mycophenolate mofetil (MMF) and prednisone
c) A triple therapy regimen with MMF, tacrolimus, and a prednisone taper
d) A triple therapy regimen with MMF, cyclosporine, and a prednisone taper
e) A triple therapy regimen with tacrolimus, everolimus, and MMF
**Answer: a**
In the context of HCC, particularly following liver transplantation with viable tumors, the use of everolimus is notable due to its immunosuppressive and potential

antitumor properties, especially concerning its antiangiogenic effects that inhibit tumor growth. Combining everolimus with low-dose tacrolimus allows for effective immunosuppression to protect the graft while minimizing the risk of recurrence associated with more potent agents.[410]

458. The immunomodulatory effect of belatacept operates by modulating which of the following signals of immune activation?
a) Signal 1
b) Signal 2
c) Signal 3
d) Signal 1 and 2
e) Signal 1, 2, and 3
**Answer: b**
Belatacept exerts its effects by blocking CTLA-4 interactions with CD80/CD86, thereby inhibiting the necessary costimulatory signaling provided by CD28 for T-cell activation. This mechanism of action results in the modulation of Signal 2, which is critical for T-cell activation and proliferation. While belatacept is currently utilized in kidney transplantation, it has been associated with an increased risk of death and graft loss in phase II clinical trial involving liver transplant recipients.[411]

459. Immunosuppressive agents can be broadly characterized as either small molecule inhibitors of intracellular pathways or biologic agents composed of larger protein molecules, such as polyclonal or monoclonal antibodies or fusion proteins, that target extracellular surface molecules. One such target molecule can be MHC class I, which is a group of cell surface receptors found on which of the following?
a) The cell surface of all nucleated cells, including red blood cells and platelets
b) The cell surface of all nucleated cells, excluding red blood cells and platelets
c) The cell surface of all nucleated cells and platelets, but not red blood cells
d) The cell surface of all nucleated cells and red blood cells, but not platelets
e) The cell surface of antigen-presenting cells, such as macrophages, B cells, and dendritic cells
**Answer: c**
MHC class I molecules are found on the cell surface of all nucleated cells and platelets, but not red blood cells.[412]

460. Among the various complications associated with transplantation, post-transplant lymphoproliferative disorder (PTLD) is a significant concern. PTLD comprises a spectrum of lymphoid malignancies that differ from lymphomas seen in immunocompetent individuals. It often presents outside of lymph nodes and may

demonstrate rapid onset and regression. Which patient population is at highest risk for developing PTLD?
a) EBV-seronegative recipients of an EBV-seropositive organ
b) EBV-seropositive recipients of an EBV-seropositive organ
c) EBV-seronegative recipients of an EBV-seronegative organ
d) EBV-seropositive, CMV-seropositive recipients
e) HIV-seropositive recipients of an HIV-seropositive organ

**Answer: a**

EBV-seronegative recipients who receive an organ from an EBV-seropositive donor are at the greatest risk for PTLD. Immunosuppressive therapy can impair the recipient's ability to control primary EBV infection, leading to unchecked B-cell proliferation and the development of PTLD.[413]

461. A 56-year-old male patient who underwent a combined heart-liver transplant for amyloidosis 2 years ago presents with malaise, fever, enlarged lymph nodes, and weight loss. The patient is EBV-positive and CMV-positive and received organs from EBV-negative and CMV-negative donors. He tolerated the procedure well; however, he experienced an episode of heart rejection 4 months ago that was resistant to high-dose steroid therapy, necessitating treatment with thymoglobulin. Laboratory findings reveal elevated LDH and EBV viremia. A lymph node biopsy indicated increased proliferation of small polytypic lymphocytes and plasma cells while preserving overall structural architecture. What is the most appropriate initial treatment?
a) Initiate IV steroids and antiviral therapy
b) Decrease immunosuppression to a minimum and initiate antiviral therapy
c) Initiate IV steroids and rituximab
d) Initiate CHOP (cyclophosphamide, hydroxydaunomycin, oncovin, and prednisone) therapy
e) Initiate antiviral therapy with close monitoring

**Answer: b**

It appears that the patient has developed posttransplantation lymphoproliferative disorder. The primary treatment involves reducing immunosuppression to enable the patient's immune response against EBV, along with initiating antiviral therapy such as ganciclovir. If the response is insufficient, additional therapies such as chemotherapy or radiation may be considered later.[413]

462. What is the best explanation for how prolonged warm ischemia and graft damage affect the immune response in liver transplantation?
a) Less rejection due to suppressed antigen presentation
b) Less rejection due to activation of only the innate immune system
c) More rejection due to increased co-stimulatory molecule expression

d) Less rejection due to immune exhaustion and T cell silencing
e) No impact on current or future rejection risk
**Answer: c**
Prolonged warm ischemia leads to tissue injury and stress, which trigger the upregulation of co-stimulatory molecules on antigen-presenting cells. This amplifies T cell activation and increases the risk of rejection.[414]

463. MHC class II is expressed on which of the following cells?
a) All nucleated cells, including platelets and red blood cells
b) All nucleated cells except platelets and red blood cells
c) All nucleated cells and red blood cells, except platelets
d) All nucleated cells and platelets, except red blood cells
e) Macrophages, dendritic cells, and B cells
**Answer: e**
MHC class II is a surface molecule expressed on antigen-presenting cells, which include macrophages, dendritic cells, and B cells.[415]

464. Possible scenarios for allosensitization include all of the following, except:
a) Pregnancy
b) Penetrating trauma
c) Previous liver transplant
d) Previous kidney transplant
e) Red blood cell transfusion
**Answer: b**
Penetrating trauma, by itself, will not cause allosensitization.[415]

465. What is the primary location of T cell activation by alloantigens?
a) Allograft
b) Bone marrow
c) Lymph nodes and spleen
d) Bloodstream and spleen
e) Bloodstream and allograft
**Answer: c**
Research indicates that donor APCs, particularly dendritic cells, are crucial for initiating an immune response against transplanted grafts, with initial activation occurring in the recipient's secondary lymphoid organs. The absence of these organs prevents T-cell activation and graft rejection, and adequate costimulatory signals are necessary for fully activating alloreactive T cells.[416]

# 12. Machine Perfusion

466. A procurement surgeon presents for organ recovery using OCS technology. The OCS liver system is primed with all of the following except:
a) Buffered electrolyte solution
b) Albumin
c) Five units of PRBC
d) Broad-spectrum antibiotics
e) Methylprednisolone
**Answer: e**
The OCS liver system is designed to preserve organs during transport and facilitate viability prior to transplantation. Methylprednisolone, a corticosteroid, is not a standard component used in the priming of the OCS liver system. However, 160 mg of methylprednisolone is added per 1 L of PlasmaLyte that is used for pre-OCS and post-OCS flush.[417]

467. A procurement surgeon presents for organ recovery using OCS technology. For the OCS liver instrumentation, which of the following is not cannulated?
a) Infrahepatic IVC
b) Suprahepatic IVC
c) Hepatic artery
d) Portal vein
e) Bile duct
**Answer: a**
In the context of liver transplantation using the OCS, the infrahepatic IVC is typically not cannulated, as the system functions as an open circuit. Blood enters the liver through the portal and arterial cannulas, exits via the open infrahepatic IVC, is collected in a chamber, and then recirculated.[417]

468. Which of the following correctly lists the main OCS liver infusion solutions?
a) TPN combined with insulin and 40,000 IU heparin, bile salts, and epoprostenol sodium
b) TPN combined with insulin and 40,000 IU heparin, bile salts, and bicarbonate
c) TPN combined with insulin and 40,000 IU heparin, bile salts, bicarbonate, and epoprostenol sodium
d) TPN combined with insulin, bicarbonate, and bile acids
e) TPN combined with insulin, bicarbonate, bile acids, and epoprostenol sodium
**Answer: a**

In the context of organ preservation using the OCS for liver transplantation, the correct infusion solutions include TPN combined with insulin, heparin, bile salts, and epoprostenol sodium. These components work together to maintain the liver's metabolic function and protect it during the organ recovery and transport process.[417]

469. What is the gas composition utilized in the OCS for liver?
a) 20% oxygen, 1% nitrogen, 2% CO2
b) 80% oxygen, 1% nitrogen, 2% CO2
c) 80% oxygen, balanced nitrogen, 0.1% CO2
d) 20% oxygen, balanced nitrogen, 2% CO2
e) 40% oxygen, 1% nitrogen, 0.1% CO2
Answer: c
The OCS utilizes a specific gas composition to ensure optimal physiological conditions for the preserved organ. The correct composition consists of 80% oxygen, with a balanced amount of nitrogen and a low concentration of carbon dioxide (0.1%).[417]

470. What are the recommended perfusion parameters for a liver graft using OCS technology in terms of portal vein flow (PVF) and hepatic artery flow (HAF), as well as the optimal PVF-to-HAF flow ratio for a standard liver weighing 1500 g?
a) 500 – 700 mL/min, 500 – 700 mL/min, 1:1
b) 700 – 1000 mL/min, 350 – 700 mL/min, 2:1
c) 1200 – 1400 mL/min, 350 – 550 mL/min, 2:1
d) 1500 – 1800 mL/min, 500 – 600 mL/min, 3:1
e) 1800 – 2100 mL/min, 300 – 350 mL/min, 6:1
Answer: c
The OCS emphasizes specific perfusion parameters to maintain liver viability during transport and preservation. For a standard liver weighing 1500 g, the recommended PVF is between 1200 and 1400 mL/min, and the HAF is between 350 and 550 mL/min, with an optimal flow ratio of 2:1 (PVF to HAF). This flow ratio helps ensure adequate perfusion and metabolic support for the liver. It is important to note that, based on liver size, the PVF can range from 700 to 1700 mL/min, and the HAF can range from 350 to 900 mL/min; however, the 2:1 ratio should remain consistent.[417]

471. What are the recommended mean perfusion pressure parameters for the portal vein and hepatic artery when using OCS technology for a liver graft?
a) <5 mmHg, <25 mmHg
b) <5 mmHg, <45 mmHg
c) <10 mmHg, <45 mmHg

d) <10 mmHg, 45 – 100 mmHg
e) 10 – 14 mmHg, >45 mmHg
**Answer: d**
For liver preservation using the OCS, the recommended mean portal vein pressure should be less than 10 mmHg, whereas the mean hepatic artery pressure should be maintained between 45 and 100 mmHg.[417]

472. What is the optimal temperature for a liver graft on the OCS while being perfused?
a) 30 °C
b) 32 °C
c) 34 °C
d) 36 °C
e) 40 °C
**Answer: c**
The optimal temperature for maintaining liver viability during perfusion with the OCS is 34°C.[417]

473. During the liver perfusion and stabilization phase on the OCS, the initial pump flow should begin at 1 L/min and gradually increase to the target rate. What is the target pump flow rate, and within what time frame should it be achieved for a standard-sized liver?
a) 1.5 L/min flow rate within the first 5 minutes
b) 2 L/min flow rate within the first 5 minutes
c) 1.6 – 2 L/min flow rate over the first 15 – 20 minutes
d) 2.5 L/min flow rate after 20 minutes
e) 2.5 – 3 L/min flow rate after 1 hour
**Answer: c**
The goal pump flow rate, defined as the sum of portal vein flow (PVF) and hepatic artery flow (HAF), for a standard-sized liver during the OCS liver perfusion should be between 1.6 and 2 L/min, this goal should be achieved within the initial 15 to 20 minutes.[417]

474. A procurement surgeon presents for organ recovery using OCS technology. As the surgeon places a standard-sized liver on the machine, he confirms that the cannula is well-positioned and that there are no kinks. After 25 minutes, the system warms up to 34 °C, with a total pump flow rate of 1.8 L/min, a portal vein flow (PVF) rate of 1.5 L/min, and a hepatic artery flow (HAF) rate of 0.3 L/min. The mean portal vein pressure (PVP) is below 4 mmHg, and the MAP is 25 mmHg. What should be done next?

a) Wait 5 minutes and draw the first blood sample
b) Increase the total pump flow rate to 2 L/min
c) Rotate the portal vein clamp anti-clockwise, thereby loosening the portal vein cannula
d) Rotate the portal vein clamp clockwise, thereby tightening the portal vein cannula
e) Initiate epoprostenol sodium infusion
Answer: d
While the total pump flow rate of 1.8 L/min is adequate for this standard-sized liver, the PVF rate is excessively high at 1.5 L/min, whereas the HAF rate is too low at 0.3 L/min. This imbalance is reflected in the decreased arterial flow rate compared to the portal vein and the low mean arterial pressure. If the MAP were elevated, initiating epoprostenol sodium infusion might have been an appropriate option. However, in this case, the surgeon should rotate the portal vein clamp clockwise to tighten the portal vein cannula.[417]

475. A procurement surgeon is recovering a liver using OCS technology. Upon initial placement of the standard-sized liver on the machine, the total flow rate gradually increases to 1.31 L/min. However, while the MAP rises to 75 mmHg, the hepatic artery flow remains low at 0.11 L/min. In contrast, the portal vein flow increases to 1.2 L/min, with mean portal vein pressure remaining low at 4 mmHg. What should be the next step?
a) Check for kinks or twists in the hepatic artery
b) Wait until the liver warms up to 34 °C
c) Initiate epoprostenol sodium infusion
d) Rotate the portal vein clamp anti-clockwise, thereby loosening the portal vein cannula
e) Look for air embolism
Answer: a
The first step should be to check for kink or twist in the hepatic artery and assess the position of the cannula. Given the presentation of increased arterial pressure without a corresponding increase in arterial flow, it is inappropriate to wait for the liver to warm up to troubleshoot the problem. The surgeon must prioritize avoiding any further damage to the artery. If there is no kink or twist present, a thorough examination of the artery should be conducted to identify any potential complications such as dissection, spasm, or air embolism.[417]

476. A procurement surgeon is recovering a liver using OCS technology. She procures a large liver weighing 3.5 kg, type 1 anatomy, and places it on the machine. The surgeon confirms that the cannula is well-positioned and there are no kinks. After 55 minutes, the system has warmed up to 34°C, with a total pump flow rate of 1.75

L/min, a portal vein flow rate of 1.20 L/min, and a hepatic artery flow rate of 0.55 L/min. The mean portal vein pressure is below 4 mmHg, and the MAP is 55 mmHg. However, repeat lactate levels continue to trend upward from 7.63 mmol/L to 7.84 mmol/L, with the last reading at 8.1 mmol/L. What should be done next?
a) Rotate the portal vein clamp anti-clockwise, thereby loosening the portal vein cannula
b) Rotate the portal vein clamp clockwise, thereby tightening the portal vein cannula
c) Initiate epoprostenol sodium infusion
d) Increase total flow rate
e) Change the target temperature setting to 36°C
**Answer: d**
This liver is large, weighing 3.5 kg, necessitating a higher than usual flow rate to effectively clear rising lactate levels. Increasing the total flow rate will enhance perfusion and facilitate better metabolic function, thereby helping to manage the elevated lactate levels indicated in the scenario.[417]

477. A procurement surgeon is recovering a liver using OCS technology. The surgeon places a standard-sized liver on the machine. After 20 minutes, the system warms up to 34°C, with a total pump flow rate of 1.4 L/min, a portal vein flow rate of 0.8 L/min, and a hepatic artery flow rate of 0.6 L/min. The mean portal vein pressure is 14 mmHg, and the MAP is 50 mmHg. What should be done next?
a) Rotate the portal vein clamp anti-clockwise, thereby loosening the portal vein cannula
b) Rotate the portal vein clamp clockwise, thereby tightening the portal vein cannula
c) Check for twist or kink in the portal vein as well as the cannula position
d) Increase the total flow rate
e) Measurements are satisfactory; draw the first blood sample
**Answer: c**
The observed portal vein pressure is elevated at 14 mmHg, which may indicate compression of the portal vein by the caudate lobe or improper cannula positioning. Given that the portal vein pressure is already high, further increasing the total pump flow is unlikely to improve perfusion. The hepatic artery appears to be adequately perfused with a good flow rate and is near the upper limit of mean arterial pressure. Tightening the portal vein clamp will further increase arterial pressure, putting stress on the artery and decreasing portal flow. While loosening the portal vein clamp may enhance flow, it could also further elevate portal vein pressure. Therefore, the first step should be to check for any twists or kinks in the portal vein and to confirm the proper positioning of the cannula to directly address the underlying issues.[417]

478. A procurement surgeon is recovering a liver using OCS technology. She procures a standard-sized liver with a truly replaced left hepatic artery and a relatively small main hepatic artery. The surgeon performs a backtable trim and places the liver on the OCS machine, confirming that the cannula is properly positioned. After 15 minutes, the system has warmed to 34°C, with a total pump flow rate of 1.7 L/min, a portal vein flow rate of 1.45 L/min, and a hepatic artery flow rate of 0.25 L/min. The mean portal vein pressure is measured at below 4 mmHg, and the MAP is 60 mmHg. The hepatic artery appears small with no kinks or twists. What should be done next?
a) Rotate the portal vein clamp anti-clockwise to loosen the portal vein cannula
b) Rotate the portal vein clamp clockwise to tighten the portal vein cannula
c) Initiate epoprostenol sodium infusion
d) Increase the total flow rate
e) Measurements are satisfactory; draw the first blood sample
**Answer: c**
Initiating an epoprostenol sodium infusion is the appropriate step in this scenario because epoprostenol is a potent vasodilator that can enhance hepatic artery blood flow without increasing hepatic artery pressure. Given that the hepatic artery flow rate is relatively low at 0.25 L/min, administering epoprostenol can help improve perfusion and increase arterial flow to the liver.[417]

479. A procurement surgeon is recovering a liver using OCS technology. The procurement process proceeds without incident, and the liver exhibits normal anatomy. The surgeon performs biopsies of the right and left lobes per the request of the accepting center. The surgeon then places the liver on the OCS machine, confirming that the cannula is correctly positioned and that there are no kinks in the system. After 30 minutes, the system has warmed to 34°C, portal and arterial flow rates, as well as pressure readings, remain within normal range; however, there is increased bleeding from the bile duct, with the bile cannula having already drained 200 ml of predominantly bloody fluid. Lactate levels are trending downwards. How should the team proceed?
a) Coagulate the biopsy site with electrocautery
b) Apply pressure to the biopsy site for 20 minutes
c) Suture the biopsy site with a 2-0 Vicryl stitch
d) Allow the bile duct cannula to drain into the main machine chamber
e) All measurements are satisfactory; the liver is ready for transportation
**Answer: d**
The bleeding observed from the bile duct suggests potential injury during the biopsy, raising concerns about hemobilia. Because the organ is on the machine and there is a high concentration of circulating heparin, intervention options are limited. In cases

of significant internal bleeding from the liver, the bile duct cannula should be positioned to allow drainage of both blood and bile into the machine chamber. Typically, the bleeding subsides following the flushing of the liver.[417]

480. A procurement surgeon presents for organ recovery utilizing OCS technology for a pediatric donor. The procurement process proceeds without incident, and the liver exhibits normal anatomy characteristic of a pediatric patient with small vessels. The surgeon successfully cannulates the proximal aorta for arterial inflow and oversees the distal end of the vessel. However, the portal vein appears small, measuring only 5 mm in diameter, and the portal vein cannula does not fit the vessel. How should the surgeon proceed?
a) This liver is too small for OCS technology; proceed with SCS
b) Proceed with cannulation of the artery and IVC only, omitting the portal vein
c) Use donor iliac vessels as an extension graft from the portal vein and connect it to the cannula
d) Use an 8Fr pediatric tube to cannulate the portal vein
e) Consider using a specialized pediatric portal vein cannula designed for smaller vessels

**Answer: c**
In the case of very small livers, such as those from pediatric donors, an extension graft may be necessary to connect the portal vein to the OCS machine. This approach allows for the continued utilization of the liver with OCS. It is important to note that standard pediatric feeding tubes are not compatible with the OCS machine for this specific connection. There is no specialized pediatric portal vein cannula designed for smaller vessels currently available.[417]

481. A procurement surgeon presents for organ recovery utilizing OCS technology from an older donor, a 68-year-old male with a history of hypertension and smoking. The procurement process proceeds without incident, and the liver exhibits normal anatomy. The surgeon successfully cannulates the vessels and places the organ on the machine. After 10 minutes, the system has warmed to 31°C, with a total pump flow rate of 1.4 L/min, a portal vein flow rate of 1.3 L/min, and a hepatic artery flow rate of 0.1 L/min. The mean portal vein pressure is measured at below 4 mmHg, while the MAP is 15 mmHg. The hepatic artery appears bluish. What should be done next?
a) Slowly increase the total flow rate
b) Wait until the liver warms up to 34°C
c) Initiate epoprostenol sodium infusion
d) Disconnect the artery from the pump and examine for arterial dissection
e) Look for air embolism

**Answer: d**

Although the temperature has not yet reached the target of 34°C, the bluish discoloration of the hepatic artery is concerning for arterial dissection. If arterial dissection is indeed present, increasing the flow rate may exacerbate the condition. Immediate action should be taken; it is inappropriate to wait. The artery must be examined, and if dissection is confirmed, the extent of the dissection should be evaluated. The liver may still be salvageable.[417]

482. A procurement surgeon is recovering a liver using OCS technology. During the procedure, the surgeon identifies a replaced/accessory right hepatic artery originating from the superior mesenteric artery (SMA) and a replaced/accessory left hepatic artery originating directly from the aorta. During backtable preparation, irrigation through the main hepatic artery yields significant backflow from the accessory left hepatic artery, with no backflow noted from the replaced right hepatic artery. What is the most optimal option for backtable reconstruction?
a) Perform an end-to-end reconstruction of the accessory left hepatic artery to the splenic artery, an end-to-end reconstruction of the gastroduodenal artery to the replaced right hepatic artery, and cannulate the celiac trunk
b) Perform an end-to-end reconstruction of the accessory left hepatic artery to the splenic artery, a sandwich reconstruction between the SMA and the celiac trunk, and cannulate the distal SMA
c) Perform an end-to-end reconstruction of the accessory left hepatic artery to the splenic artery, an end-to-end reconstruction between the proximal SMA and the celiac trunk, and cannulate the distal SMA
d) Perform an end-to-end reconstruction of the left hepatic artery to the splenic artery, ligate the replaced right hepatic artery, and cannulate the celiac trunk
e) Ligate the accessory left hepatic artery, perform a sandwich reconstruction between the SMA and the celiac trunk, and cannulate the distal SMA
**Answer: e**
The arterial anatomy of this liver is consistent with the presence of an accessory left hepatic artery, as evidenced by backflow from the vessel and the identification of a truly replaced right hepatic artery. To minimize the complexity of arterial reconstructions and reduce backtable time, ligation of the accessory left hepatic artery is an appropriate strategy in this scenario. However, it is essential to reconstruct the truly replaced right hepatic artery, which can be achieved through various surgical methods.[418]

483. A procurement surgeon is preparing for organ recovery using OCS technology for a pediatric donor. The procurement proceeds without incident, and the liver exhibits normal anatomical characteristics common to pediatric patients, including smaller vessels. The surgeon aims to cannulate the proximal aorta for arterial inflow

but discovers an arterial dissection within the main aorta. The surgeon divides the celiac trunk at the aortic takeoff, and while the vessels appear intact, their length is insufficient for cannulation. How should the surgeon proceed?
a) This liver is no longer suitable for OCS technology; therefore, proceed with SCS
b) Utilize the donor iliac vein due to its extensibility as an extension graft to connect to the cannula
c) Use the donor iliac artery as an extension graft to connect to the cannula
d) Employ a synthetic graft to establish a connection between the celiac trunk and the cannula for arterial inflow
e) Proceed with cannulation of the IVC and portal vein only, omitting arterial cannulation altogether

**Answer: c**

In cases where a pediatric liver is placed on OCS and the main aorta is not available for cannulation for various reasons, it is still possible to utilize extension grafts from the celiac trunk to facilitate connection to the cannula. The ideal conduit material is donor iliac arteries.[417]

484. Which of the following statements best reflects the expected advantages of the OCS compared to SCS in liver transplantation?
a) Although OCS reduces ischemic injury, it has no impact on the incidence of early allograft dysfunction
b) OCS decreases histologic signs of ischemia-reperfusion injury and lobular inflammation but does not improve hemodynamic stability during reperfusion
c) OCS reduces ischemic injury and is associated with improved short-term and midterm transplant outcomes
d) OCS improves reperfusion stability but has no effect on patient or graft survival
e) While OCS reduces ischemic injury, it does not influence ICU or hospital length of stay

**Answer: c**

A randomized controlled trial demonstrated that the use of OCS significantly reduces ischemic injury and is associated with better short- and midterm outcomes in liver transplantation. By preserving the liver in normothermic conditions, OCS improves graft viability and reduces complications such as early allograft dysfunction.[417]

485. A 59-year-old male with a history of obesity and mild liver steatosis is evaluated for organ donation following a massive stroke. His donor profile indicates characteristics associated with an increased risk of early allograft dysfunction, primary nonfunction, and ischemic biliary complications. His liver is considered for transplantation using the OCS. Which of the following statements most accurately reflects the advantages of utilizing the OCS for this donor?

a) This donor poses a high risk for complications and should not be utilized, even with OCS technology
b) OCS liver perfusion significantly increases the transplantation of marginal liver grafts, enabling greater utilization of donor organs
c) OCS perfusion primarily benefits liver grafts from DBD donors by eliminating concerns about prolonged cold ischemia time
d) OCS increases the availability of grafts in the region and reduces the need for organ retrieval teams to travel long distances
e) OCS does not improve clinical outcomes for DCD grafts compared to traditional organ preservation methods

**Answer: b**

Findings from a randomized controlled trial demonstrate that OCS technology significantly enhances the utilization of DCD donors, particularly those considered marginal due to factors such as advanced age or moderate steatosis. By facilitating ex vivo clinical optimization and assessment of these livers, OCS improves graft viability evaluation, leading to a higher rate of successful transplantation compared to SCS.[417]

486. A transplant team is comparing liver perfusion devices for organ preservation in transplantation. They are particularly interested in the OrganOx metra liver perfusion device and how it differs from the OCS by Tranmedics. Which of the following statements accurately characterizes the OrganOx device in comparison to the OCS Liver?
a) The OrganOx operates as a closed-circuit system
b) It maintains a temperature of 32°C during perfusion
c) The device does not utilize supplementary oxygen
d) Heparin is not used in the perfusion process
e) The machine is lighter and more transportable than the OCS

**Answer: a**

The OrganOx metra liver perfusion device functions as a closed-circuit system, providing automated pumping, oxygen delivery, and heat exchange to maintain the perfusate at physiological conditions. While it keeps the liver at normal temperature (37°C) and regulates parameters such as pO2, pCO2, and pH. It is notably larger and less transportable than the OCS. The device continuously monitors hemodynamic parameters and bile production, while also infusing essential substances like bile salts, insulin, heparin and glucose to support liver function during preservation.[419]

487. A procurement surgeon is preparing for liver graft recovery using the OrganOx metra liver perfusion device. As he procures the liver and conducts the backtable

preparation, he connects the organ to the machine. What are the optimal parameters for perfusion during this process?
a) Hepatic artery pressure of 20 to 25 mmHg; IVC pressure of 0 to 2 mmHg
b) Hepatic artery pressure of 40 to 45 mmHg; IVC pressure of 2 to 6 mmHg
c) Hepatic artery pressure of 60 to 75 mmHg; IVC pressure of −1 to 2 mmHg
d) Hepatic artery pressure of 80 to 95 mmHg; IVC pressure of −1 to 2 mmHg
e) Hepatic artery pressure of 40 to 45 mmHg; IVC pressure of −1 to 2 mmHg
Answer: c
The optimal parameters for perfusion using the OrganOx metra liver perfusion device include maintaining a hepatic artery pressure between 60 to 75 mmHg and an IVC pressure between −1 to 2 mmHg.[419]

488. Based on a recent randomized controlled trial assessing the OrganOx normothermic preservation technology in liver transplantation, which of the following statements best summarizes the implications of using this technology?
a) OrganOx was not superior to SCS in terms of peak AST levels and acute early dysfunction
b) OrganOx is linked to a significantly higher rate of bile duct complications while improving graft survival
c) OrganOx leads to a significant reduction in graft injury and a lower rate of organ discards, with extended preservation time
d) OrganOx improves both graft and patient survival
e) OrganOx increases the mean preservation time, consequently resulting in higher rates of graft loss and complications
Answer: c
The recent randomized controlled trial demonstrated that the use of OrganOx significantly reduces graft injury levels and lowers the rate of organ discards while extending preservation time. Importantly, this extended preservation did not pose additional risks to either patient or graft survival.[420]

489. Based on a recent randomized controlled trial evaluating OrganOx preservation technology in liver transplantation, which statement best summarizes its implications?
a) OrganOx reduces histological markers of ischemia-reperfusion injury but does not significantly improve reperfusion syndrome stability
b) OrganOx prevents hepatic ischemic injury and reduces ICU and hospital stay durations
c) OrganOx decreases hemodynamic instability post-reperfusion, reducing the need for renal replacement therapy
d) OrganOx demonstrates superior hemodynamic characteristics post-reperfusion compared to SCS

e) OrganOx improves long-term graft function and reduces acute rejection rates compared to SCS
**Answer: d**
The trial showed that OrganOx provides superior hemodynamic stability post-reperfusion compared to SCS. However, this did not significantly reduce ICU or hospital stay durations or the need for renal replacement therapy. While OrganOx reduces graft injury during preservation, it lacks definitive evidence of improved long-term graft function or reduced acute rejection rates.[420]

490. A procurement surgeon presents for liver graft recovery utilizing hypothermic oxygenated perfusion (HOPE) technology. Upon placing the liver graft on the HOPE system, the graft is cannulated for perfusion. In this context, which anatomical structure is primarily utilized for the perfusion of the liver graft?
a) Suprahepatic IVC
b) Infrahepatic IVC
c) Portal vein
d) Hepatic artery
e) Portal vein and hepatic artery
**Answer: c**
In the HOPE methodology, the liver graft is typically perfused through the portal vein only. However, in dual hypothermic oxygenated perfusion (D-HOPE), both the hepatic artery and the portal vein are cannulated.[421]

491. What is the temperature used for liver preservation with hypothermic oxygenated perfusion (HOPE) technology?
a) 4°C
b) 10°C
c) 15°C
d) 20°C
**Answer: b**
In HOPE, the perfusate is cooled to approximately 10°C, optimizing metabolic suppression while preserving cellular viability.[421]

492. When preserving a liver graft using hypothermic oxygenated perfusion (HOPE) with a perfusion flow rate of 0.1 to 0.15 mL/min/g of liver weight, what is the appropriate pressure control for perfusion?
a) < 1 mmHg
b) < 3 mmHg
c) < 7 mmHg
d) < 10 mmHg

e) < 15 mmHg
**Answer: b**
In HOPE, the perfusion flow rate is maintained at 0.1 to 0.15 mL/min/g of liver weight under a pressure control of less than 3 mmHg. This low pressure ensures gentle and effective perfusion. For a 1.5 kg liver, typical flow rates range from 150 to 225 mL/min. Continuous monitoring is essential, and perfusion must be stopped immediately if the flow exceeds 400 mL/min to protect graft integrity.[421]

493. Based on the results of a randomized controlled trial, what is the most accurate expectation regarding the use of hypothermic oxygenated perfusion (HOPE) technology for DBD livers?
a) HOPE significantly improves one-year patient survival rates
b) HOPE significantly reduces the incidence of grade ≥III complications compared to SCS
c) HOPE significantly improves post-transplantation laboratory values compared to SCS
d) HOPE does not significantly improve patient outcomes compared to SCS
e) HOPE significantly reduces ICU and hospital stay durations compared to SCS
**Answer: d**
The trial demonstrated that HOPE for DBD livers does not significantly improve key patient outcomes, including survival rates, severe complication rates, laboratory values, or ICU and hospital stay durations, compared to SCS. Thus, HOPE does not offer a clear advantage over SCS for DBD livers based on the evaluated endpoints.[421]

494. Experimental studies show that hypothermic oxygenated perfusion (HOPE) enhances liver graft preservation through adequate perfusate oxygenation under hypothermic conditions. Which of the following is not a benefit of HOPE?
a) Promotes mitochondrial metabolic shift, reducing accumulated citric acid cycle intermediates
b) Facilitates mitochondrial metabolic conversion, decreasing electron donors like succinate and NADH
c) Preserves mitochondrial ATP production with minimal oxidative stress, maintaining low lactate and succinate levels and intact complex I-IV function
d) The benefits of HOPE are expected to enhance as the degree of graft injury increases
e) Reduces mitochondrial metabolic activity, conserving electron donors such as succinate and NADH
**Answer: e**

HOPE supports mitochondrial metabolic improvements, enabling efficient ATP production while minimizing oxidative stress and harmful metabolite accumulation. Its benefits are most significant in grafts with greater injury, promoting immediate function and recovery post-transplantation. However, HOPE does not reduce mitochondrial metabolic activity to conserve electron donors, as this contradicts its mechanism.[421]

495. A 42-year-old male with end-stage liver disease secondary to autoimmune hepatitis successfully receives a liver transplant from a DBD donor. The liver was stored using the hypothermic oxygenated perfusion (HOPE) preservation method. Which of the following statements is correct?
a) The risk of anastomotic biliary complications is decreased in the HOPE compared to SCS
b) The risk of anastomotic biliary complications is decreased in the dual HOPE (D-HOPE), but not in the HOPE preservation method
c) The risk of anastomotic biliary complications is not reduced in either the HOPE or D-HOPE compared to SCS
d) HOPE is capable of protecting the extrahepatic bile duct epithelium, including the common bile duct, from ischemic injury
e) The hypothermic oxygenated perfusion significantly improves overall graft survival rates

**Answer: c**

Despite the known biochemical advantages of HOPE liver treatment, it has not succeeded in preventing anastomotic biliary complications, such as IIIa complications, even when implemented via the hepatic artery through the D-HOPE method. The protection of the extrahepatic bile duct epithelium, including the common bile duct, proves to be more challenging compared to intrahepatic cholangiocytes and hepatocytes.[421]

# 13. Liver Transplant Survival and Results

496. What are the current five-year survival rates for liver transplantation in adults and children in the U.S.?
a) 52% and 76%
b) 76% for both
c) 90% and 76%
d) 76% and 90%
e) 96% for both
**Answer: d**
Five-year survival rates for liver transplantation now approach 76% for adults and 90% for children, reflecting continued improvement in graft survival despite changing recipient characteristics, such as older age and higher rates of obesity.[422]

497. Given the worse long-term outcomes for older patients receiving liver transplants, what is the specific age cutoff based on the UNOS Ethics Committee recommendation?
a) 70 years
b) 75 years
c) 80 years
d) 85 years
e) No specific age cutoff
**Answer: e**
The UNOS Ethics Committee does not endorse a specific age cutoff when selecting transplant candidates. However, the committee has previously emphasized that a candidate's age should be considered as a selection factor to ensure that the recipient's life expectancy is not significantly shorter than the expected lifespan of the transplanted organ.[423]

498. Based on recent data, what percentage of patients aged 18–65 return to work within 2 years after a liver transplant?
a) 20%
b) 34%
c) 50%
d) 65%
e) 80%
**Answer: b**

Valeria Ripa, MD and Fady M. Kaldas, MD

According to a study of 35,340 liver transplant recipients aged 18–65 from 2010–2018, 34.2% were employed within 2 years post-transplant. This includes 70.4% of those working pre-transplant and 18.2% of those not working pre-transplant.[424]

499. A 45-year-old male patient with a history of cirrhosis due to hepatitis B underwent a liver transplant 18 months ago. Prior to the transplant, he was full-time employed as a software engineer but had to stop working 6 months before the procedure due to declining health. He has a college degree, reports good functional status post-transplant, and is motivated to return to work. All of the following factors are associated with a higher probability of returning to employment except:
a) Younger age
b) Male sex
c) College degree
d) Employment before transplant
e) Local job conditions
**Answer: e**
Overall employment post-liver transplant has improved, and 70% of recipients with employment pre-transplant returned to work within 2 years. New employment among recipients not working before transplant is much less common, however. The factors associated with returning to employment include younger age, male sex, greater educational attainment, and prior employment before transplant. Local job conditions are also likely important, and changes in the job landscape as a result of the COVID-19 pandemic and the rise in remote work may impact transplant recipients as well; however, current data are lacking.[424]

500. With advancements in transplantation techniques and rising demand for donor organs, steatotic donor livers are increasingly used in liver transplantation. Studies show that mildly steatotic donor livers do not significantly increase the risk of poor outcomes post-transplantation. What is the outcome for moderately and severely steatotic donor livers compared to non-steatotic livers?
a) Higher primary nonfunction and 1-year mortality
b) Higher primary nonfunction, trend toward increased 1-month mortality, less impact on long-term outcomes
c) No impact on primary nonfunction or short-term mortality, worse 1-year graft function
d) Similar rate of primary nonfunction, higher short- and long-term mortality
e) Equivalent primary nonfunction and 1-year mortality
**Answer: b**

Moderately and severely steatotic livers have a significantly increased risk of primary nonfunction and a trend toward higher 1-month mortality. Long-term outcomes, like 1-year mortality, are less affected.[425]

501. Given the shortage of deceased donor organs for liver transplantation, accurate prediction of graft outcomes is critical for optimizing allocation decisions. Recent studies have explored artificial intelligence (AI) techniques to predict graft survival compared to traditional models like the Donor Risk Index (DRI), MELD, and Survival Outcome Following Liver Transplantation (SOFT). What is the outcome of using AI techniques for predicting graft survival after deceased donor liver transplantation compared to standard predictive models?
a) Lower predictive accuracy, better explainability
b) Higher predictive accuracy, reduced explainability
c) Equivalent predictive accuracy, similar explainability
d) Lower predictive accuracy, reduced explainability
e) Higher predictive accuracy, improved explainability
**Answer: b**
AI techniques, particularly artificial neural networks, demonstrated higher predictive accuracy compared to standard models. However, AI methods are less explainable to clinicians and patients.[426]

502. An 18-year-old Hispanic male with a history of pediatric liver transplantation is transitioning from pediatric to adult care. He has a documented psychiatric illness, polysubstance abuse, diabetes mellitus, and did not complete high school. Which of the following factors in this patient is not associated with an increased mortality rate after transfer to adult care?
a) Hispanic race
b) Failure to graduate high school
c) Polysubstance abuse
d) Psychiatric illness
e) Diabetes mellitus
**Answer: a**
Recent studies identified several risk factors for mortality after transfer to adult care: Black race, psychiatric illness, substance use, failure to graduate high school, tacrolimus variability >2.5, nonadherence, acute rejection, diabetes mellitus, and chronic kidney disease.[427]

503. A 29-year-old male who underwent liver transplantation for alcohol-related liver disease 18 months ago presents for a follow-up visit. His pretransplant history includes a psychiatric diagnosis of depression, a single episode of alcohol relapse

before transplantation, and an abstinence period of 1 year prior to transplantation. Posttransplantation, he developed a chronic complication requiring a prolonged hospital stay (45 days). Which of the following factors in this patient is not associated with an increased risk of posttransplantation alcohol relapse?
a) Age younger than 30 years
b) Psychiatric comorbidity
c) Posttransplantation chronic complications
d) History of previous alcohol relapse
e) Abstinence period less than 1.5 years

**Answer: a**

Recent studies identified posttransplantation chronic complications, psychiatric comorbidity, history of alcohol relapse before transplantation, and an abstinence period of less than 1.5 years as independent risk factors for alcohol relapse after liver transplantation.[428]

# References

[1] Thomas Starzl, The Puzzle People: Memories of a Transplant Surgeon, 1st edition, University of Pittsburgh Press, 1992.
[2] R.Y. Calne, K. Rolles, S. Thiru, P. McMaster, G.N. Craddock, S. Aziz, D.J.G. White, D.B. Evans, D.C. Dunn, R.G. Henderson, P. Lewis, Cyclosporin A initially as the only immunosuppressant in 34 recipients of cadaveric organs: 32 kidneys, 2 pancreases, and 2 livers, The Lancet 314 (1979) 1033–1036. https://doi.org/10.1016/S0140-6736(79)92440-1.
[3] M. Yoglu, R. Stratta, R. Hoffmann, H. Sollinger, A. D'Alessandro, J. Pirsch, F. Belzer, Extended preservation of the liver for clinical transplantation, The Lancet 331 (1988) 617–619. https://doi.org/10.1016/S0140-6736(88)91416-X.
[4] T. Starzl, S. Todo, A. Demetris, J. Fung, Tacrolimus (FK506) and the pharmaceutical/academic/regulatory gauntlet, American Journal of Kidney Diseases 31 (1998) S7–S14. https://doi.org/10.1053/ajkd.1998.v31.pm9631858.
[5] R. Wiesner, E. Edwards, R. Freeman, A. Harper, R. Kim, P. Kamath, W. Kremers, J. Lake, T. Howard, R.M. Merion, R.A. Wolfe, R. Krom, P.M. Colombani, P.C. Cottingham, S.P. Dunn, J.J. Fung, D.W. Hanto, S. V. McDiarmid, J.M. Rabkin, L.W. Teperman, J.G. Turcotte, L.R. Wegman, Model for end-stage liver disease (MELD) and allocation of donor livers, Gastroenterology 124 (2003) 91–96. https://doi.org/10.1053/gast.2003.50016.
[6] T.M. Van Gulik, J.W. Van Den Esschert, James Cantlie's early messages for hepatic surgeons: how the concept of pre-operative portal vein occlusion was defined, HPB 12 (2010) 81–83. https://doi.org/10.1111/j.1477-2574.2009.00124.x.
[7] J.C. Emond, J.F. Renz, Surgical anatomy of the liver and its application to hepatobiliary surgery and transplantation, Semin Liver Dis 14 (1994). https://doi.org/10.1055/s-2007-1007308.
[8] J. Healey, P. Schroy, Anatomy of the biliary ducts within the human liver; analysis of the prevailing pattern of branchings and the major variations of the biliary ducts, AMA Arch Surg 66 (1953) 599. https://doi.org/10.1001/archsurg.1953.01260030616008.
[9] P.R. Reichert, J.F. Renz, L.A.C. D'Albuquerque, P. Rosenthal, R.C. Lim, J.P. Roberts, N.L. Ascher, J.C. Emond, Surgical anatomy of the left lateral segment as applied to living-donor and split-liver transplantation: a clinicopathologic study, Ann Surg 232 (2000) 658–664. https://doi.org/10.1097/00000658-200011000-00007.
[10] J.F. Renz, P.R. Reichert, J.C. Emond, Biliary anatomy as applied to pediatric living donor and split-liver transplantation, Liver Transpl 6 (2000) 801–4. https://doi.org/10.1053/jlts.2000.19365.
[11] R. Jalan, P. Gines, J.C. Olson, R.P. Mookerjee, R. Moreau, G. Garcia-Tsao, V. Arroyo, P.S. Kamath, Acute-on chronic liver failure, J Hepatol 57 (2012) 1336–1348. https://doi.org/10.1016/j.jhep.2012.06.026.
[12] W.M. Lee, R.H. Squires, S.L. Nyberg, E. Doo, J.H. Hoofnagle, Acute liver failure: Summary of a workshop, Hepatology 47 (2007) 1401–1415. https://doi.org/10.1002/hep.22177.
[13] L. Atzori, G. Poli, A. Perra, Hepatic stellate cell: A star cell in the liver, Int J Biochem Cell Biol 41 (2009) 1639–1642. https://doi.org/10.1016/j.biocel.2009.03.001.
[14] H. Gilgenkrantz, A. Collin de l'Hortet, New insights into liver regeneration, Clin Res Hepatol Gastroenterol 35 (2011) 623–629. https://doi.org/10.1016/j.clinre.2011.04.002.
[15] A.W. Duncan, C. Dorrell, M. Grompe, Stem cells and liver regeneration, Gastroenterology 137 (2009) 466–481. https://doi.org/10.1053/j.gastro.2009.05.044.
[16] D.Q. Huang, N.A. Terrault, F. Tacke, L.L. Gluud, M. Arrese, E. Bugianesi, R. Loomba, Global epidemiology of cirrhosis — aetiology, trends and predictions, Nat Rev Gastroenterol Hepatol 20 (2023) 388–398. https://doi.org/10.1038/s41575-023-00759-2.
[17] S.L. Friedman, Mechanisms of hepatic fibrogenesis, Gastroenterology 134 (2008) 1655–1669. https://doi.org/10.1053/j.gastro.2008.03.003.
[18] M.E. Guicciardi, H. Malhi, J.L. Mott, G.J. Gores, Apoptosis and necrosis in the liver, in: Compr Physiol, Wiley, 2013: pp. 977–1010. https://doi.org/10.1002/cphy.c120020.
[19] Z. Du, C.M. Lovly, Mechanisms of receptor tyrosine kinase activation in cancer, Mol Cancer 17 (2018) 58. https://doi.org/10.1186/s12943-018-0782-4.

[20] J. Belghiti, R. Noun, R. Malafosse, P. Jagot, A. Sauvanet, F. Pierangeli, J. Marty, O. Farges, Continuous versus intermittent portal triad clamping for liver resection: a controlled study, Ann Surg 229 (1999) 369–375. https://doi.org/10.1097/00000658-199903000-00010.
[21] J.M. Sims, A brief review of the Belmont report, Dimensions of Critical Care Nursing 29 (2010) 173–174. https://doi.org/10.1097/DCC.0b013e3181de9ec5.
[22] R. Wiesner, E. Edwards, R. Freeman, A. Harper, R. Kim, P. Kamath, W. Kremers, J. Lake, T. Howard, R.M. Merion, R.A. Wolfe, R. Krom, Model for end-stage liver disease (MELD) and allocation of donor livers, Gastroenterology 124 (2003) 91–96. https://doi.org/10.1053/gast.2003.50016.
[23] S. V. McDiarmid, R. Anand, A.S. Lindblad, Development of a pediatric end-stage liver disease score to predict poor outcome in children awaiting liver transplantation1, Transplantation 74 (2002) 173–181. https://doi.org/10.1097/00007890-200207270-00006.
[24] N.L. Latt, M. Niazi, N.T. Pyrsopoulos, Liver transplant allocation policies and outcomes in United States: A comprehensive review, World J Methodol 12 (2022) 32–42. https://doi.org/10.5662/wjm.v12.i1.32.
[25] Richard.J. Howard, D.L. Cornell, L. Cochran, History of deceased organ donation, organ procurement, and organ procurement organizations, Progress in Transplantation 22 (2012) 6–17. https://doi.org/10.7182/pit2012157.
[26] R.D. Truog, F.G. Miller, Counterpoint: are donors after circulatory death really dead, and does it matter? No and not really, Chest 138 (2010) 16–18. https://doi.org/10.1378/chest.10-0657.
[27] B. Victorian, Organ donation after cardiac death lawsuit underscores need for better communication of policies, Nephrology Times 2 (2009) 9–10. https://doi.org/10.1097/01.NEP.0000346567.61667.e4.
[28] W. Spears, A. Mian, D. Greer, Brain death: a clinical overview, J Intensive Care 10 (2022) 16. https://doi.org/10.1186/s40560-022-00609-4.
[29] N.R. Mazumder, R.J. Fontana, MELD 3.0 in Advanced Chronic Liver Disease, Annu Rev Med 75 (2024) 233–245. https://doi.org/10.1146/annurev-med-051322-122539.
[30] S.A. Alqahtani, Update in liver transplantation, Curr Opin Gastroenterol 28 (2012) 230–238. https://doi.org/10.1097/MOG.0b013e3283527f16.
[31] K.F. Murray, R.L. Carithers, AASLD practice guidelines: Evaluation of the patient for liver transplantation, Hepatology 41 (2005) 1407–1432. https://doi.org/10.1002/hep.20704.
[32] B. Roche, D. Samuel, Prevention of hepatitis B virus reinfection in liver transplant recipients, Intervirology 57 (2014) 196–201. https://doi.org/10.1159/000360944.
[33] E. Loggi, S. Gitto, F. Gabrielli, E. Franchi, H. Seferi, C. Cursaro, P. Andreone, Virological Treatment Monitoring for Chronic Hepatitis B, Viruses 14 (2022) 1376. https://doi.org/10.3390/v14071376.
[34] A. Marzano, S. Gaia, V. Ghisetti, S. Carenzi, A. Premoli, W. Debernardi-Venon, C. Alessandria, A. Franchello, M. Salizzoni, M. Rizzetto, Viral load at the time of liver transplantation and risk of hepatitis B virus recurrence, Liver Transplantation 11 (2005) 402–409. https://doi.org/10.1002/lt.20402.
[35] D. Samuel, R. Muller, G. Alexander, L. Fassati, B. Ducot, J.-P. Benhamou, H. Bismuth, Liver transplantation in European patients with the hepatitis B surface antigen, New England Journal of Medicine 329 (1993) 1842–1847. https://doi.org/10.1056/NEJM199312163292503.
[36] P. Simmonds, Genetic diversity and evolution of hepatitis C virus – 15 years on, Journal of General Virology 85 (2004) 3173–3188. https://doi.org/10.1099/vir.0.80401-0.
[37] E.A. Nabatchikova, D.T. Abdurakhmanov, T.P. Rozina, E.N. Nikulkina, E.L. Tanaschuk, S. V. Moiseev, Delisting and clinical outcomes of liver transplant candidates after hepatitis C virus eradication: A long-term single-center experience, Clin Res Hepatol Gastroenterol 45 (2021) 101714. https://doi.org/10.1016/j.clinre.2021.101714.
[38] B. Myers, Y. Bekki, A. Kozato, J.F. Crismale, T.D. Schiano, S. Florman, DCD hepatitis C virus-positive donor livers can achieve favorable outcomes with liver transplantation and are underutilized, Transplantation 107 (2023) 670–679. https://doi.org/10.1097/TP.0000000000004401.
[39] N.R. Barshes, T.C. Lee, R. Balkrishnan, S.J. Karpen, B.A. Carter, J.A. Goss, Risk stratification of adult patients undergoing orthotopic liver transplantation for fulminant hepatic failure, Transplantation 81 (2006) 195–201. https://doi.org/10.1097/01.tp.0000188149.90975.63.
[40] J. Neuberger, A. Gimson, M. Davies, M. Akyol, J. O'Grady, A. Burroughs, M. Hudson, Selection of patients for liver transplantation and allocation of donated livers in the UK, Gut 57 (2008) 252–257. https://doi.org/10.1136/gut.2007.131730.
[41] J. Trivella, B. V. John, C. Levy, Primary biliary cholangitis: Epidemiology, prognosis, and treatment, Hepatol Commun 7 (2023). https://doi.org/10.1097/HC9.0000000000000179.

# Liver Transplantation and Hepatobiliary Surgery: 500 Practice Questions

[42] S. Solá, M.M. Aranha, C.J. Steer, C.M.P. Rodrigues, Game and players: mitochondrial apoptosis and the therapeutic potential of ursodeoxycholic acid., Curr Issues Mol Biol 9 (2007) 123–38.
[43] K.D. Lindor, M.E. Gershwin, R. Poupon, M. Kaplan, N. V. Bergasa, E.J. Heathcote, Primary biliary cirrhosis, Hepatology 50 (2009) 291–308. https://doi.org/10.1002/hep.22906.
[44] N. Guañabens, A. Monegal, D. Cerdá, Á. Muxí, L. Gifre, P. Peris, A. Parés, Randomized trial comparing monthly ibandronate and weekly alendronate for osteoporosis in patients with primary biliary cirrhosis, Hepatology 58 (2013) 2070–2078. https://doi.org/10.1002/hep.26466.
[45] E. V Loftus, PSC-IBD: a unique form of inflammatory bowel disease associated with primary sclerosing cholangitis, Gut 54 (2005) 91–96. https://doi.org/10.1136/gut.2004.046615.
[46] A. Tanaka, X. Ma, A. Takahashi, J.M. Vierling, Primary biliary cholangitis, The Lancet 404 (2024) 1053–1066. https://doi.org/10.1016/S0140-6736(24)01303-5.
[47] A. Michaels, C. Levy, The medical management of primary sclerosing cholangitis., Medscape J Med 10 (2008) 61.
[48] B. Lindberg, U. Arnelo, A. Bergquist, A. Thörne, A. Hjerpe, S. Granqvist, L.-O. Hansson, B. Tribukait, B. Persson, U. Broomé, Diagnosis of biliary strictures in conjunction with endoscopic retrograde cholangiopancreaticography, with special reference to patients with primary sclerosing cholangitis, Endoscopy 34 (2002) 909–916. https://doi.org/10.1055/s-2002-35298.
[49] R.C. Verdonk, G. Dijkstra, E.B. Haagsma, V.K. Shostrom, A.P. Van den Berg, J.H. Kleibeuker, A.N. Langnas, D.L. Sudan, Inflammatory bowel disease after liver transplantation: risk factors for recurrence and de novo disease, American Journal of Transplantation 6 (2006) 1422–1429. https://doi.org/10.1111/j.1600-6143.2006.01333.x.
[50] J.K. Heimbach, G.J. Gores, M.G. Haddock, S.R. Alberts, R. Pedersen, W. Kremers, S.L. Nyberg, M.B. Ishitani, C.B. Rosen, Predictors of disease recurrence following neoadjuvant chemoradiotherapy and liver transplantation for unresectable perihilar cholangiocarcinoma, Transplantation 82 (2006) 1703–1707. https://doi.org/10.1097/01.tp.0000253551.43583.d1.
[51] A. Shamsaeefar, M. Shafiee, S. Nikeghbalian, K. Kazemi, M. Mansorian, N. Motazedian, F. Afshinnia, B. Geramizadeh, S.A. Malekhosseini, Biliary reconstruction in liver transplant patients with primary sclerosing cholangitis, duct‐to‐duct or Roux‐en‐Y?, Clin Transplant 31 (2017). https://doi.org/10.1111/ctr.12964.
[52] T. Visseren, N.S. Erler, J.K. Heimbach, J.E. Eaton, N. Selzner, A. Gulamhusein, F. van der Heide, R.J. Porte, B. van Hoek, I.P.J. Alwayn, H.J. Metselaar, J.N.M. IJzermans, S. Darwish Murad, Inflammatory conditions play a role in recurrence of PSC after liver transplantation: An international multicentre study, JHEP Reports 4 (2022) 100599. https://doi.org/10.1016/j.jhepr.2022.100599.
[53] S.D. Murad, W.R. Kim, T. Therneau, G.J. Gores, C.B. Rosen, J.A. Martenson, S.R. Alberts, J.K. Heimbach, Predictors of pretransplant dropout and posttransplant recurrence in patients with perihilar cholangiocarcinoma, Hepatology 56 (2012) 972–981. https://doi.org/10.1002/hep.25629.
[54] I.W. Graziadei, R.H. Wiesner, P.J. Marotta, M.K. Porayko, J.E. Hay, M.R. Charlton, J.J. Poterucha, C.B. Rosen, G.J. Gores, N.F. LaRusso, R.A.F. Krom, Long-term results of patients undergoing liver transplantation for primary sclerosing cholangitis, Hepatology 30 (1999) 1121–1127. https://doi.org/10.1002/hep.510300501.
[55] E. Alabraba, P. Nightingale, B. Gunson, S. Hubscher, S. Olliff, D. Mirza, J. Neuberger, A re-evaluation of the risk factors for the recurrence of primary sclerosing cholangitis in liver allografts, Liver Transplantation 15 (2009) 330–340. https://doi.org/10.1002/lt.21619.
[56] L. Muratori, A.W. Lohse, M. Lenzi, Diagnosis and management of autoimmune hepatitis, BMJ (2023) e070201. https://doi.org/10.1136/bmj-2022-070201.
[57] P. Milkiewicz, B. Gunson, S. Saksena, M. Hathaway, S.G. Hubscher, E. Elias, Increased incidence of chronic rejection in adult patients transplanted for autoimmune hepatitis: assessment of risk factors, Transplantation 70 (2000) 477–480. https://doi.org/10.1097/00007890-200008150-00014.
[58] P.V. Nayantara, S. Kamath, K.N. Manjunath, K.V. Rajagopal, Computer-aided diagnosis of liver lesions using CT images: A systematic review, Comput Biol Med 127 (2020) 104035. https://doi.org/10.1016/j.compbiomed.2020.104035.
[59] B. Müllhaupt, F. Durand, T. Roskams, P. Dutkowski, M. Heim, Is tumor biopsy necessary?, Liver Transplantation 17 (2011) S14–S25. https://doi.org/10.1002/lt.22374.
[60] B. Müllhaupt, F. Durand, T. Roskams, P. Dutkowski, M. Heim, Is tumor biopsy necessary?, Liver Transplantation 17 (2011) S14–S25. https://doi.org/10.1002/lt.22374.

[61] Q. Wang, W. Luan, G.A. Villanueva, N.N. Rahbari, H.T. Yee, F. Manizate, S.P. Hiotis, Clinical prognostic variables in young patients (under 40 years) with hepatitis B virus-associated hepatocellular carcinoma, J Dig Dis 13 (2012) 214–218. https://doi.org/10.1111/j.1751-2980.2012.00577.x.
[62] M. Schmelzle, F. Krenzien, W. Schöning, J. Pratschke, Treatment of hepatocellular carcinoma in the cirrhotic and non-cirrhotic liver, Der Chirurg 89 (2018) 851–857. https://doi.org/10.1007/s00104-018-0690-6.
[63] J.M. Llovet, J. Bruix, J. Fuster, A. Castells, J.C. Garcia-Valdecasas, L. Grande, A. França, C. Brú, M. Navasa, M. del Ayuso, M. Solé, M.I. Real, R. Vilana, A. Rimola, J. Visa, J. Rodés, Liver transplantation for small hepatocellular carcinoma: The tumor-node-metastasis classification does not have prognostic power, Hepatology 27 (1998) 1572–1577. https://doi.org/10.1002/hep.510270616.
[64] V. Mazzaferro, G.F. Rondinara, G. Rossi, E. Regalia, L. De Carlis, L. Caccamo, R. Doci, C. V Sansalone, L.S. Belli, E. Armiraglio, Milan multicenter experience in liver transplantation for hepatocellular carcinoma., Transplant Proc 26 (1994) 3557–60.
[65] T. Decaens, F. Roudot-Thoraval, S. Hadni-Bresson, C. Meyer, J. Gugenheim, F. Durand, P.-H. Bernard, O. Boillot, L. Sulpice, Y. Calmus, J. Hardwigsen, C. Ducerf, G.-P. Pageaux, S. Dharancy, O. Chazouilleres, D. Cherqui, C. Duvoux, Impact of UCSF criteria according to pre- and post-OLT tumor features: Analysis of 479 patients listed for HCC with a short waiting time, Liver Transplantation 12 (2006) 1761–1769. https://doi.org/10.1002/lt.20884.
[66] F.Y. Yao, R.K. Kerlan, R. Hirose, T.J. Davern, N.M. Bass, S. Feng, M. Peters, N. Terrault, C.E. Freise, N.L. Ascher, J.P. Roberts, Excellent outcome following down-staging of hepatocellular carcinoma prior to liver transplantation: An intention-to-treat analysis, Hepatology 48 (2008) 819–827. https://doi.org/10.1002/hep.22412.
[67] F. Santopaolo, I. Lenci, M. Milana, T.M. Manzia, L. Baiocchi, Liver transplantation for hepatocellular carcinoma: Where do we stand?, World J Gastroenterol 25 (2019) 2591–2602. https://doi.org/10.3748/wjg.v25.i21.2591.
[68] V. Mazzaferro, A. Gorgen, S. Roayaie, M. Droz dit Busset, G. Sapisochin, Liver resection and transplantation for intrahepatic cholangiocarcinoma, J Hepatol 72 (2020) 364–377. https://doi.org/10.1016/j.jhep.2019.11.020.
[69] A.P. Loehrer, M.G. House, A. Nakeeb, M.E. Kilbane, H.A. Pitt, Cholangiocarcinoma: are North American surgical outcomes optimal?, J Am Coll Surg 216 (2013) 192–200. https://doi.org/10.1016/j.jamcollsurg.2012.11.002.
[70] S.S. Raman, D.S.K. Lu, S.C. Chen, J. Sayre, F. Eilber, J. Economou, Hepatic MR imaging using ferumoxides: prospective evaluation with surgical and intraoperative sonographic confirmation in 25 cases, American Journal of Roentgenology 177 (2001) 807–812. https://doi.org/10.2214/ajr.177.4.1770807.
[71] G.K. Bonney, C.A. Chew, P. Lodge, J. Hubbard, K.J. Halazun, P. Trunecka, P. Muiesan, D.F. Mirza, J. Isaac, R.W. Laing, S.G. Iyer, C.E. Chee, W.P. Yong, M.D. Muthiah, F. Panaro, J. Sanabria, A. Grothey, K. Moodley, I. Chau, A.C.Y. Chan, C.C. Wang, K. Menon, G. Sapisochin, M. Hagness, S. Dueland, P.-D. Line, R. Adam, Liver transplantation for non-resectable colorectal liver metastases: the International Hepato-Pancreato-Biliary Association consensus guidelines, Lancet Gastroenterol Hepatol 6 (2021) 933–946. https://doi.org/10.1016/S2468-1253(21)00219-3.
[72] A. Taylor, Primrose, W. Langeberg, Kelsh, F. Mowat, D. Alexander, M. Choti, G. Poston, Gena Kanas, Survival after liver resection in metastatic colorectal cancer: review and meta-analysis of prognostic factors, Clin Epidemiol (2012) 283. https://doi.org/10.2147/CLEP.S34285.
[73] T.M. Smedman, P.-D. Line, M. Hagness, T. Syversveen, H. Grut, S. Dueland, Liver transplantation for unresectable colorectal liver metastases in patients and donors with extended criteria (SECA-II arm D study), BJS Open 4 (2020) 467–477. https://doi.org/10.1002/bjs5.50278.
[74] V. Mazzaferro, A. Pulvirenti, J. Coppa, Neuroendocrine tumors metastatic to the liver: How to select patients for liver transplantation?, J Hepatol 47 (2007) 460–466. https://doi.org/10.1016/j.jhep.2007.07.004.
[75] R. Hörnsten, U. Wiklund, B.-O. Olofsson, S.M. Jensen, O.B. Suhr, Liver transplantation does not prevent the development of life-threatening arrhythmia in familial amyloidotic polyneuropathy, Portuguese-type (ATTR Val30Met) patients, Transplantation 78 (2004) 112–116. https://doi.org/10.1097/01.TP.0000133517.20972.27.
[76] G. Herlenius, H.E. Wilczek, M. Larsson, B.-G. Ericzon, Ten years of international experience with liver transplantation for familial amyloidotic polyneuropathy: results from the familial amyloidotic polyneuropathy world transplant registry, Transplantation 77 (2004) 64–71. https://doi.org/10.1097/01.TP.0000092307.98347.CB.

[77] A. Tefferi, Polycythemia vera and essential thrombocythemia: 2012 update on diagnosis, risk stratification, and management, Am J Hematol 87 (2012) 284–293. https://doi.org/10.1002/ajh.23135.
[78] Z.-Y. Chen, L.-N. Yan, Y. Zeng, T.-F. Wen, B. Li, J.-C. Zhao, W.-T. Wang, J.-Y. Yang, M.-Q. Xu, Transdiaphragmatic exposure for direct atrioatrial anastomosis in liver transplantation., Chin Med J (Engl) 123 (2010) 3515–8.
[79] P. Yarra, W. Dunn, Z. Younossi, Y.-F. Kuo, A.K. Singal, Association of previous gastric bypass surgery and patient outcomes in alcohol-associated cirrhosis hospitalizations, Dig Dis Sci 68 (2023) 1026–1034. https://doi.org/10.1007/s10620-022-07591-9.
[80] J.L. Mellinger, K. Shedden, G.S. Winder, A.C. Fernandez, B.P. Lee, J. Waljee, R. Fontana, M.L. Volk, F.C. Blow, A.S.F. Lok, Bariatric surgery and the risk of alcohol-related cirrhosis and alcohol misuse, Liver International 41 (2021) 1012–1019. https://doi.org/10.1111/liv.14805.
[81] D. Vanjak, D. Samuel, F. Gosset, S. Derrida, R. Moreau, T. Soupison, A. Soulier, H. Bismuth, C. Sicot, [Fulminant hepatitis induced by disulfiram in a patient with alcoholic cirrhosis. Survival after liver transplantation]., Gastroenterol Clin Biol 13 (1989) 1075–8.
[82] B. Sureka, K. Bansal, Y. Patidar, S. Rajesh, A. Mukund, A. Arora, Neurologic manifestations of chronic liver disease and liver cirrhosis, Curr Probl Diagn Radiol 44 (2015) 449–461. https://doi.org/10.1067/j.cpradiol.2015.03.004.
[83] K. Houston, N. Duong, R.K. Sterling, A. Asgharpour, S. Bullock, S. Weinland, N. Keller, E. Smirnova, H. Khan, S. Matherly, J. Wedd, H. Lee, M. Siddiqui, V. Patel, A. Arias, V. Kumaran, S. Lee, A. Sharma, A. Khan, D. Imai, M. Levy, D. Bruno, Utility of scores to predict alcohol use after liver transplant: Take them with a grain of salt, Liver Transplantation 30 (2024) 1281–1288. https://doi.org/10.1097/LVT.0000000000000407.
[84] L.L. Jophlin, A.K. Singal, R. Bataller, R.J. Wong, B.G. Sauer, N.A. Terrault, V.H. Shah, ACG clinical guideline: Alcohol-associated liver disease, American Journal of Gastroenterology 119 (2024) 30–54. https://doi.org/10.14309/ajg.0000000000002572.
[85] Y. Li, P. Yang, J. Ye, Q. Xu, J. Wu, Y. Wang, Updated mechanisms of MASLD pathogenesis, Lipids Health Dis 23 (2024) 117. https://doi.org/10.1186/s12944-024-02108-x.
[86] A. Shetty, F. Giron, M.K. Divatia, M.I. Ahmad, S. Kodali, D. Victor, Nonalcoholic fatty liver disease after liver transplant, J Clin Transl Hepatol 000 (2021) 000–000. https://doi.org/10.14218/JCTH.2020.00072.
[87] R. Idriss, J. Hasse, T. Wu, F. Khan, G. Saracino, G. McKenna, G. Testa, J. Trotter, G. Klintmalm, S.K. Asrani, Impact of prior bariatric surgery on perioperative liver transplant outcomes, Liver Transplantation 25 (2019) 217–227. https://doi.org/10.1002/lt.25368.
[88] L. Pestana, J. Swain, R. Dierkhising, M.L. Kendrick, P.S. Kamath, K.D. Watt, Bariatric surgery in patients with cirrhosis with and without portal hypertension: a single-center experience, Mayo Clin Proc 90 (2015) 209–215. https://doi.org/10.1016/j.mayocp.2014.11.012.
[89] R.A. Bhanji, P. Narayanan, M.R. Moynagh, N. Takahashi, M. Angirekula, C.C. Kennedy, K.C. Mara, R.A. Dierkhising, K.D. Watt, Differing impact of Sarcopenia and frailty in nonalcoholic steatohepatitis and alcoholic liver disease, Liver Transplantation 25 (2019) 14–24. https://doi.org/10.1002/lt.25346.
[90] F. Brinkert, R. Ganschow, K. Helmke, E. Harps, L. Fischer, B. Nashan, B. Hoppe, S. Kulke, D.E. Müller-Wiefel, M.J. Kemper, Transplantation procedures in children with primary hyperoxaluria type 1: outcome and longitudinal growth, Transplantation 87 (2009) 1415–1421. https://doi.org/10.1097/TP.0b013e3181a27939.
[91] H. Ruder, G. Otto, R.B.H. Schutgens, U. Querfeld, R.J.A. Wanders, K.-H. Herzog, P. Wölfel, S. Pomer, K. Schärer, G.A. Rose, Excessive urinary oxalate excretion after combined renal and hepatic transplantation for correction of hyperoxaluria type 1, Eur J Pediatr 150 (1990) 56–58. https://doi.org/10.1007/BF01959482.
[92] F.H. Saner, J. Treckmann, J. Pratschke, H. Arbogast, A. Rahmel, U. Vester, A. Paul, Early renal failure after domino liver transplantation using organs from donors with primary hyperoxaluria type 1, Transplantation 90 (2010) 782–785. https://doi.org/10.1097/TP.0b013e3181eefe1f.
[93] J.A. Castilla Cabezas, P. López-Cillero, J. Jiménez, E. Fraga, J.M. Arizón, J. Briceño, G. Solórzano, M. De la Mata, C. Pera, Role of orthotopic liver transplant in the treatment of homozygous familial hypercholesterolemia., Revista Espanola de Enfermedades Digestivas 92 (2000) 601–8.
[94] I. Popescu, N. Habib, S. Dima, N. Hancu, L. Gheorghe, S. Iacob, M. Mihaila, B. Dorobantu, E. Matei, F. Botea, Domino liver transplantation using a graft from a donor with familial hypercholesterolemia: seven-yr follow-up, Clin Transplant 23 (2009) 565–570. https://doi.org/10.1111/j.1399-0012.2008.00935.x.
[95] A. Link, B. Kaplan, M. Böhm, [21-year-old woman with Reye's syndrome after influenza], DMW - Deutsche Medizinische Wochenschrift 137 (2012) 1853–1856. https://doi.org/10.1055/s-0032-1305311.

[96] T. Hasegawa, A.G. Tzakis, S. Todo, J. Reyes, B. Nour, D.N. Finegold, T.E. Starzl, Orthotopic liver transplantation for ornithine transcarbamylase deficiency with hyperammonemic encephalopathy, J Pediatr Surg 30 (1995) 863–865. https://doi.org/10.1016/0022-3468(95)90766-1.

[97] D. Katarey, S. Verma, Drug-induced liver injury, Clinical Medicine 16 (2016) s104–s109. https://doi.org/10.7861/clinmedicine.16-6-s104.

[98] H.R. Makhlouf, K.G. Ishak, Z.D. Goodman, Epithelioid hemangioendothelioma of the liver, Cancer 85 (1999) 562–582. https://doi.org/10.1002/(SICI)1097-0142(19990201)85:3<562::AID-CNCR7>3.0.CO;2-T.

[99] A. Mehrabi, A. Kashfi, H. Fonouni, P. Schemmer, B.M. Schmied, P. Hallscheidt, P. Schirmacher, J. Weitz, H. Friess, M.W. Buchler, J. Schmidt, Primary malignant hepatic epithelioid hemangioendothelioma, Cancer 107 (2006) 2108–2121. https://doi.org/10.1002/cncr.22425.

[100] J.P. Lerut, G. Orlando, R. Adam, M. Schiavo, J. Klempnauer, D. Mirza, E. Boleslawski, A. Burroughs, C.F. Sellés, D. Jaeck, R. Pfitzmann, M. Salizzoni, G. Söderdahl, R. Steininger, A. Wettergren, V. Mazzaferro, Y.P. Le Treut, V. Karam, The place of liver transplantation in the treatment of hepatic epiteloid hemangioendothelioma: report of the European liver transplant registry, Ann Surg 246 (2007) 949–957. https://doi.org/10.1097/SLA.0b013e31815c2a70.

[101] G. Ercolani, G.L. Grazi, A.D. Pinna, Liver transplantation for benign hepatic tumors: a systematic review, Dig Surg 27 (2010) 68–75. https://doi.org/10.1159/000268628.

[102] L. De Kerckhove, M. De Meyer, C. Verbaandert, M. Mourad, E. Sokal, P. Goffette, A. Geubel, V. Karam, R. Adam, J. Lerut, The place of liver transplantation in Caroli's disease and syndrome, Transplant International 19 (2006) 381–388. https://doi.org/10.1111/j.1432-2277.2006.00292.x.

[103] F.A. Alharbi, N.R. Al-Shammari, K.M. Aloqeely, Liver transplantation in a child with Crigler-Najjar syndrome type I: A case report with review of the literature., Cureus 15 (2023) e42064. https://doi.org/10.7759/cureus.42064.

[104] J. Menon, A. Rammohan, M. Vij, N. Shanmugam, M. Rela, Current perspectives on the role of liver transplantation for Langerhans cell histiocytosis: A narrative review., World J Gastroenterol 28 (2022) 4044–4052. https://doi.org/10.3748/wjg.v28.i30.4044.

[105] H. Ismail, D. Broniszczak, P. Kaliciński, B. Dembowska-Bagińska, D. Perek, J. Teisseyre, P. Kluge, A. Kościesza, A. Lembas, M. Markiewicz, Changing treatment and outcome of children with hepatoblastoma: analysis of a single center experience over the last 20 years, J Pediatr Surg 47 (2012) 1331–1339. https://doi.org/10.1016/j.jpedsurg.2011.11.073.

[106] J.M. Boster, R. Superina, G. V. Mazariegos, G.M. Tiao, J.P. Roach, M.A. Lovell, B.S. Greffe, G. Yanni, D.H. Leung, S.A. Elisofon, S. V. McDiarmid, N.A. Gupta, S.J. Lobritto, C. Lemoine, J.M. Stoll, B.E. Vitola, J.F. Daniel, B.A. Sayed, D.M. Desai, A.E. Martin, A. Amin, R. Anand, S.G. Anderson, S.S. Sundaram, Predictors of survival following liver transplantation for pediatric hepatoblastoma and hepatocellular carcinoma: Experience from the Society of Pediatric Liver Transplantation (SPLIT), American Journal of Transplantation 22 (2022) 1396–1408. https://doi.org/10.1111/ajt.16945.

[107] E. Hoti, R. Adam, Liver transplantation for primary and metastatic liver cancers, Transplant International 21 (2008) 1107–1117. https://doi.org/10.1111/j.1432-2277.2008.00735.x.

[108] Y. Toyoki, K. Hakamada, S. Narumi, M. Nara, M. Sugai, H. Munakata, M. Sasaki, Timing for orthotopic liver transplantation in children with biliary atresia: a single-center experience, Transplant Proc 40 (2008) 2494–2496. https://doi.org/10.1016/j.transproceed.2008.08.043.

[109] M. Kasai, I. Watanabe, R. Ohi, Follow-up studies of long-term survivors after hepatic portoenterostomy for "noncorrectable" biliary atresia, J Pediatr Surg 10 (1975) 173–182. https://doi.org/10.1016/0022-3468(75)90275-4.

[110] O. Madadi-Sanjani, M. Uecker, G. Thomas, L. Fischer, B. Hegen, J. Herrmann, K. Reinshagen, C. Tomuschat, Optimizing post-Kasai management in biliary atresia: Balancing native liver survival and transplant timing, European Journal of Pediatric Surgery (2024). https://doi.org/10.1055/a-2507-8270.

[111] P. Baliga, S. Alvarez, A. Lindblad, L. Zeng, Posttransplant survival in pediatric fulminant hepatic failure: The SPLIT experience, Liver Transplantation 10 (2004) 1364–1371. https://doi.org/10.1002/lt.20252.

[112] K.A. Strauss, V.J. Carson, K. Soltys, M.E. Young, L.E. Bowser, E.G. Puffenberger, K.W. Brigatti, K.B. Williams, D.L. Robinson, C. Hendrickson, K. Beiler, C.M. Taylor, B. Haas-Givler, S. Chopko, J. Hailey, E.R. Muelly, D.A. Shellmer, Z. Radcliff, A. Rodrigues, K. Loeven, A.D. Heaps, G. V. Mazariegos, D.H. Morton, Branched-chain α-ketoacid dehydrogenase deficiency (maple syrup urine disease): Treatment, biomarkers, and outcomes, Mol Genet Metab 129 (2020) 193–206. https://doi.org/10.1016/j.ymgme.2020.01.006.

[113] S.M. Vandriel, L. Li, H. She, J. Wang, M.A. Gilbert, I. Jankowska, P. Czubkowski, D. Gliwicz-Miedzińska, E.M. Gonzales, E. Jacquemin, J. Bouligand, N.B. Spinner, K.M. Loomes, D.A. Piccoli, L. D'Antiga, E. Nicastro, É. Sokal, T. Demaret, N.H. Ebel, J.A. Feinstein, R. Fawaz, S. Nastasio, F. Lacaille, D. Debray, H. Arnell, B. Fischler, S. Siew, M. Stormon, S.J. Karpen, R. Romero, K.M. Kim, W.Y. Baek, W. Hardikar, S. Shankar, A.J. Roberts, H.M. Evans, M.K. Jensen, M. Kavan, S.S. Sundaram, A. Chaidez, P. Karthikeyan, M.C. Sanchez, M.L. Cavalieri, H.J. Verkade, W.S. Lee, J.E. Squires, C. Hajinicolaou, C. Lertudomphonwanit, R.T. Fischer, C. Larson-Nath, Y. Mozer-Glassberg, C. Arikan, H.C. Lin, J.Q. Bernabeu, S. Alam, D.A. Kelly, E. Carvalho, C.T. Ferreira, G. Indolfi, R.E. Quiros-Tejeira, P. Bulut, P.L. Calvo, Z. Önal, P.L. Valentino, D.M. Desai, J. Eshun, M. Rogalidou, A. Dezsőfi, S. Wiecek, G. Nebbia, R.B. Pinto, V.M. Wolters, M.L. Tamara, A.N. Zizzo, J. Garcia, K. Schwarz, M. Beretta, T.D. Sandahl, C. Jimenez-Rivera, N. Kerkar, J. Brecelj, Q. Mujawar, N. Rock, C.M. Busoms, W. Karnsakul, E. Lurz, E. Santos-Silva, N. Blondet, L. Bujanda, U. Shah, R.J. Thompson, B.E. Hansen, B.M. Kamath, Natural history of liver disease in a large international cohort of children with Alagille syndrome: Results from the GALA study, Hepatology 77 (2023) 512–529. https://doi.org/10.1002/hep.32761.

[114] G. Maggiore, O. Bernard, C.A. Riely, M. Hadchouel, A. Lemonnier, D. Alagille, Normal serum γ-glutamyl-transpeptidase activity identifies groups of infants with idiopathic cholestasis with poor prognosis, J Pediatr 111 (1987) 251–252. https://doi.org/10.1016/S0022-3476(87)80079-3.

[115] F.J. Suchy, Another form of familial intrahepatic cholestasis, another new gene, Hepatology 29 (1999) 1911–1912. https://doi.org/10.1002/hep.510290642.

[116] R. Thompson, S. Strautnieks, BSEP: function and role in progressive familial intrahepatic cholestasis, Semin Liver Dis 21 (2001) 545–550. https://doi.org/10.1055/s-2001-19038.

[117] S.S. Strautnieks, L.N. Bull, A.S. Knisely, S.A. Kocoshis, N. Dahl, H. Arnell, E. Sokal, K. Dahan, S. Childs, V. Ling, M.S. Tanner, A.F. Kagalwalla, A. Németh, J. Pawlowska, A. Baker, G. Mieli-Vergani, N.B. Freimer, R.M. Gardiner, R.J. Thompson, A gene encoding a liver-specific ABC transporter is mutated in progressive familial intrahepatic cholestasis, Nat Genet 20 (1998) 233–238. https://doi.org/10.1038/3034.

[118] V. Keitel, M. Burdelski, Z. Vojnisek, L. Schmitt, D. Häussinger, R. Kubitz, De novo bile salt transporter antibodies as a possible cause of recurrent graft failure after liver transplantation, Hepatology 50 (2009) 510–517. https://doi.org/10.1002/hep.23083.

[119] J.M.L. de Vree, E. Jacquemin, E. Sturm, D. Cresteil, P.J. Bosma, J. Aten, J.-F. Deleuze, M. Desrochers, M. Burdelski, O. Bernard, R.P.J.O. Elferink, M. Hadchouel, Mutations in the MDR3 gene cause progressive familial intrahepatic cholestasis, Proceedings of the National Academy of Sciences 95 (1998) 282–287. https://doi.org/10.1073/pnas.95.1.282.

[120] J.J.M. Smit, A.H. Schinkel, R.P.J.O. Elferink, A.K. Groen, E. Wagenaar, L. van Deemter, C.A.A.M. Mol, R. Ottenhoff, N.M.T. van der Lugt, M.A. van Roon, M.A. van der Valk, G.J.A. Offerhaus, A.J.M. Berns, P. Borst, Homozygous disruption of the murine MDR2 P-glycoprotein gene leads to a complete absence of phospholipid from bile and to liver disease, Cell 75 (1993) 451–462. https://doi.org/10.1016/0092-8674(93)90380-9.

[121] E. Drouin, P. Russo, B. Tuchweber, G. Mitchell, A. Rasquin-Weber, North American Indian cirrhosis in children: a review of 30 cases, J Pediatr Gastroenterol Nutr 31 (2000) 395–404. https://doi.org/10.1097/00005176-200010000-00013.

[122] L.W.J. Klomp, L.N. Bull, A.S. Knisely, M.A.M. van der Doelen, J.A. Juijn, R. Berger, S. Forget, I.-M. Nielsen, H. Eiberg, R.H.J. Houwen, A missense mutation in FIC1 is associated with greenland familial cholestasis, Hepatology 32 (2000) 1337–1341. https://doi.org/10.1053/jhep.2000.20520.

[123] V.A. Luketic, M.L. Shiffman, Benign recurrent intrahepatic cholestasis, Clin Liver Dis 8 (2004) 133–149. https://doi.org/10.1016/S1089-3261(03)00133-8.

[124] J. V. Gutierrez, L. Johnson, K. Desai, B. Tabak, R.K. Woo, Timing of Kasai procedure for biliary atresia: An analysis of the pediatric national surgical quality improvement program database, Journal of Surgical Research 301 (2024) 681–685. https://doi.org/10.1016/j.jss.2024.07.002.

[125] Y.-H. Ni, H.-Y. Hsu, E.-T. Wu, H.-L. Chen, P.-I. Lee, M.-H. Chang, H.-S. Lai, Bacterial cholangitis in patients with biliary atresia: impact on short-term outcome, Pediatr Surg Int 17 (2001) 390–395. https://doi.org/10.1007/s003830000573.

[126] R. Ohi, Surgery for biliary atresia, Liver 21 (2001) 175–182. https://doi.org/10.1034/j.1600-0676.2001.021003175.x.

[127] A.A. Darwish, C. Bourdeaux, H.A. Kader, M. Janssen, E. Sokal, J. Lerut, O. Ciccarelli, F. Veyckemans, J. Otte, J. de V. de Goyet, R. Reding, Pediatric liver transplantation using left hepatic segments from living related

donors: Surgical experience in 100 recipients at Saint-Luc University Clinics, Pediatr Transplant 10 (2006) 345–353. https://doi.org/10.1111/j.1399-3046.2005.00477.x.

[128] J. Häberle, N. Boddaert, A. Burlina, A. Chakrapani, M. Dixon, M. Huemer, D. Karall, D. Martinelli, P. Crespo, R. Santer, A. Servais, V. Valayannopoulos, M. Lindner, V. Rubio, C. Dionisi-Vici, Suggested guidelines for the diagnosis and management of urea cycle disorders, Orphanet J Rare Dis 7 (2012) 32. https://doi.org/10.1186/1750-1172-7-32.

[129] H. Sharp, Alpha-1-antitrypsin: an ignored protein in understanding liver disease, Semin Liver Dis 2 (1982) 314–328. https://doi.org/10.1055/s-2008-1040718.

[130] Y. Wang, D.H. Perlmutter, Targeting intracellular degradation pathways for treatment of liver disease caused by α1-antitrypsin deficiency, Pediatr Res 75 (2014) 133–139. https://doi.org/10.1038/pr.2013.190.

[131] R. Francavilla, S.P. Castellaneta, N. Hadzic, S.M. Chambers, B. Portmann, J. Tung, P. Cheeseman, M. Rela, N.D. Heaton, G. Mieli-Vergani, Prognosis of alpha-1-antitrypsin deficiency-related liver disease in the era of paediatric liver transplantion, J Hepatol 32 (2000) 986–992. https://doi.org/10.1016/S0168-8278(00)80103-8.

[132] R. Ohi, J.R. Lilly, Copper kinetics in infantile hepatobiliary disease, J Pediatr Surg 15 (1980) 509–512. https://doi.org/10.1016/S0022-3468(80)80763-9.

[133] G. Loudianos, M.B. Lepori, E. Mameli, V. Dessì, A. Zappu, Wilson's disease., Pril (Makedon Akad Nauk Umet Odd Med Nauki) 35 (2014) 93–8.

[134] R. Srinivasan, S. Dominic, A. George, Clinical and laboratory profile and outcome in children with Wilson disease: an observational study in South India, Paediatr Int Child Health 44 (2024) 131–140. https://doi.org/10.1080/20469047.2024.2396716.

[135] R.T. Bax, A. Hässler, W. Luck, H. Hefter, I. Krägeloh-Mann, P. Neuhaus, P. Emmrich, Cerebral manifestation of Wilson's disease successfully treated with liver transplantation, Neurology 51 (1998) 863–865. https://doi.org/10.1212/WNL.51.3.863.

[136] J.M. Croffie, S.K. Gupta, S.K.F. Chong, J.F. Fitzgerald, Tyrosinemia type 1 should be suspected in infants with severe coagulopathy even in the absence of other signs of liver failure, Pediatrics 103 (1999) 675–678. https://doi.org/10.1542/peds.103.3.675.

[137] G. Mitchell, J. Larochelle, M. Lambert, J. Michaud, A. Grenier, H. Ogier, M. Gauthier, J. Lacroix, M. Vanasse, A. Larbrisseau, K. Paradis, A. Weber, Y. Lefevre, S. Melançon, L. Dallaire, Neurologic crises in hereditary tyrosinemia, New England Journal of Medicine 322 (1990) 432–437. https://doi.org/10.1056/NEJM199002153220704.

[138] L.A. Mieles, C.O. Esquivel, D.H. Van Thiel, B. Koneru, L. Makowka, A.G. Tzakis, T.E. Starzl, Liver transplantation for tyrosinemia, Dig Dis Sci 35 (1990) 153–157. https://doi.org/10.1007/BF01537237.

[139] P.M. Campeau, P.J. Pivalizza, G. Miller, K. McBride, S. Karpen, J. Goss, B.H. Lee, Early orthotopic liver transplantation in urea cycle defects: Follow up of a developmental outcome study, Mol Genet Metab 100 (2010) S84–S87. https://doi.org/10.1016/j.ymgme.2010.02.012.

[140] M. Deon, G. Guerreiro, J. Girardi, G. Ribas, C.R. Vargas, Treatment of maple syrup urine disease: Benefits, risks, and challenges of liver transplantation, International Journal of Developmental Neuroscience 83 (2023) 489–504. https://doi.org/10.1002/jdn.10283.

[141] E. Mayatepek, B. Hoffmann, T. Meissner, Inborn errors of carbohydrate metabolism, Best Pract Res Clin Gastroenterol 24 (2010) 607–618. https://doi.org/10.1016/j.bpg.2010.07.012.

[142] D. Matern, T.E. Starzl, W. Arnaout, J. Barnard, J.S. Bynon, A. Dhawan, J. Emond, E.B. Haagsma, G. Hug, A. Lachaux, G.P.A. Smit, Y.-T. Chen, Liver transplantation for glycogen storage disease types I, III, and IV, Eur J Pediatr 158 (1999) S043–S048. https://doi.org/10.1007/PL00014320.

[143] H.-R. Qiu, L. Zhang, Z.-J. Zhu, Perioperative management and clinical outcomes of liver transplantation for children with homozygous familial hypercholesterolemia, Medicina (B Aires) 58 (2022) 1430. https://doi.org/10.3390/medicina58101430.

[144] J.C. Gartner, I. Bergman, J.J. Malatack, B.J. Zitelli, R. Jaffe, J.B. Watkins, B.W. Shaw, S. Iwatsuki, T.E. Starzl, Progression of neurovisceral storage disease with supranuclear ophthalmoplegia following orthotopic liver transplantation., Pediatrics 77 (1986) 104–6.

[145] K. Schultz, T. Dizseri, M. Kardos, M. Tóth, [Crigler-Najjar syndrome. Successful home-care phototherapy with good results]., Orv Hetil 121 (1980) 2457–9.

[146] A. Dhawan, M.W. Lawlor, G. V Mazariegos, P. McKiernan, J.E. Squires, K.A. Strauss, D. Gupta, E. James, S. Prasad, Disease burden of Crigler–Najjar syndrome: Systematic review and future perspectives, J Gastroenterol Hepatol 35 (2020) 530–543. https://doi.org/10.1111/jgh.14853.

[147] V. Sambati, S. Laudisio, M. Motta, S. Esposito, Therapeutic options for Crigler–Najjar syndrome: A scoping review, Int J Mol Sci 25 (2024) 11006. https://doi.org/10.3390/ijms252011006.
[148] R. Shapiro, I. Weismann, H. Mandel, B. Eisenstein, Z. Ben-Ari, N. Bar-Nathan, I. Zehavi, G. Dinari, E. Mor, Primary hyperoxaluria type 1: improved outcome with timely liver transplantation: a single-center report of 36 children, Transplantation 72 (2001) 428–432. https://doi.org/10.1097/00007890-200108150-00012.
[149] B. Behnke, M.J. Kemper, H. Kruse, D.E. Müller-Wiefel, Bone mineral density in children with primary hyperoxaluria type I, Nephrology Dialysis Transplantation 16 (2001) 2236–2239. https://doi.org/10.1093/ndt/16.11.2236.
[150] A. Munnich, A. Rötig, D. Chretien, V. Cormier, T. Bourgeron, J. -P. Bonnefont, J. -M. Saudubray, P. Rustin, Clinical presentation of mitochondrial disorders in childhood, J Inherit Metab Dis 19 (1996) 521–527. https://doi.org/10.1007/BF01799112.
[151] W. Lee, R. Sokol, Liver disease in mitochondrial disorders, Semin Liver Dis 27 (2007) 259–273. https://doi.org/10.1055/s-2007-985071.
[152] A.J. Towbin, R.L. Meyers, H. Woodley, O. Miyazaki, C.B. Weldon, B. Morland, E. Hiyama, P. Czauderna, D.J. Roebuck, G.M. Tiao, 2017 PRETEXT: radiologic staging system for primary hepatic malignancies of childhood revised for the Paediatric Hepatic International Tumour Trial (PHITT), Pediatr Radiol 48 (2018) 536–554. https://doi.org/10.1007/s00247-018-4078-z.
[153] A.P. Pimpalwar, K. Sharif, P. Ramani, M. Stevens, R. Grundy, B. Morland, C. Lloyd, D.A. Kelly, J.A.C. Buckles, J. de Ville de Goyet, Strategy for hepatoblastoma management: Transplant versus nontransplant surgery, J Pediatr Surg 37 (2002) 240–245. https://doi.org/10.1053/jpsu.2002.30264.
[154] J.D. Reyes, B. Carr, I. Dvorchik, S. Kocoshis, R. Jaffe, D. Gerber, G. V Mazariegos, J. Bueno, R. Selby, Liver transplantation and chemotherapy for hepatoblastoma and hepatocellular cancer in childhood and adolescence., J Pediatr 136 (2000) 795–804.
[155] L.M. Franco, V. Krishnamurthy, D. Bali, D.A. Weinstein, P. Arn, B. Clary, A. Boney, J. Sullivan, D.P. Frush, Y. -T. Chen, P.S. Kishnani, Hepatocellular carcinoma in glycogen storage disease type Ia: A case series, J Inherit Metab Dis 28 (2005) 153–162. https://doi.org/10.1007/s10545-005-7500-2.
[156] A.-N. Elzouki, S. Eriksson, Risk of hepatobiliary disease in adults with severe ??1-antitrypsin deficiency (PiZZ): is chronic viral hepatitis B or C an additional risk factor for cirrhosis and hepatocellular carcinoma?, Eur J Gastroenterol Hepatol 8 (1996) 989–994. https://doi.org/10.1097/00042737-199610000-00010.
[157] E. Bonaccorsi-Riani, J.P. Lerut, Liver transplantation and vascular tumours, Transplant International 23 (2010) 686–691. https://doi.org/10.1111/j.1432-2277.2010.01107.x.
[158] J.A. Rodriguez, N.S. Becker, C.A. O'Mahony, J.A. Goss, T.A. Aloia, Long-term outcomes following liver transplantation for hepatic hemangioendothelioma: the UNOS experience from 1987 to 2005, Journal of Gastrointestinal Surgery 12 (2008) 110–116. https://doi.org/10.1007/s11605-007-0247-3.
[159] R. Kumar, U. Anand, R.N. Priyadarshi, Liver transplantation in acute liver failure: Dilemmas and challenges, World J Transplant 11 (2021) 187–202. https://doi.org/10.5500/wjt.v11.i6.187.
[160] K.I. Kroeker, V.G. Bain, T. Shaw-Stiffel, T. Fong, E.M. Yoshida, Adult liver transplant survey: policies towards eligibility criteria in Canada and the United States 2007, Liver International 28 (2008) 1250–1255. https://doi.org/10.1111/j.1478-3231.2008.01807.x.
[161] K. Berry, J.M. Ruck, F. Barry, A.M. Shui, A. Cortella, D. Kent, S. Seetharaman, R. Wong, L. VandeVrede, J.C. Lai, Prevalence of cognitive impairment in liver transplant recipients, Clin Transplant 38 (2024). https://doi.org/10.1111/ctr.15249.
[162] B. Lima, E.R. Nowicki, C.M. Miller, K. Hashimoto, N.G. Smedira, G. V. Gonzalez-Stawinski, Outcomes of simultaneous liver transplantation and elective cardiac surgical procedures, Ann Thorac Surg 92 (2011) 1580–1584. https://doi.org/10.1016/j.athoracsur.2011.06.056.
[163] R. Lavi, S. Lavi, E. Daghini, L.O. Lerman, D.C. Warltier, New frontiers in the evaluation of cardiac patients for noncardiac surgery, Anesthesiology 107 (2007) 1018–1028. https://doi.org/10.1097/01.anes.0000287613.49204.94.
[164] A. Hameed, R. Condliffe, A.J. Swift, S. Alabed, D.G. Kiely, A. Charalampopoulos, Assessment of right ventricular function—a state of the art, Curr Heart Fail Rep 20 (2023) 194–207. https://doi.org/10.1007/s11897-023-00600-6.
[165] P. Maggiore, J. Bellinge, D. Chieng, D. White, N.S.R. Lan, B. Jaltotage, U. Ali, M. Gordon, K. Chung, P. Stobie, J. Ng, G.J. Hankey, B. McQuillan, Ischaemic stroke and the echocardiographic "Bubble Study": Are we screening the right patients?, Heart Lung Circ 28 (2019) 1183–1189. https://doi.org/10.1016/j.hlc.2018.07.007.

[166] L. Castello, M. Pirisi, P.P. Sainaghi, E. Bartoli, Hyponatremia in liver cirrhosis: pathophysiological principles of management, Digestive and Liver Disease 37 (2005) 73–81. https://doi.org/10.1016/j.dld.2004.09.012.
[167] Y. Ozier, J.R. Klinck, Anesthetic management of hepatic transplantation, Curr Opin Anaesthesiol 21 (2008) 391–400. https://doi.org/10.1097/ACO.0b013e3282ff85f4.
[168] L. Dubourg, S. Lemoine, B. Joannard, L. Chardon, V. de Souza, P. Cochat, J. Iwaz, M. Rabilloud, L. Selistre, Comparison of iohexol plasma clearance formulas vs. inulin urinary clearance for measuring glomerular filtration rate, Clinical Chemistry and Laboratory Medicine (CCLM) 59 (2021) 571–579. https://doi.org/10.1515/cclm-2020-0770.
[169] F. Wong, M.K. Nadim, J.A. Kellum, F. Salerno, R. Bellomo, A. Gerbes, P. Angeli, R. Moreau, A. Davenport, R. Jalan, C. Ronco, Y. Genyk, V. Arroyo, Working Party proposal for a revised classification system of renal dysfunction in patients with cirrhosis, Gut 60 (2011) 702–709. https://doi.org/10.1136/gut.2010.236133.
[170] D.A. Simonetto, P. Gines, P.S. Kamath, Hepatorenal syndrome: pathophysiology, diagnosis, and management, BMJ (2020) m2687. https://doi.org/10.1136/bmj.m2687.
[171] S. Fasolato, P. Angeli, L. Dallagnese, G. Maresio, E. Zola, E. Mazza, F. Salinas, S. Donà, S. Fagiuoli, A. Sticca, G. Zanus, U. Cillo, I. Frasson, C. Destro, A. Gatta, Renal failure and bacterial infections in patients with cirrhosis: Epidemiology and clinical features, Hepatology 45 (2007) 223–229. https://doi.org/10.1002/hep.21443.
[172] T. Tanaka, K.L. Lentine, Q. Shi, M. Vander Weg, D.A. Axelrod, Differential impact of the UNOS simultaneous liver-kidney transplant policy change among patients with sustained acute kidney injury, Transplantation (2023). https://doi.org/10.1097/TP.0000000000004774.
[173] R. Mounzer, S.M. Malik, J. Nasr, B. Madani, M.E. Devera, J. Ahmad, Spontaneous bacterial peritonitis before liver transplantation does not affect patient survival., Clin Gastroenterol Hepatol 8 (2010) 623-628.e1. https://doi.org/10.1016/j.cgh.2010.04.013.
[174] M.A. Huaman, V. Vilchez, X. Mei, M.B. Shah, M.F. Daily, J. Berger, R. Gedaly, Decreased graft survival in liver transplant recipients of donors with positive blood cultures: a review of the United Network for Organ Sharing dataset, Transplant International 30 (2017) 558–565. https://doi.org/10.1111/tri.12900.
[175] M.I. Morris, J.S. Daly, E. Blumberg, D. Kumar, M. Sester, N. Schluger, S.-H. Kim, B.S. Schwartz, M.G. Ison, A. Humar, N. Singh, M. Michaels, J.P. Orlowski, F. Delmonico, T. Pruett, G.T. John, C.N. Kotton, Diagnosis and management of tuberculosis in transplant donors: a donor-derived infections consensus conference report, American Journal of Transplantation 12 (2012) 2288–2300. https://doi.org/10.1111/j.1600-6143.2012.04205.x.
[176] L. Danziger-Isakov, D. Kumar, Vaccination of solid organ transplant candidates and recipients: Guidelines from the American society of transplantation infectious diseases community of practice, Clin Transplant 33 (2019). https://doi.org/10.1111/ctr.13563.
[177] I. Cruite, M. Schroeder, E.M. Merkle, C.B. Sirlin, Gadoxetate disodium-enhanced MRI of the liver: part 2, protocol optimization and lesion appearance in the cirrhotic liver, American Journal of Roentgenology 195 (2010) 29–41. https://doi.org/10.2214/AJR.10.4538.
[178] J.C. García-Pagán, S. Saffo, M. Mandorfer, G. Garcia-Tsao, Where does TIPS fit in the management of patients with cirrhosis?, JHEP Reports 2 (2020) 100122. https://doi.org/10.1016/j.jhepr.2020.100122.
[179] R.A. Hawkins, T. Hall, S.S. Gambhir, R.W. Busuttil, S. Huang, S. Glickman, D. Marciano, R.K.J. Brown, M.E. Phelps, Radionuclide evaluation of liver transplants, Semin Nucl Med 18 (1988) 199–212. https://doi.org/10.1016/S0001-2998(88)80028-X.
[180] E.M. Teegen, B. Globke, T. Denecke, A. Pascher, R. Öllinger, J. Pratschke, S.S. Chopra, Vascular anomalies of the extrahepatic artery as a predictable risk factor for complications after liver transplant, Experimental and Clinical Transplantation 17 (2019). https://doi.org/10.6002/ect.2018.0201.
[181] N. Ohkohchi, H. Katoh, T. Orii, K. Fujimori, S. Shimaoka, S. Satomi, Complications and treatments of donors and recipients in living-related liver transplantation, Transplant Proc 30 (1998) 3218–3220. https://doi.org/10.1016/S0041-1345(98)01002-1.
[182] J. Bekker, S. Ploem, K.P. De Jong, Early hepatic artery thrombosis after liver transplantation: a systematic review of the incidence, outcome and risk factors, American Journal of Transplantation 9 (2009) 746–757. https://doi.org/10.1111/j.1600-6143.2008.02541.x.
[183] Z. Xue, X. Zhang, Z. Li, R. Deng, L. Wu, Y. Ma, Analysis of portal vein thrombosis after liver transplantation, ANZ J Surg 89 (2019) 1075–1079. https://doi.org/10.1111/ans.15242.

[184] G. Gheorghe, C. Diaconu, S. Bungau, N. Bacalbasa, N. Motas, V.-A. Ionescu, Biliary and vascular complications after liver transplantation–from diagnosis to treatment, Medicina (B Aires) 59 (2023) 850. https://doi.org/10.3390/medicina59050850.
[185] S.B. Kaplan, A.B. Zajko, B. Koneru, Hepatic bilomas due to hepatic artery thrombosis in liver transplant recipients: percutaneous drainage and clinical outcome, Radiology 174 (1990) 1031–1035. https://doi.org/10.1148/radiology.174.3.174-3-1031.
[186] J. Ward, M.B. Sheridan, J.A. Guthrie, M.H. Davies, C.E. Millson, J.P.A. Lodge, S.G. Pollard, K.R. Prasad, G.J. Toogood, P.J. Robinson, Bile duct strictures after hepatobiliary surgery: assessment with MR cholangiography, Radiology 231 (2004) 101–108. https://doi.org/10.1148/radiol.2311030017.
[187] T.R. Glowka, C. Karlstetter, T.J. Weismüller, T.O. Vilz, C.P. Strassburg, J.C. Kalff, S. Manekeller, Intensified endoscopic evaluation for biliary complications after orthotopic liver transplantation, Ann Transplant 26 (2021). https://doi.org/10.12659/AOT.928907.
[188] M. Fasullo, M. Patel, L. Khanna, T. Shah, Post-transplant biliary complications: advances in pathophysiology, diagnosis, and treatment, BMJ Open Gastroenterol 9 (2022) e000778. https://doi.org/10.1136/bmjgast-2021-000778.
[189] P.A. Cortesi, L.S. Belli, R. Facchetti, C. Mazzarelli, G. Perricone, S. De Nicola, G. Cesana, C. Duvoux, L.G. Mantovani, M. Strazzabosco, The optimal timing of hepatitis C therapy in liver transplant-eligible patients: Cost-effectiveness analysis of new opportunities, J Viral Hepat 25 (2018) 791–801. https://doi.org/10.1111/jvh.12877.
[190] C. Levy, M. Manns, G. Hirschfield, New treatment paradigms in primary biliary cholangitis, Clinical Gastroenterology and Hepatology 21 (2023) 2076–2087. https://doi.org/10.1016/j.cgh.2023.02.005.
[191] D.N. Assis, C.L. Bowlus, Recent advances in the management of primary sclerosing cholangitis, Clinical Gastroenterology and Hepatology 21 (2023) 2065–2075. https://doi.org/10.1016/j.cgh.2023.04.004.
[192] J. Bosch, J.C. García-Pagán, Prevention of variceal rebleeding, The Lancet 361 (2003) 952–954. https://doi.org/10.1016/S0140-6736(03)12778-X.
[193] G. Sahagun, K.G. Benner, R. Saxon, R.E. Barton, J. Rabkin, F.S. Keller, J. Rosch, Outcome of 100 patients after transjugular intrahepatic portosystemic shunt for variceal hemorrhage., Am J Gastroenterol 92 (1997) 1444–52.
[194] P. Schindler, L. Seifert, M. Masthoff, A. Riegel, M. Köhler, C. Wilms, H.H. Schmidt, H. Heinzow, M. Wildgruber, TIPS modification in the management of shunt-induced hepatic encephalopathy: analysis of predictive factors and outcome with shunt modification., J Clin Med 9 (2020). https://doi.org/10.3390/jcm9020567.
[195] S. Singh, S. Chandan, R. Vinayek, G. Aswath, A. Facciorusso, M. Maida, Comprehensive approach to esophageal variceal bleeding: From prevention to treatment, World J Gastroenterol 30 (2024) 4602–4608. https://doi.org/10.3748/wjg.v30.i43.4602.
[196] B.A. Runyon, Management of adult patients with ascites due to cirrhosis, Hepatology 49 (2009) 2087–2107. https://doi.org/10.1002/hep.22853.
[197] S. Saab, J.M. Nieto, S.K. Lewis, B.A. Runyon, TIPS versus paracentesis for cirrhotic patients with refractory ascites, Cochrane Database of Systematic Reviews 2010 (2006). https://doi.org/10.1002/14651858.CD004889.pub2.
[198] B.C. Sharma, P. Sharma, M.K. Lunia, S. Srivastava, R. Goyal, S.K. Sarin, A randomized, double-blind, controlled trial comparing rifaximin plus lactulose with lactulose alone in treatment of overt hepatic encephalopathy, American Journal of Gastroenterology 108 (2013) 1458–1463. https://doi.org/10.1038/ajg.2013.219.
[199] Y. Lv, D. Fan, Hepatopulmonary syndrome, Dig Dis Sci 60 (2015) 1914–1923. https://doi.org/10.1007/s10620-015-3593-0.
[200] M.M. Düll, A.E. Kremer, Evaluation and management of pruritus in primary biliary cholangitis, Clin Liver Dis 26 (2022) 727–745. https://doi.org/10.1016/j.cld.2022.06.009.
[201] T. Yatabe, Strategies for optimal calorie administration in critically ill patients, J Intensive Care 7 (2019) 15. https://doi.org/10.1186/s40560-019-0371-7.
[202] M. Ryan-Harshman, W. Aldoori, New dietary reference intakes for macronutrients and fibre., Can Fam Physician 52 (2006) 177–9.
[203] R. de Franchis, Revising consensus in portal hypertension: Report of the Baveno V consensus workshop on methodology of diagnosis and therapy in portal hypertension, J Hepatol 53 (2010) 762–768. https://doi.org/10.1016/j.jhep.2010.06.004.

[204] Y. Liu, S. Wu, S. Cai, B. Xie, The prognostic evaluation of ALBI score in endoscopic treatment of esophagogastric varices hemorrhage in liver cirrhosis, Sci Rep 14 (2024) 780. https://doi.org/10.1038/s41598-023-50629-9.
[205] F.P. Gómez, G. Martínez-Pallí, J.A. Barberà, J. Roca, M. Navasa, R. Rodríguez-Roisin, Gas exchange mechanism of orthodeoxia in hepatopulmonary syndrome, Hepatology 40 (2004) 660–666. https://doi.org/10.1002/hep.20358.
[206] R. Rodríguez-Roisin, M.J. Krowka, Ph. Hervé, M.B. Fallon, Pulmonary–Hepatic vascular Disorders (PHD), European Respiratory Journal 24 (2004) 861–880. https://doi.org/10.1183/09031936.04.00010904.
[207] K.L. Swanson, R.H. Wiesner, M.J. Krowka, Natural history of hepatopulmonary syndrome, Hepatology 41 (2005) 1122–1129. https://doi.org/10.1002/hep.20658.
[208] H.M. DuBrock, Portopulmonary hypertension: Management and liver transplantation evaluation, Chest 164 (2023) 206–214. https://doi.org/10.1016/j.chest.2023.01.009.
[209] A. Hadengue, M.K. Benhayoun, D. Lebrec, J.-P. Benhamou, Pulmonary hypertension complicating portal hypertension: Prevalence and relation to splanchnic hemodynamics, Gastroenterology 100 (1991) 520–528. https://doi.org/10.1016/0016-5085(91)90225-A.
[210] S. Provencher, P. Herve, X. Jais, D. Lebrec, M. Humbert, G. Simonneau, O. Sitbon, Deleterious effects of beta-blockers on exercise capacity and hemodynamics in patients with portopulmonary hypertension, Gastroenterology 130 (2006) 120–126. https://doi.org/10.1053/j.gastro.2005.10.013.
[211] M.J. Krowka, R.H. Wiesner, J.K. Heimbach, Pulmonary contraindications, indications and MELD exceptions for liver transplantation: A contemporary view and look forward, J Hepatol 59 (2013) 367–374. https://doi.org/10.1016/j.jhep.2013.03.026.
[212] M.J.J. Chu, A.J. Dare, A.R.J. Phillips, A.S.J.R. Bartlett, Donor hepatic steatosis and outcome after liver transplantation: A systematic review, Journal of Gastrointestinal Surgery 19 (2015) 1713–1724. https://doi.org/10.1007/s11605-015-2832-1.
[213] S. Huprikar, L. Danziger-Isakov, J. Ahn, S. Naugler, E. Blumberg, R.K. Avery, C. Koval, E.D. Lease, A. Pillai, K.E. Doucette, J. Levitsky, M.I. Morris, K. Lu, J.K. McDermott, T. Mone, J.P. Orlowski, D.M. Dadhania, K. Abbott, S. Horslen, B.L. Laskin, A. Mougdil, V.L. Venkat, K. Korenblat, V. Kumar, P. Grossi, R.D. Bloom, K. Brown, C.N. Kotton, D. Kumar, Solid organ transplantation from hepatitis B virus–positive donors: Consensus guidelines for recipient management, American Journal of Transplantation 15 (2015) 1162–1172. https://doi.org/10.1111/ajt.13187.
[214] J.F. Crismale, J. Ahmad, Expanding the donor pool: Hepatitis C, hepatitis B and human immunodeficiency virus-positive donors in liver transplantation, World J Gastroenterol 25 (2019) 6799–6812. https://doi.org/10.3748/wjg.v25.i47.6799.
[215] K. Mils, L. Lladó, J. Fabregat, C. Baliellas, E. Ramos, L. Secanella, J. Busquets, N. Pelaez, Outcomes of liver transplant with donors over 70 years of age, Cirugía Española (English Edition) 93 (2015) 516–521. https://doi.org/10.1016/j.cireng.2015.04.008.
[216] L.M. Kucirka, R. Namuyinga, C. Hanrahan, R.A. Montgomery, D.L. Segev, Formal policies and special informed consent are associated with higher provider utilization of CDC high-risk donor organs, American Journal of Transplantation 9 (2009) 629–635. https://doi.org/10.1111/j.1600-6143.2008.02523.x.
[217] D.P. Al-Adra, L. Hammel, J. Roberts, E.S. Woodle, D. Levine, D. Mandelbrot, E. Verna, J. Locke, J. D'Cunha, M. Farr, D. Sawinski, P.K. Agarwal, J. Plichta, S. Pruthi, D. Farr, R. Carvajal, J. Walker, F. Zwald, T. Habermann, M. Gertz, P. Bierman, D.S. Dizon, C. Langstraat, T. Al-Qaoud, S. Eggener, J.P. Richgels, G.J. Chang, C. Geltzeiler, G. Sapisochin, R. Ricciardi, A.S. Krupnick, C. Kennedy, N. Mohindra, D.P. Foley, K.D. Watt, Pretransplant solid organ malignancy and organ transplant candidacy: A consensus expert opinion statement, American Journal of Transplantation 21 (2021) 460–474. https://doi.org/10.1111/ajt.16318.
[218] W.H. Kitchens, Domino liver transplantation: indications, techniques, and outcomes, Transplant Rev 25 (2011) 167–177. https://doi.org/10.1016/j.trre.2011.04.002.
[219] S.A. Wisel, J.A. Steggerda, I.K. Kim, Use of machine perfusion in the United States increases organ utilization and improves DCD graft survival in liver transplantation, Transplant Direct 10 (2024) e1726. https://doi.org/10.1097/TXD.0000000000001726.
[220] K.P. Croome, Should advanced perfusion be the standard of care for donation after circulatory death liver transplant?, American Journal of Transplantation 24 (2024) 1127–1131. https://doi.org/10.1016/j.ajt.2024.03.021.
[221] Y. Bekki, C. Rocha, B. Myers, R. Wang, N. Smith, P. Tabrizian, J. DiNorcia, J. Moon, A. Arvelakis, M.E. Facciuto, S. DeMaria, S. Florman, Asystolic donor warm ischemia time is associated with development of

postreperfusion syndrome in donation after circulatory death liver transplant, Clin Transplant 38 (2024). https://doi.org/10.1111/ctr.15336.

[222] M.S. Reddy, J. Varghese, J. Venkataraman, M. Rela, Matching donor to recipient in liver transplantation: Relevance in clinical practice, World J Hepatol 5 (2013) 603. https://doi.org/10.4254/wjh.v5.i11.603.

[223] S. Elde, A.L. Brubaker, P.A. Than, D. Rinewalt, J.W. MacArthur, A. Alassar, C.A. Bonham, C.O. Esquivel, Y. Shudo, W. Concepcion, Y.J. Woo, Operative technique of donor organ procurement for en bloc heart-liver transplantation, Transplantation 105 (2021) 2661–2665. https://doi.org/10.1097/TP.0000000000003697.

[224] H.P. Hwang, J.M. Kim, S. Shin, H.J. Ahn, S. Lee, D.J. Joo, S.Y. Han, S.J. Haam, J.K. Hwang, H.C. Yu, Organ procurement in a deceased donor, Korean Journal of Transplantation 34 (2020) 134–150. https://doi.org/10.4285/kjt.2020.34.3.134.

[225] M. Pavlakis, M.G. Michaels, S. Tlusty, N. Turgeon, G. Vece, C. Wolfe, R.P. Wood, M.A. Nalesnik, Renal cell carcinoma suspected at time of organ donation 2008-2016: A report of the OPTN ad hoc Disease Transmission Advisory Committee Registry, Clin Transplant 33 (2019). https://doi.org/10.1111/ctr.13597.

[226] D.J. Reich, D.C. Mulligan, P.L. Abt, T.L. Pruett, M.M.I. Abecassis, A. D'Alessandro, E.A. Pomfret, R.B. Freeman, J.F. Markmann, D.W. Hanto, A.J. Matas, J.P. Roberts, R.M. Merion, G.B.G. Klintmalm, ASTS recommended practice guidelines for controlled donation after cardiac death organ procurement and transplantation, American Journal of Transplantation 9 (2009) 2004–2011. https://doi.org/10.1111/j.1600-6143.2009.02739.x.

[227] J.H. Kaplan, L.J. Kenney, Temperature effects on sodium pump phosphoenzyme distribution in human red blood cells., J Gen Physiol 85 (1985) 123–136. https://doi.org/10.1085/jgp.85.1.123.

[228] N. Askenasy, A. Vivi, M. Tassini, G. Navon, Efficient limitation of intracellular edema and sodium accumulation by cardioplegia is dissociated from recovery of rat hearts from cold ischemic storage, J Mol Cell Cardiol 31 (1999) 1795–1808. https://doi.org/10.1006/jmcc.1999.1009.

[229] J. Liu, K. Man, Mechanistic insight and clinical implications of ischemia/reperfusion injury post liver transplantation, Cell Mol Gastroenterol Hepatol 15 (2023) 1463–1474. https://doi.org/10.1016/j.jcmgh.2023.03.003.

[230] J.H. Southard, T.M. van Gulik, M.S. Ametani, P.K. Vreugdenhil, S.L. Lindell, B.L. PIENAAR, F.O. BELZER, Important components of the UW solution, Transplantation 49 (1990) 251–257. https://doi.org/10.1097/00007890-199002000-00004.

[231] K. Kotsch, F. Ulrich, A. Reutzel-Selke, A. Pascher, W. Faber, P. Warnick, S. Hoffman, M. Francuski, C. Kunert, O. Kuecuek, G. Schumacher, C. Wesslau, A. Lun, S. Kohler, S. Weiss, S.G. Tullius, P. Neuhaus, J. Pratschke, Methylprednisolone therapy in deceased donors reduces inflammation in the donor liver and improves outcome after liver transplantation: a prospective randomized controlled trial, Ann Surg 248 (2008) 1042–1050. https://doi.org/10.1097/SLA.0b013e318190e70c.

[232] J.P. Duffy, J.C. Hong, D.G. Farmer, R.M. Ghobrial, H. Yersiz, J.R. Hiatt, R.W. Busuttil, Vascular complications of orthotopic liver transplantation: experience in more than 4,200 patients, J Am Coll Surg 208 (2009) 896–903. https://doi.org/10.1016/j.jamcollsurg.2008.12.032.

[233] K.L. Thomsen, P.L. Eriksen, A.JC. Kerbert, F. De Chiara, R. Jalan, H. Vilstrup, Role of ammonia in NAFLD: An unusual suspect, JHEP Reports 5 (2023) 100780. https://doi.org/10.1016/j.jhepr.2023.100780.

[234] A.S. Basile, R.D. Hughes, P.M. Harrison, Y. Murata, L. Pannell, E.A. Jones, R. Williams, P. Skolnick, Elevated brain concentrations of 1,4-benzodiazepines in fulminant hepatic failure, New England Journal of Medicine 325 (1991) 473–478. https://doi.org/10.1056/NEJM199108153250705.

[235] M. Dursun, M. Caliskan, F. Canoruc, U. Aluclu, N. Canoruc, A. Tuzcu, S. Yilmaz, A. Isikdogan, M. Ertem, The efficacy of flumazenil in subclinical to mild hepatic encephalopathic ambulatory patients, Swiss Med Wkly (2003). https://doi.org/10.4414/smw.2003.10107.

[236] C. Ichai, C. Vinsonneau, B. Souweine, F. Armando, E. Canet, C. Clec'h, J.-M. Constantin, M. Darmon, J. Duranteau, T. Gaillot, A. Garnier, L. Jacob, O. Joannes-Boyau, L. Juillard, D. Journois, A. Lautrette, L. Muller, M. Legrand, N. Lerolle, T. Rimmelé, E. Rondeau, F. Tamion, Y. Walrave, L. Velly, Acute kidney injury in the perioperative period and in intensive care units (excluding renal replacement therapies), Ann Intensive Care 6 (2016) 48. https://doi.org/10.1186/s13613-016-0145-5.

[237] F. Salerno, A. Gerbes, P. Ginès, F. Wong, V. Arroyo, Diagnosis, prevention and treatment of hepatorenal syndrome in cirrhosis, Postgrad Med J 84 (2008) 662–670. https://doi.org/10.1136/gut.2006.107789.

[238] S. Stanford, B. Stanford, P. Gillman, Risk of severe serotonin toxicity following co-administration of methylene blue and serotonin reuptake inhibitors: an update on a case report of post-operative delirium, Journal of Psychopharmacology 24 (2010) 1433–1438. https://doi.org/10.1177/0269881109105450.

[239] A.E. Schmidt, A.K. Israel, M.A. Refaai, The utility of thromboelastography to guide blood product transfusion, Am J Clin Pathol 152 (2019) 407–422. https://doi.org/10.1093/ajcp/aqz074.
[240] J.C. George, W. Zafar, I.D. Bucaloiu, A.R. Chang, Risk factors and outcomes of rapid correction of severe hyponatremia, Clinical Journal of the American Society of Nephrology 13 (2018) 984–992. https://doi.org/10.2215/CJN.13061117.
[241] V.J. Aijtink, V.C. Rutten, B.E.M. Meijer, R. de Jong, J.L. Isaac, W.G. Polak, M.T.P.R. Perera, D. Sneiders, H. Hartog, Safety of intraoperative blood salvage during liver transplantation in patients with hepatocellular carcinoma, Ann Surg 276 (2022) 239–245. https://doi.org/10.1097/SLA.0000000000005476.
[242] T. Liang, J. Li, D. Li, L. Liang, X. Bai, S. Zheng, Intraoperative blood salvage and leukocyte depletion during liver transplantation with bacterial contamination, Clin Transplant 24 (2010) 265–272. https://doi.org/10.1111/j.1399-0012.2009.01091.x.
[243] D. Fabbroni, M. Bellamy, Anaesthesia for hepatic transplantation, Continuing Education in Anaesthesia Critical Care & Pain 6 (2006) 171–175. https://doi.org/10.1093/bjaceaccp/mkl040.
[244] G. Guarino, G. Licitra, D. Ghinolfi, P. Desimone, F. Forfori, M.L. Bindi, G. Biancofiore, Use of an intraoperative veno-venous bypass during liver transplantation: an observational, single center, cohort study, Minerva Anestesiol 88 (2022). https://doi.org/10.23736/S0375-9393.22.15749-4.
[245] P. Limanond, S.S. Raman, C. Lassman, J. Sayre, R.M. Ghobrial, R.W. Busuttil, S. Saab, D.S.K. Lu, Macrovesicular hepatic steatosis in living related liver donors: correlation between CT and histologic findings, Radiology 230 (2004) 276–280. https://doi.org/10.1148/radiol.2301021176.
[246] N.A. Michels, Newer anatomy of the liver and its variant blood supply and collateral circulation, The American Journal of Surgery 112 (1966) 337–347. https://doi.org/10.1016/0002-9610(66)90201-7.
[247] M. Kasahara, J.C. Hong, A. Dhawan, Evaluation of living donors for hereditary liver disease (siblings, heterozygotes), J Hepatol 78 (2023) 1147–1156. https://doi.org/10.1016/j.jhep.2022.10.013.
[248] T. Kiuchi, M. Kasahara, K. Uryuhara, Y. Inomata, S. Uemoto, K. Asonuma, H. Egawa, S. Fujita, M. Hayashi, K. Tanaka, Impact of graft size mismatching on graft prognosis in liver transplantation from living donors, Transplantation 67 (1999) 321–327. https://doi.org/10.1097/00007890-199901270-00024.
[249] H. Kamei, F. Oike, Y. Fujimoto, H. Yamamoto, K. Tanaka, T. Kiuchi, Fatal graft-versus-host disease after living donor liver transplantation: Differential impact of donor-dominant one-way HLA matching, Liver Transplantation 12 (2006) 140–145. https://doi.org/10.1002/lt.20573.
[250] I.K. Marwan, A.T. Fawzy, H. Egawa, Y. Inomata, S. Uemoto, K. Asonuma, T. Kiuchi, M. Hayashi, S. Fujita, Y. Ogura, K. Tanaka, Innovative techniques for and results of portal vein reconstruction in living-related liver transplantation. Surgery 125 (1999) 265–70.
[251] C.P. Lemoine, K.A. Brandt, M. Keswani, R. Superina, Outcomes after ABO incompatible pediatric liver transplantation are comparable to ABO identical/compatible transplant, Front Pediatr 11 (2023). https://doi.org/10.3389/fped.2023.1092412.
[252] Y. Sarigol Ordin, A.K. Harmanci Seren, O. Karayurt, G. Aksu Kul, M. Kilic, C.A. Bozoklar, Y. Tokat, Evaluation of psychosocial outcomes of living liver donors in liver transplantation, Turkish Journal of Gastroenterology 33 (2022) 346–355. https://doi.org/10.5152/tjg.2022.21262.
[253] G.-C. Park, G.-W. Song, D.-B. Moon, S.-G. Lee, A review of current status of living donor liver transplantation., Hepatobiliary Surg Nutr 5 (2016) 107–17. https://doi.org/10.3978/j.issn.2304-3881.2015.08.04.
[254] M. Ben-Haim, Critical graft size in adult-to-adult living donor liver transplantation: Impact of the recipient's disease, Liver Transplantation 7 (2001) 948–953. https://doi.org/10.1053/jlts.2001.29033.
[255] K. Oshita, S. Kuroda, T. Kobayashi, G. Aoki, H. Mashima, T. Onoe, N. Shigemoto, T. Hirata, H. Tashiro, H. Ohdan, A multicenter, open-label, single-arm phase I trial of d-wield parenchymal transection: A new technique of liver resection using the cavitron ultrasonic surgical aspirator and water-jet scalpel simultaneously (HiSCO-14 Trial)., Cureus 15 (2023) e49428. https://doi.org/10.7759/cureus.49428.
[256] I.D. Vellar, Preliminary study of the anatomy of the venous drainage of the intrahepatic and extrahepatic bile ducts and its relevance to the practice of hepatobiliary surgery, ANZ J Surg 71 (2001) 418–422. https://doi.org/10.1046/j.1440-1622.2001.02150.x.
[257] D. Bezinover, A. Mukhtar, G. Wagener, C. Wray, A. Blasi, K. Kronish, J. Zerillo, D. Tomescu, A. Pustavoitau, M. Gitman, A. Singh, F.H. Saner, Hemodynamic instability during liver transplantation in patients with end-stage liver disease: A consensus document from ILTS, LICAGE, and SATA, Transplantation 105 (2021) 2184–2200. https://doi.org/10.1097/TP.0000000000003642.
[258] S. Yagi, A. Singhal, D.-H. Jung, K. Hashimoto, Living-donor liver transplantation: Right versus left, International Journal of Surgery 82 (2020) 128–133. https://doi.org/10.1016/j.ijsu.2020.06.022.

# Liver Transplantation and Hepatobiliary Surgery: 500 Practice Questions

[259] M.G. Bowring, A.B. Massie, K.B. Schwarz, A.M. Cameron, E.A. King, D.L. Segev, D.B. Mogul, Survival benefit of split-liver transplantation for pediatric and adult candidates, Liver Transplantation 28 (2022) 969–982. https://doi.org/10.1002/lt.26393.

[260] M.I. Rodriguez-Davalos, A. Arvelakis, V. Umman, V. Tanjavur, P.S. Yoo, S. Kulkarni, S.M. Luczycki, M. Schilsky, S. Emre, Segmental grafts in adult and pediatric liver transplantation, JAMA Surg 149 (2014) 63. https://doi.org/10.1001/jamasurg.2013.3384.

[261] E. Chaib, M.M. Morales, M.B. Bordalo, L.G. Antonio, L.F. Feijo, R.Y. Ishida, J. Lima Júnior, P.A. Nunes, Predicting the donor liver lobe weight from body weight for split-liver transplantation., Braz J Med Biol Res 28 (1995) 759–60.

[262] A. Humar, T. Ramcharan, T.D. Sielaff, R. Kandaswamy, R.W. Gruessner, J.R. Lake, W.D. Payne, Split liver transplantation for two adult recipients: an initial experience, American Journal of Transplantation 1 (2001) 366–372. https://doi.org/10.1034/j.1600-6143.2001.10413.x.

[263] K. Sano, M. Makuuchi, K. Miki, A. Maema, Y. Sugawara, H. Imamura, H. Matsunami, T. Takayama, Evaluation of hepatic venous congestion: proposed indication criteria for hepatic vein reconstruction, Ann Surg 236 (2002) 241–247. https://doi.org/10.1097/00000658-200208000-00013.

[264] S. Hwang, S.-G. Lee, C.-S. Ahn, K.-H. Kim, D.-B. Moon, T.-Y. Ha, G.-W. Song, D.-H. Jung, J.-H. Ryu, K.-H. Ko, N.-K. Choi, K.-W. Kim, Technique and outcome of autologous portal Y-graft interposition for anomalous right portal veins in living donor liver transplantation, Liver Transplantation 15 (2009) 427–434. https://doi.org/10.1002/lt.21697.

[265] Y. Sugawara, S. Tamura, J. Kaneko, T. Iida, M. Mihara, M. Makuuchi, I. Koshima, N. Kokudo, Single artery reconstruction in left liver transplantation, Surgery 149 (2011) 841–845. https://doi.org/10.1016/j.surg.2010.11.016.

[266] P. Cheng, Z. Li, Z. Fu, Q. Jian, R. Deng, Y. Ma, Small-for-size syndrome and graft inflow modulation techniques in liver transplantation, Digestive Diseases 41 (2023) 250–258. https://doi.org/10.1159/000525540.

[267] A.J. Demetris, D.M. Kelly, B. Eghtesad, P. Fontes, J. Wallis Marsh, K. Tom, H.P. Tan, T. Shaw-Stiffel, L. Boig, P. Novelli, R. Planinsic, J.J. Fung, A. Marcos, Pathophysiologic observations and histopathologic recognition of the portal hyperperfusion or small-for-size syndrome, Am J Surg Pathol 30 (2006) 986–993. https://doi.org/10.1097/00000478-200608000-00009.

[268] K. Man, S.-T. Fan, C.-M. Lo, C.-L. Liu, P.C.-W. Fung, T.-B. Liang, T.K.-W. Lee, S.H.-T. Tsui, I.O.-L. Ng, Z.-W. Zhang, J. Wong, Graft injury in relation to graft size in right lobe live donor liver transplantation: a study of hepatic sinusoidal injury in correlation with portal hemodynamics and intragraft gene expression, Ann Surg 237 (2003) 256–264. https://doi.org/10.1097/01.SLA.0000048976.11824.67.

[269] C.D. Kakos, A. Papanikolaou, I.A. Ziogas, G. Tsoulfas, Global dissemination of minimally invasive living donor hepatectomy: What are the barriers?, World J Gastrointest Surg 15 (2023) 776–787. https://doi.org/10.4240/wjgs.v15.i5.776.

[270] Y. Xu, H. Chen, H. Yeh, H. Wang, J. Leng, J. Dong, Living donor liver transplantation using dual grafts: Experience and lessons learned from cases worldwide, Liver Transplantation 21 (2015) 1438–1448. https://doi.org/10.1002/lt.24315.

[271] J.F. Trotter, R. Adam, C.M. Lo, J. Kenison, Documented deaths of hepatic lobe donors for living donor liver transplantation, Liver Transplantation 12 (2006) 1485–1488. https://doi.org/10.1002/lt.20875.

[272] L. Shazi, Z. Abbas, Ethical dilemmas related to living donor liver transplantation in Asia, Irish Journal of Medical Science (1971 -) 188 (2019) 1185–1189. https://doi.org/10.1007/s11845-019-01989-7.

[273] J.P. Duffy, J.C. Hong, D.G. Farmer, R.M. Ghobrial, H. Yersiz, J.R. Hiatt, R.W. Busuttil, Vascular complications of orthotopic liver transplantation: experience in more than 4,200 patients, J Am Coll Surg 208 (2009) 896–903. https://doi.org/10.1016/j.jamcollsurg.2008.12.032.

[274] H.K. Pannu, W.R. Maley, E.K. Fishman, Liver transplantation: Preoperative CT evaluation, RadioGraphics 21 (2001) S133–S146. https://doi.org/10.1148/radiographics.21.suppl_1.g01oc03s133.

[275] M. Vilatobá, D. Zamora-Valdés, M. Guerrero-Hernández, H. Romero-Talamás, R.P. Leal-Villalpando, M.A. Mercado, Arcuate ligament compression as a cause of early-onset thrombosis of the hepatic artery after liver transplantation., Ann Hepatol 10 (2011) 88–92.

[276] Y. Imaoka, M. Ohira, R. Nakano, S. Shimizu, S. Kuroda, H. Tahara, K. Ide, T. Kobayashi, H. Ohdan, Impact of abdominal aortic calcification among liver transplantation recipients, Liver Transplantation 25 (2019) 79–87. https://doi.org/10.1002/lt.25311.

[277] P. Bhangui, E.S.M. Fernandes, F. Di Benedetto, D.-J. Joo, S. Nadalin, Current management of portal vein thrombosis in liver transplantation, International Journal of Surgery 82 (2020) 122–127. https://doi.org/10.1016/j.ijsu.2020.04.068.
[278] A. Anton, G. Campreciós, V. Pérez-Campuzano, L. Orts, J.C. García-Pagán, V. Hernández-Gea, The pathophysiology of portal vein thrombosis in cirrhosis: Getting deeper into Virchow's triad, J Clin Med 11 (2022) 800. https://doi.org/10.3390/jcm11030800.
[279] M.A. Zocco, E. Di Stasio, R. De Cristofaro, M. Novi, M.E. Ainora, F. Ponziani, L. Riccardi, S. Lancellotti, A. Santoliquido, R. Flore, M. Pompili, G.L. Rapaccini, P. Tondi, G.B. Gasbarrini, R. Landolfi, A. Gasbarrini, Thrombotic risk factors in patients with liver cirrhosis: Correlation with MELD scoring system and portal vein thrombosis development, J Hepatol 51 (2009) 682–689. https://doi.org/10.1016/j.jhep.2009.03.013.
[280] F. Turon, E.G. Driever, A. Baiges, E. Cerda, Á. García-Criado, R. Gilabert, C. Bru, A. Berzigotti, I. Nuñez, L. Orts, J.C. Reverter, M. Magaz, G. Camprecios, P. Olivas, F. Betancourt-Sanchez, V. Perez-Campuzano, A. Blasi, S. Seijo, E. Reverter, J. Bosch, R. Borràs, V. Hernandez-Gea, T. Lisman, J.C. Garcia-Pagan, Predicting portal thrombosis in cirrhosis: A prospective study of clinical, ultrasonographic and hemostatic factors, J Hepatol 75 (2021) 1367–1376. https://doi.org/10.1016/j.jhep.2021.07.020.
[281] J.G. O'Leary, H.M. Gebel, R. Ruiz, R.A. Bray, J.D. Marr, X.J. Zhou, S.M. Shiller, B.M. Susskind, A.D. Kirk, G.B. Klintmalm, Class II alloantibody and mortality in simultaneous liver-kidney transplantation, American Journal of Transplantation 13 (2013) 954–960. https://doi.org/10.1111/ajt.12817.
[282] J. DiNorcia, M.K. Lee, M.P. Harlander-Locke, V. Xia, F.M. Kaldas, A. Zarrinpar, D.G. Farmer, H. Yersiz, J.R. Hiatt, R.W. Busuttil, V.G. Agopian, Damage control as a strategy to manage postreperfusion hemodynamic instability and coagulopathy in liver transplant, JAMA Surg 150 (2015) 1066. https://doi.org/10.1001/jamasurg.2015.1853.
[283] T.A. Gonwa, M.A. McBride, M.L. Mai, H.M. Wadei, Kidney transplantation after previous liver transplantation: analysis of the organ procurement transplant network database, Transplantation 92 (2011) 31–35. https://doi.org/10.1097/TP.0b013e31821c1e54.
[284] S.M. Strasberg, T.K. Howard, E.P. Molmenti, M. Hertl, Selecting the donor liver: risk factors for poor function after orthotopic liver transplantation, Hepatology 20 (1994) 829–838. https://doi.org/10.1002/hep.1840200410.
[285] N. Goldaracena, J.M. Cullen, D.-S. Kim, B. Ekser, K.J. Halazun, Expanding the donor pool for liver transplantation with marginal donors, International Journal of Surgery 82 (2020) 30–35. https://doi.org/10.1016/j.ijsu.2020.05.024.
[286] M. Facciuto, D. Heidt, J. Guarrera, C.A. Bodian, C.M. Miller, S. Emre, S.R. Guy, T.M. Fishbein, M.E. Schwartz, P.A. Sheiner, Retransplantation for late liver graft failure: Predictors of mortality, Liver Transplantation 6 (2000) 174–179. https://doi.org/10.1002/lt.500060222.
[287] G.D. Dodd, D.S. Memel, A.B. Zajko, R.L. Baron, L.A. Santaguida, Hepatic artery stenosis and thrombosis in transplant recipients: Doppler diagnosis with resistive index and systolic acceleration time., Radiology 192 (1994) 657–661. https://doi.org/10.1148/radiology.192.3.8058930.
[288] A.E. Handschin, M. Weber, E. Renner, P.-A. Clavien, Abdominal compartment syndrome after liver transplantation, Liver Transplantation 11 (2005) 98–100. https://doi.org/10.1002/lt.20295.
[289] M.J. Guirl, J.S. Weinstein, R.M. Goldstein, M.F. Levy, G.B. Klintmalm, Two-stage total hepatectomy and liver transplantation for acute deterioration of chronic liver disease: A new bridge to transplantation, Liver Transplantation 10 (2004) 564–570. https://doi.org/10.1002/lt.20134.
[290] S. Hoyos, C. Guzmán, G. Correa, J. Carlos Restrepo, H. Franco, A. Cárdenas, Orthotopic liver transplantation in an adult with situs inversus: an easy way to fit the liver, Ann Hepatol 5 (2006) 53–55. https://doi.org/10.1016/S1665-2681(19)32042-3.
[291] I. Rajput, K.R. Prasad, M.C. Bellamy, M. Davies, M.S. Attia, J.P.A. Lodge, Subtotal hepatectomy and whole graft auxiliary transplantation for acetaminophen-associated acute liver failure, HPB 16 (2014) 220–228. https://doi.org/10.1111/hpb.12124.
[292] C. Jerusalem, M.N. van der Heyde, W.J. Schmidt, F.A. Tjebbes, Heterotopic liver transplantation. II. Unfavorable outflow conditions as a possible cause for late graft failure, European Surgical Research 4 (1972) 186–197. https://doi.org/10.1159/000127614.
[293] M. Kasahara, Y. Takada, H. Egawa, Y. Fujimoto, Y. Ogura, K. Ogawa, K. Kozaki, H. Haga, M. Ueda, K. Tanaka, Auxiliary partial orthotopic living donor liver transplantation: Kyoto University experience, American Journal of Transplantation 5 (2005) 558–565. https://doi.org/10.1111/j.1600-6143.2005.00717.x.
[294] J.H. Levy, M.D. Neal, J.H. Herman, Bacterial contamination of platelets for transfusion: strategies for prevention, Crit Care 22 (2018) 271. https://doi.org/10.1186/s13054-018-2212-9.

[295] M.T. Giglio, M. Marucci, M. Testini, N. Brienza, Goal-directed haemodynamic therapy and gastrointestinal complications in major surgery: a meta-analysis of randomized controlled trials, Br J Anaesth 103 (2009) 637–646. https://doi.org/10.1093/bja/aep279.
[296] M.R. Rudnick, Hemodynamic monitoring during liver transplantation: A state of the art review, World J Hepatol 7 (2015) 1302. https://doi.org/10.4254/wjh.v7.i10.1302.
[297] A. Fedoravicius, M. Charlton, Abnormal liver tests after liver transplantation, Clin Liver Dis (Hoboken) 7 (2016) 73–79. https://doi.org/10.1002/cld.540.
[298] J. Bekker, S. Ploem, K.P. De Jong, Early hepatic artery thrombosis after liver transplantation: a systematic review of the incidence, outcome and risk factors, American Journal of Transplantation 9 (2009) 746–757. https://doi.org/10.1111/j.1600-6143.2008.02541.x.
[299] K. Nitta, K. Okamoto, H. Imamura, K. Mochizuki, H. Takayama, H. Kamijo, M. Okada, K. Takeshige, Y. Kashima, T. Satou, A comprehensive protocol for ventilator weaning and extubation: a prospective observational study, J Intensive Care 7 (2019) 50. https://doi.org/10.1186/s40560-019-0402-4.
[300] F.H. Saner, S.W.M. Olde Damink, G. Pavlaković, G.C. Sotiropoulos, A. Radtke, J. Treckmann, S. Beckebaum, V. Cicinnati, A. Paul, How far can we go with positive end-expiratory pressure (PEEP) in liver transplant patients?, J Clin Anesth 22 (2010) 104–109. https://doi.org/10.1016/j.jclinane.2009.03.015.
[301] J. Ng, S.J. Finney, R. Shulman, G.J. Bellingan, M. Singer, P.A. Glynne, Treatment of pulmonary hypertension in the general adult intensive care unit: a role for oral sildenafil?, Br J Anaesth 94 (2005) 774–777. https://doi.org/10.1093/bja/aei114.
[302] J.M. von Vital, A. Karachristos, A. Singhal, R. Thomas, A. Jain, Acute amiodarone hepatotoxicity after liver transplantation, Transplantation 91 (2011) e62–e64. https://doi.org/10.1097/TP.0b013e3182115bc1.
[303] G. Lindner, G.-C. Funk, Hypernatremia in critically ill patients, J Crit Care 28 (2013) 216.e11-216.e20. https://doi.org/10.1016/j.jcrc.2012.05.001.
[304] L.S. Weisberg, Management of severe hyperkalemia, Crit Care Med 36 (2008) 3246–3251. https://doi.org/10.1097/CCM.0b013e31818f222b.
[305] K.A. Abraham, M.A. Little, A.M. Dorman, J.J. Walshe, Hemolytic-uremic syndrome in association with both cyclosporine and tacrolimus, Transplant International 13 (2000) 443–447. https://doi.org/10.1007/s001470050727.
[306] A. Dilibe, L. Subramanian, T.-A. Poyser, O. Oriaifo, R. Brady, S. Srikanth, O. Adabale, O.A. Bolaji, H. Ali, Tacrolimus-induced posterior reversible encephalopathy syndrome following liver transplantation, World J Transplant 14 (2024). https://doi.org/10.5500/wjt.v14.i2.91146.
[307] G.A. Glass, J. Stankiewicz, A. Mithoefer, R. Freeman, P.R. Bergethon, Levetiracetam for seizures after liver transplantation, Neurology 64 (2005) 1084–1085. https://doi.org/10.1212/01.WNL.0000154598.03596.40.
[308] J. Seifter, M. Samuels, Uremic encephalopathy and other brain disorders associated with renal failure, Semin Neurol 31 (2011) 139–143. https://doi.org/10.1055/s-0031-1277984.
[309] R. Bilik, M. Yellen, R.A. Superina, Surgical complications in children after liver transplantation, J Pediatr Surg 27 (1992) 1371–1375. https://doi.org/10.1016/0022-3468(92)90179-B.
[310] R. Bilik, M. Yellen, R.A. Superina, Surgical complications in children after liver transplantation, J Pediatr Surg 27 (1992) 1371–1375. https://doi.org/10.1016/0022-3468(92)90179-B.
[311] M.J. Mihatsch, M. Kyo, K. Morozumi, Y. Yamaguchi, V. Nickeleit, B. Ryffel, The side-effects of ciclosporine-A and tacrolimus., Clin Nephrol 49 (1998) 356–63.
[312] M. Eugenia Rinella, Pregnancy after liver transplantation, Ann Hepatol 5 (2006) 212–215. https://doi.org/10.1016/S1665-2681(19)32014-9.
[313] H. Hartog, A. Hann, M.T.P.R. Perera, Primary nonfunction of the liver allograft, Transplantation 106 (2022) 117–128. https://doi.org/10.1097/TP.0000000000003682.
[314] E.B. Rand, K.M. Olthoff, Overview of pediatric liver transplantation, Gastroenterol Clin North Am 32 (2003) 913–929. https://doi.org/10.1016/S0889-8553(03)00048-7.
[315] L. Penninga, A. Wettergren, A.-W. Chan, D.A. Steinbrüchel, C. Gluud, Calcineurin inhibitor minimisation versus continuation of calcineurin inhibitor treatment for liver transplant recipients, Cochrane Database of Systematic Reviews 2012 (2012). https://doi.org/10.1002/14651858.CD008852.pub2.
[316] W.C. Cooley, P.J. Sagerman, Supporting the health care transition from adolescence to adulthood in the medical home, Pediatrics 128 (2011) 182–200. https://doi.org/10.1542/peds.2011-0969.
[317] T.A. Gonwa, L. Jennings, M.L. Mai, P.C. Stark, A.S. Levey, G.B. Klintmalm, Estimation of glomerular filtration rates before and after orthotopic liver transplantation: Evaluation of current equations, Liver Transplantation 10 (2004) 301–309. https://doi.org/10.1002/lt.20017.

[318] V. Dong, M.K. Nadim, C.J. Karvellas, Post–Liver transplant acute kidney injury, Liver Transplantation 27 (2021) 1653–1664. https://doi.org/10.1002/lt.26094.
[319] N. Singh, K. Washburn, A. Schenk, B. Hill, T. Hardy, S. Black, C. Sims, M. Alebrahim, A. El-Hinnawi, Rescue hepatectomy and anhepatic phase management after primary nonfunction in a liver transplant, Experimental and Clinical Transplantation 20 (2022) 776–779. https://doi.org/10.6002/ect.2020.0129.
[320] E. Levesque, E. Hoti, M. Khalfallah, C. Salloum, L. Ricca, E. Vibert, D. Azoulay, Impact of reversible cardiac arrest in the brain-dead organ donor on the outcome of adult liver transplantation, Liver Transplantation 17 (2011) 1159–1166. https://doi.org/10.1002/lt.22372.
[321] G. Testa, M. Malagò, C.E. Broelsch, Complications of biliary tract in liver transplantation, World J Surg 25 (2001) 1296–1299. https://doi.org/10.1007/s00268-001-0113-5.
[322] S. Chatterjee, D. Das, M. Hudson, M.F. Bassendine, J. Scott, K.E. Oppong, G. Sen, J.J. French, Mucocele of the cystic duct remnant after orthotopic liver transplant: a problem revisited., Exp Clin Transplant 9 (2011) 214–6.
[323] A.C. Westerkamp, K.S. Korkmaz, J.T. Bottema, J. Ringers, W.G. Polak, A. van den Berg, B. van Hoek, H.J. Metselaar, R.J. Porte, Elderly donor liver grafts are not associated with a higher incidence of biliary complications after liver transplantation: results of a national multicenter study, Clin Transplant 29 (2015) 636–643. https://doi.org/10.1111/ctr.12569.
[324] M.M. Mourad, C. Liossis, B.K. Gunson, H. Mergental, J. Isaac, P. Muiesan, D.F. Mirza, T.M.P.R. Perera, S.R. Bramhall, Etiology and management of hepatic artery thrombosis after adult liver transplantation, Liver Transplantation 20 (2014) 713–723. https://doi.org/10.1002/lt.23874.
[325] D.P. St. Michel, N. Goussous, N.L. Orr, R.N. Barth, S.H. Gray, J.C. LaMattina, D.A. Bruno, Hepatic artery pseudoaneurysm in the liver transplant recipient: A case series, Case Rep Transplant 2019 (2019) 1–6. https://doi.org/10.1155/2019/9108903.
[326] J.M. Zamora-Olaya, R. Tejero-Jurado, P.E. Alañón-Martínez, M. Prieto-Torre, C. Rodríguez-Medina, J.L. Montero, M. Sánchez-Frías, J. Briceño, R. Ciria, P. Barrera, A. Poyato, M. De la Mata, M.L. Rodríguez-Perálvarez, Donor atheromatous disease is a risk factor for hepatic artery thrombosis after liver transplantation, Clin Transplant 38 (2024). https://doi.org/10.1111/ctr.15405.
[327] D. Zamora, S. Dasgupta, T. Stevens-Ayers, B. Edmison, D.J. Winston, R.R. Razonable, A.K. Mehta, G.M. Lyon, M. Boeckh, N. Singh, D.M. Koelle, A.P. Limaye, Cytomegalovirus immunity in high-risk liver transplant recipients following preemptive antiviral therapy versus prophylaxis, JCI Insight 9 (2024). https://doi.org/10.1172/jci.insight.180115.
[328] B.C. Lizaola-Mayo, E.A. Rodriguez, Cytomegalovirus infection after liver transplantation, World J Transplant 10 (2020) 183–190. https://doi.org/10.5500/wjt.v10.i7.183.
[329] D. Vucicevic, E.J. Carey, J.E. Blair, Coccidioidomycosis in liver transplant recipients in an endemic area, American Journal of Transplantation 11 (2011) 111–119. https://doi.org/10.1111/j.1600-6143.2010.03328.x.
[330] M.R. Jorgenson, A.S. Gracon, B. Hanlon, G.E. Leverson, S. Parajuli, J.A. Smith, D.P. Al-Adra, Pre-transplant bariatric surgery is associated with increased fungal infection after liver transplant, Transplant Infectious Disease 23 (2021). https://doi.org/10.1111/tid.13484.
[331] N.C. Issa, J.A. Fishman, Infectious complications of antilymphocyte therapies in solid organ transplantation, Clinical Infectious Diseases 48 (2009) 772–786. https://doi.org/10.1086/597089.
[332] M. Sahathevan, F.A.H. Harvey, G. Forbes, J. O'Grady, A. Gimson, S. Bragman, R. Jensen, J. Philpott-Howard, R. Williams, M.W. Casewell, Epidemiology, bacteriology and control of an outbreak of Nocardia asteroides infection on a liver unit, Journal of Hospital Infection 18 (1991) 473–480. https://doi.org/10.1016/0195-6701(91)90059-H.
[333] N.M. Ampel, E.J. Wing, Legionella infection in transplant patients., Semin Respir Infect 5 (1990) 30–7.
[334] L. Radoshevich, P. Cossart, Listeria monocytogenes: towards a complete picture of its physiology and pathogenesis, Nat Rev Microbiol 16 (2018) 32–46. https://doi.org/10.1038/nrmicro.2017.126.
[335] A. Shetty, F. Giron, M.K. Divatia, M.I. Ahmad, S. Kodali, D. Victor, Nonalcoholic fatty liver disease after liver transplant, J Clin Transl Hepatol 000 (2021) 000–000. https://doi.org/10.14218/JCTH.2020.00072.
[336] A.J. Montano-Loza, A.L. Mason, M. Ma, R.J. Bastiampillai, V.G. Bain, P. Tandon, Risk factors for recurrence of autoimmune hepatitis after liver transplantation, Liver Transplantation 15 (2009) 1254–1261. https://doi.org/10.1002/lt.21796.
[337] P.B. Sylvestre, K.P. Batts, L.J. Burgart, J.J. Poterucha, R.H. Wiesner, Recurrence of primary biliary cirrhosis after liver transplantation: Histologic estimate of incidence and natural history, Liver Transplantation 9 (2003) 1086–1093. https://doi.org/10.1053/jlts.2003.50213.

[338] E. Alabraba, P. Nightingale, B. Gunson, S. Hubscher, S. Olliff, D. Mirza, J. Neuberger, A re-evaluation of the risk factors for the recurrence of primary sclerosing cholangitis in liver allografts, Liver Transplantation 15 (2009) 330–340. https://doi.org/10.1002/lt.21679.
[339] R. Garcia-Martinez, A. Rovira, J. Alonso, C. Jacas, M. Simón-Talero, L. Chavarria, V. Vargas, J. Córdoba, Hepatic encephalopathy is associated with posttransplant cognitive function and brain volume, Liver Transplantation 17 (2011) 38–46. https://doi.org/10.1002/lt.22197.
[340] G. Walker, T. Hussaini, R. Stowe, S. Cresswell, E.M. Yoshida, Liver transplant can resolve severe neuropsychiatric manifestations of Wilson disease: A case report., Exp Clin Transplant 16 (2018) 620–624. https://doi.org/10.6002/ect.2016.0053.
[341] H.-W. Shin, H.K. Park, Recent updates on acquired hepatocerebral degeneration., Tremor Other Hyperkinet Mov (N Y) 7 (2017) 463. https://doi.org/10.7916/D8TB1K44.
[342] J. Henssler, Y. Schmidt, U. Schmidt, G. Schwarzer, T. Bschor, C. Baethge, Incidence of antidepressant discontinuation symptoms: a systematic review and meta-analysis, Lancet Psychiatry 11 (2024) 526–535. https://doi.org/10.1016/S2215-0366(24)00133-0.
[343] S.B. Venkateshiah, N.A. Collop, Sleep and sleep disorders in the hospital, Chest 141 (2012) 1337–1345. https://doi.org/10.1378/chest.11-2591.
[344] G. Vassallo, A. Mirijello, T. Dionisi, C. Tarli, G. Augello, A. Gasbarrini, G. Addolorato, Wernicke's encephalopathy in alcohol use disorder patients after liver transplantation: A case series and review of literature, J Clin Med 9 (2020) 3809. https://doi.org/10.3390/jcm9123809.
[345] F.J. Mateen, R. Muralidharan, M. Carone, D. van de Beek, D.M. Harrison, A.J. Aksamit, M.S. Gould, D.B. Clifford, A. Nath, Progressive multifocal leukoencephalopathy in transplant recipients, Ann Neurol 70 (2011) 305–322. https://doi.org/10.1002/ana.22408.
[346] A. Rastogi, N.S. Ashwini, I. Rath, C. Bihari, S. V. Sasturkar, V. Pamecha, Utility and diagnostic accuracy of intraoperative frozen sections in hepato-pancreato-biliary surgical pathology, Langenbecks Arch Surg 408 (2023) 390. https://doi.org/10.1007/s00423-023-03124-8.
[347] S. Kakizoe, K. Yanaga, T.E. Starzl, J.A. Demetris, Evaluation of protocol before transplantation and after reperfusion biopsies from human orthotopic liver allografts: considerations of preservation and early immunological injury, Hepatology 11 (1990) 932–941. https://doi.org/10.1002/hep.1840110605.
[348] A.J. Demetris, Distinguishing between recurrent primary sclerosing cholangitis and chronic rejection, Liver Transplantation 12 (2006) S68–S72. https://doi.org/10.1002/lt.20947.
[349] J. Lunz, K.M. Ruppert, M.M. Cajaiba, K. Isse, C.A. Bentlejewski, M. Minervini, M.A. Nalesnik, P. Randhawa, E. Rubin, E. Sasatomi, M.E. de Vera, P. Fontes, A. Humar, A. Zeevi, A.J. Demetris, Re-examination of the lymphocytotoxic crossmatch in liver transplantation: can C4d stains help in monitoring?, American Journal of Transplantation 12 (2012) 171–182. https://doi.org/10.1111/j.1600-6143.2011.03786.x.
[350] S.G. Hubscher, E. Elias, J.A.C. Buckels, A.D. Mayer, P. McMaster, J.M. Neuberger, Primary biliary cirrhosis. Histological evidence of disease recurrence after liver transplantation, J Hepatol 18 (1993) 173–184. https://doi.org/10.1016/S0168-8278(05)80244-2.
[351] J. Lerut, A. Sanchez-Fueyo, An appraisal of tolerance in liver transplantation, American Journal of Transplantation 6 (2006) 1774–1780. https://doi.org/10.1111/j.1600-6143.2006.01396.x.
[352] A. Demetris, Importance of liver biopsy findings in immunosuppression management: Biopsy monitoring and working criteria for patients with operational tolerance, Liver Transplantation 18 (2012) 1154–1170. https://doi.org/10.1002/lt.23481.
[353] O. Adeyi, S.E. Fischer, M. Guindi, Liver allograft pathology: approach to interpretation of needle biopsies with clinicopathological correlation, J Clin Pathol 63 (2010) 47–74. https://doi.org/10.1136/jcp.2009.068254.
[354] B.F. Banner, L. Savas, J. Zivny, K. Tortorelli, H.L. Bonkovsky, Ubiquitin as a marker of cell injury in nonalcoholic steatohepatitis, Am J Clin Pathol 114 (2000) 860–866. https://doi.org/10.1309/4UBB-BF78-F55V-50KA.
[355] T.K. Friman, S. Jäämaa-Holmberg, F. Åberg, I. Helanterä, M. Halme, M.O. Pentikäinen, A. Nordin, K.B. Lemström, T. Jahnukainen, R. Räty, B. Salmela, Cancer risk and mortality after solid organ transplantation: A population-based 30-year cohort study in Finland, Int J Cancer 150 (2022) 1779–1791. https://doi.org/10.1002/ijc.33934.
[356] M.M.M. Copeland, J. Trainor, W.J. Cash, C. Braniff, Fatal donor-derived Kaposi sarcoma following liver transplantation, BMJ Case Rep 14 (2021) e236061. https://doi.org/10.1136/bcr-2020-236061.

Valeria Ripa, MD and Fady M. Kaldas, MD

[357] K.D.S. Watt, R.A. Pedersen, W.K. Kremers, J.K. Heimbach, W. Sanchez, G.J. Gores, Long-term probability of and mortality from de novo malignancy after liver transplantation, Gastroenterology 137 (2009) 2010–2017. https://doi.org/10.1053/j.gastro.2009.08.070.
[358] K. Mumtaz, N. Faisal, M. Marquez, A. Healey, L.B. Lilly, E.L. Renner, Post-transplant lymphoproliferative disorder in liver recipients: Characteristics, management, and outcome from a single-centre experience with >1000 liver transplantations, Can J Gastroenterol Hepatol 29 (2015) 417–422. https://doi.org/10.1155/2015/517359.
[359] M.-W. Welker, W.-O. Bechstein, S. Zeuzem, J. Trojan, Recurrent hepatocellular carcinoma after liver transplantation - an emerging clinical challenge, Transplant International 26 (2013) 109–118. https://doi.org/10.1111/j.1432-2277.2012.01562.x.
[360] S.D. Murad, R.W. Kim, T. Therneau, G.J. Gores, C.B. Rosen, J.A. Martenson, S.R. Alberts, J.K. Heimbach, Predictors of pretransplant dropout and posttransplant recurrence in patients with perihilar cholangiocarcinoma, Hepatology 56 (2012) 972–981. https://doi.org/10.1002/hep.25629.
[361] V. Ronca, G. Wootton, C. Milani, O. Cain, The immunological basis of liver allograft rejection, Front Immunol 11 (2020). https://doi.org/10.3389/fimmu.2020.02155.
[362] M. Rodríguez-Perálvarez, G. Germani, E. Tsochatzis, N. Rolando, T.V. Luong, A.P. Dhillon, D. Thorburn, J. O'Beirne, D. Patch, A.K. Burroughs, Predicting severity and clinical course of acute rejection after liver transplantation using blood eosinophil count, Transplant International 25 (2012) 555–563. https://doi.org/10.1111/j.1432-2277.2012.01457.x.
[363] A.W. Thomson, J. Vionnet, A. Sanchez-Fueyo, Understanding, predicting and achieving liver transplant tolerance: from bench to bedside, Nat Rev Gastroenterol Hepatol 17 (2020) 719–739. https://doi.org/10.1038/s41575-020-0334-4.
[364] R.G. de la Garza, P. Sarobe, J. Merino, J.J. Lasarte, D. D'Avola, V. Belsue, J.A. Delgado, L. Silva, M. Iñarrairaegui, B. Sangro, J.J. Sola, F. Pardo, J. Quiroga, I.J. Herrero, Trial of complete weaning from immunosuppression for liver transplant recipients: Factors predictive of tolerance, Liver Transplantation 19 (2013) 937–944. https://doi.org/10.1002/lt.23686.
[365] T.E. Starzl, N. Murase, S. Ildstad, C. Ricordi, A.J. Demetris, M. Trucco, Cell migration, chimerism, and graft acceptance, The Lancet 339 (1992) 1579–1582. https://doi.org/10.1016/0140-6736(92)91840-5.
[366] H. Egawa, H. Ohdan, K. Saito, Current status of ABO-incompatible liver transplantation, Transplantation 107 (2023) 313–325. https://doi.org/10.1097/TP.0000000000004250.
[367] J.G. O'Leary, H. Kaneku, B.M. Susskind, L.W. Jennings, M.A. Neri, G.L. Davis, G.B. Klintmalm, P.I. Terasaki, High mean fluorescence intensity donor-specific anti-HLA antibodies associated with chronic rejection Postliver transplant, American Journal of Transplantation 11 (2011) 1868–1876. https://doi.org/10.1111/j.1600-6143.2011.03593.x.
[368] K.K. Renganathan, A. Ramamurthy, S. Jacob, A. Tharigopula, A. Vaidya, M. Gopashetty, A. Khakar, Acute graft versus host disease following liver transplantation: Case report with review of current literature, J Clin Exp Hepatol 12 (2022) 1244–1251. https://doi.org/10.1016/j.jceh.2022.03.009.
[369] R. Domiati-Saad, G.B. Klintmalm, G. Netto, E.D. Agura, S. Chinnakotla, D.M. Smith, Acute graft versus host disease after liver transplantation: patterns of lymphocyte chimerism, American Journal of Transplantation 5 (2005) 2968–2973. https://doi.org/10.1111/j.1600-6143.2005.01110.x.
[370] A. Corthay, A three-cell model for activation of naïve T helper cells, Scand J Immunol 64 (2006) 93–96. https://doi.org/10.1111/j.1365-3083.2006.01782.x.
[371] S.A. Hunt, F. Haddad, The changing face of heart transplantation, J Am Coll Cardiol 52 (2008) 587–598. https://doi.org/10.1016/j.jacc.2008.05.020.
[372] S. Mukherjee, J. Botha, U. Mukherjee, Immunosuppression in liver transplantation, Curr Drug Targets 10 (2009) 557–574. https://doi.org/10.2174/138945009788488477.
[373] T.E. Starzl, G.B.G. Klintmalm, K.A. Porter, S. Iwatsuki, G.P.J. Schröter, Liver transplantation with use of cyclosporin a and prednisone, New England Journal of Medicine 305 (1981) 266–269. https://doi.org/10.1056/NEJM198107303050507.
[374] R.Y. Calne, S. Thiru, P. Mcmaster, G.N. Craddock, D.J.G. White, D.B. Evans, D.C. Dunn, B.D. Pentlow, K. Rolles, Cyclosporin A in patients receiving renal allografts from cadaver donors, The Lancet 312 (1978) 1323–1327. https://doi.org/10.1016/S0140-6736(78)91970-0.
[375] Y. Murakami, T. Tanaka, H. Murakami, M. Tsujimoto, H. Ohtani, Y. Sawada, Pharmacokinetic modelling of the interaction between St John's wort and ciclosporin A, Br J Clin Pharmacol 61 (2006) 671–676. https://doi.org/10.1111/j.1365-2125.2006.02606.x.

[376] M.G. Choc, Bioavailability and pharmacokinetics of cyclosporine formulations: Neoral® vs Sandimmune®, Int J Dermatol 36 (1997) 1–6. https://doi.org/10.1046/j.1365-4362.36.s1.2.x.
[377] A.L. Taylor, C.J.E. Watson, J.A. Bradley, Immunosuppressive agents in solid organ transplantation: Mechanisms of action and therapeutic efficacy, Crit Rev Oncol Hematol 56 (2005) 23–46. https://doi.org/10.1016/j.critrevonc.2005.03.012.
[378] R. Venkataramanan, A. Swaminathan, T. Prasad, A. Jain, S. Zuckerman, V. Warty, J. McMichael, J. Lever, G. Burckart, T. Starzl, Clinical Pharmacokinetics of Tacrolimus, Clin Pharmacokinet 29 (1995) 404–430. https://doi.org/10.2165/00003088-199529060-00003.
[379] M. Naesens, D.R.J. Kuypers, M. Sarwal, Calcineurin inhibitor nephrotoxicity, Clinical Journal of the American Society of Nephrology 4 (2009) 481–508. https://doi.org/10.2215/CJN.04800908.
[380] A.O. Ojo, P.J. Held, F.K. Port, R.A. Wolfe, A.B. Leichtman, E.W. Young, J. Arndorfer, L. Christensen, R.M. Merion, Chronic renal failure after transplantation of a nonrenal organ, New England Journal of Medicine 349 (2003) 931–940. https://doi.org/10.1056/NEJMoa021744.
[381] S.A. Živković, Neurologic complications after liver transplantation, World J Hepatol 5 (2013) 409. https://doi.org/10.4254/wjh.v5.i8.409.
[382] G. Vizzini, M. Asaro, R. Miraglia, S. Gruttadauria, D. Filì, A. D'Antoni, I. Petridis, G. Marrone, D. Pagano, B. Gridelli, Changing picture of central nervous system complications in liver transplant recipients, Liver Transplantation 17 (2011) 1279–1285. https://doi.org/10.1002/lt.22383.
[383] J. Li, S.G. Kim, J. Blenis, Rapamycin: one drug, many effects, Cell Metab 19 (2014) 373–379. https://doi.org/10.1016/j.cmet.2014.01.001.
[384] L. Bäckman, H. Kreis, J.M. Morales, H. Wilczek, R. Taylor, J.T. Burke, Sirolimus steady-state trough concentrations are not affected by bolus methylprednisolone therapy in renal allograft recipients, Br J Clin Pharmacol 54 (2002) 65–68. https://doi.org/10.1046/j.1365-2125.2002.01594.x.
[385] J.M. Cruzado, R. Poveda, M. Ibernon, M. Diaz, X. Fulladosa, M. Carrera, J. Torras, O. Bestard, I. Navarro, J. Ballarin, R. Romero, J.M. Grinyo, Low-dose sirolimus combined with angiotensin-converting enzyme inhibitor and statin stabilizes renal function and reduces glomerular proliferation in poor prognosis IgA nephropathy, Nephrology Dialysis Transplantation 26 (2011) 3596–3602. https://doi.org/10.1093/ndt/gfr072.
[386] S.N. Sehgal, Rapamune® (RAPA, rapamycin, sirolimus): mechanism of action immunosuppressive effect results from blockade of signal transduction and inhibition of cell cycle progression, Clin Biochem 31 (1998) 335–340. https://doi.org/10.1016/S0009-9120(98)00045-9.
[387] Y. Akselband, M.W. Harding, P.A. Nelson, Rapamycin inhibits spontaneous and fibroblast growth factor beta-stimulated proliferation of endothelial cells and fibroblasts., Transplant Proc 23 (1991) 2833–6.
[388] D. Shegogue, M. Trojanowska, Mammalian target of rapamycin positively regulates collagen type I production via a phosphatidylinositol 3-kinase-independent pathway, Journal of Biological Chemistry 279 (2004) 23166–23175. https://doi.org/10.1074/jbc.M401238200.
[389] K. Budde, L. Fritsche, J. Waiser, P. Glander, T. Slowinski, H.-H. Neumayer, RADW 102 Renal Transplant Study Group, Pharmacokinetics of the immunosuppressant everolimus in maintenance renal transplant patients., Eur J Med Res 10 (2005) 169–74.
[390] M.D. Sintchak, M.A. Fleming, O. Futer, S.A. Raybuck, S.P. Chambers, P.R. Caron, M.A. Murcko, K.P. Wilson, Structure and mechanism of inosine monophosphate dehydrogenase in complex with the immunosuppressant mycophenolic acid, Cell 85 (1996) 921–930. https://doi.org/10.1016/S0092-8674(00)81275-1.
[391] C.E. Staatz, S.E. Tett, Clinical pharmacokinetics and pharmacodynamics of mycophenolate in solid organ transplant recipients, Clin Pharmacokinet 46 (2007) 13–58. https://doi.org/10.2165/00003088-200746010-00002.
[392] R. Bullingham, S. Monroe, A. Nicholls, M. Hale, Pharmacokinetics and bioavailability of mycophenolate mofetil in healthy subjects after single-dose oral and intravenous administration, The Journal of Clinical Pharmacology 36 (1996) 315–324. https://doi.org/10.1002/j.1552-4604.1996.tb04207.x.
[393] H.W. Sollinger, Mycophenolates in transplantation, Clin Transplant 18 (2004) 485–492. https://doi.org/10.1111/j.1399-0012.2004.00203.x.
[394] C.N. Pisoni, D.P. D'Cruz, The safety of mycophenolate mofetil in pregnancy, Expert Opin Drug Saf 7 (2008) 219–222. https://doi.org/10.1517/14740338.7.3.219.
[395] A.L. Lundquist, R.S. Chari, J.H. Wood, G.G. Miller, H.M. Schaefer, D.S. Raiford, K.J. Wright, D.L. Gorden, Serum sickness following rabbit antithymocyte-globulin induction in a liver transplant recipient: case report and literature review, Liver Transplantation 13 (2007) 647–650. https://doi.org/10.1002/lt.21098.

[396] A.G. Tzakis, P. Tryphonopoulos, T. Kato, S. Nishida, D.M. Levi, J.R. Madariaga, J.J. Gaynor, W. De Faria, A. Regev, V. Esquenazi, D. Weppler, P. Ruiz, J. Miller, Preliminary experience with alemtuzumab (Campath-1H) and low-dose tacrolimus immunosuppression in adult liver transplantation, Transplantation 77 (2004) 1209–1214. https://doi.org/10.1097/01.TP.0000116562.15920.43.
[397] T. Cerny, B. Borisch, M. Introna, P. Johnson, A.L. Rose, Mechanism of action of rituximab, Anticancer Drugs 13 (2002) S3–S10. https://doi.org/10.1097/00001813-200211002-00002.
[398] J. Merola, A. Shamim, J. Weiner, Update on immunosuppressive strategies in intestinal transplantation, Curr Opin Organ Transplant 27 (2022) 119–125. https://doi.org/10.1097/MOT.0000000000000958.
[399] J.M. Kovarik, B.D. Kahan, P.R. Rajagopalan, W. Bennett, L.L. Mulloy, C. Gerbeau, M.L. Hall, Population pharmacokinetics and exposure-response relationships for basiliximab in kidney transplantation. The U.S. Simulect Renal Transplant Study Group, Transplantation 68 (1999) 1288–1294. https://doi.org/10.1097/00007890-199911150-00012.
[400] R.A. McDonald, J.M. Smith, M. Ho, R. Lindblad, D. Ikle, P. Grimm, R. Wyatt, M. Arar, D. Liereman, N. Bridges, W. Harmon, Incidence of PTLD in pediatric renal transplant recipients receiving basiliximab, calcineurin inhibitor, sirolimus and steroids, American Journal of Transplantation 8 (2008) 984–989. https://doi.org/10.1111/j.1600-6143.2008.02167.x.
[401] S.J. Pacini-Edelstein, M. Mehra, M.E. Ament, J.H. Vargas, M.G. Martin, S. V. McDiarmid, Varicella in pediatric liver transplant patients: a retrospective analysis of treatment and outcome, J Pediatr Gastroenterol Nutr 37 (2003) 183–186. https://doi.org/10.1097/00005176-200308000-00018.
[402] C.D. Ericsson, Travellers with pre-existing medical conditions, Int J Antimicrob Agents 21 (2003) 181–188. https://doi.org/10.1016/S0924-8579(02)00288-1.
[403] F.M. Blodgett, L. Burgin, D. Iezzoni, D. Gribetz, N.B. Talbot, Effects of prolonged cortisone therapy on the statural growth, skeletal maturation and metabolic status of children, New England Journal of Medicine 254 (1956) 636–641. https://doi.org/10.1056/NEJM195604052541402.
[404] A.J. Pennisi, G. Costin, L.S. Phillips, M.M. Malekzadeh, C. Uittenbogaart, R.B. Ettenger, R.N. Fine, Somatomedin and growth hormone studies in pediatric renal allograft recipients who receive daily prednisone., Am J Dis Child 133 (1979) 950–4.
[405] Y. Toyoki, J.F. Renz, C. Mudge, N.L. Ascher, J.P. Roberts, P. Rosenthal, Allograft rejection in pediatric liver transplantation: Comparison between cadaveric and living related donors, Pediatr Transplant 6 (2002) 301–307. https://doi.org/10.1034/j.1399-3046.2002.02013.x.
[406] R. Moreno, M. Berenguer, Post-liver transplantation medical complications, Ann Hepatol 5 (2006) 77–85. https://doi.org/10.1016/S1665-2681(19)32022-8.
[407] R.H. Wiesner, J. Ludwig, R.A.F. Krom, J.L. Steers, M.K. Porayko, G.J. Gores, J.E. Hay, Treatment of early cellular rejection following liver transplantation with intravenous methylprednisolone. The effect of dose on response, Transplantation 58 (1994) 1053–1056. https://doi.org/10.1097/00007890-199411150-00015.
[408] B. Van Hoek, R. Wiesner, R. Krom, J. Ludwig, S. Moore, Severe ductopenic rejection following liver transplantation: incidence, time of onset, risk factors, treatment, and outcome, Semin Liver Dis 12 (1992) 41–50. https://doi.org/10.1055/s-2007-1007375.
[409] B.T. Lee, M.I. Fiel, T.D. Schiano, Antibody-mediated rejection of the liver allograft: An update and a clinico-pathological perspective, J Hepatol 75 (2021) 1203–1216. https://doi.org/10.1016/j.jhep.2021.07.027.
[410] I. Kang, J.G. Lee, S.H. Choi, H.J. Kim, D.H. Han, G.H. Choi, M.S. Kim, J.S. Choi, S. Il Kim, D.J. Joo, Impact of everolimus on survival after liver transplantation for hepatocellular carcinoma, Clin Mol Hepatol 27 (2021) 589–602. https://doi.org/10.3350/cmh.2021.0038.
[411] G.B. Klintmalm, S. Feng, J.R. Lake, H.E. Vargas, T. Wekerle, S. Agnes, K.A. Brown, B. Nashan, L. Rostaing, S. Meadows-Shropshire, M. Agarwal, M.B. Harler, J.-C. García-Valdecasas, Belatacept-based immunosuppression in de novo liver transplant recipients: 1-year experience from a phase II randomized study, American Journal of Transplantation 14 (2014) 1817–1827. https://doi.org/10.1111/ajt.12810.
[412] M.G. Rudolph, R.L. Stanfield, I.A. Wilson, How TCRs bind MHCs, peptides, and coreceptors, Annu Rev Immunol 24 (2006) 419–466. https://doi.org/10.1146/annurev.immunol.23.021704.115658.
[413] W.K. Kremers, H.C. Devarbhavi, R.H. Wiesner, R.A.F. Krom, W.R. Macon, T.M. Habermann, Post-transplant lymphoproliferative disorders following liver transplantation: incidence, risk factors and survival, American Journal of Transplantation 6 (2006) 1017–1024. https://doi.org/10.1111/j.1600-6143.2006.01294.x.
[414] P. Muiesan, R. Girlanda, W. Jassem, H.V. Melendez, J. O??Grady, M. Bowles, M. Rela, N. Heaton, Single-center experience with liver transplantation from controlled non-heartbeating donors: a viable source of grafts, Ann Surg 242 (2005) 732–738. https://doi.org/10.1097/01.sla.0000186177.26112.d2.

# Liver Transplantation and Hepatobiliary Surgery: 500 Practice Questions

[415] A. Zeevi, J.G. Lunz, R. Shapiro, P. Randhawa, G. Mazariegos, S. Webber, A. Girnita, Emerging role of donor-specific anti–human leukocyte antigen antibody determination for clinical management after solid organ transplantation, Hum Immunol 70 (2009) 645–650. https://doi.org/10.1016/j.humimm.2009.06.009.

[416] P.S. Heeger, T-cell allorecognition and transplant rejection: a summary and update, American Journal of Transplantation 3 (2003) 525–533. https://doi.org/10.1034/j.1600-6143.2003.00123.x.

[417] J.F. Markmann, M.S. Abouljoud, R.M. Ghobrial, C.S. Bhati, S.J. Pelletier, A.D. Lu, S. Ottmann, T. Klair, C. Eymard, G.R. Roll, J. Magliocca, T.L. Pruett, J. Reyes, S.M. Black, C.L. Marsh, G. Schnickel, M. Kinkhabwala, S.S. Florman, S. Merani, A.J. Demetris, S. Kimura, M. Rizzari, A. Saharia, M. Levy, A. Agarwal, F.G. Cigarroa, J.D. Eason, S. Syed, W.K. Washburn, J. Parekh, J. Moon, A. Maskin, H. Yeh, P.A. Vagefi, M.P. MacConmara, Impact of portable normothermic blood-based machine perfusion on outcomes of liver transplant, JAMA Surg 157 (2022) 189. https://doi.org/10.1001/jamasurg.2021.6781.

[418] H.J. Merhav, L.A. Mieles, Y. Ye, R.R. Selby, G. Snowden, Alternative procedure for failed reconstruction of a right replaced hepatic artery in liver transplantation, Transplant International 8 (1995) 414–417. https://doi.org/10.1007/BF00337178.

[419] R. Ravikumar, W. Jassem, H. Mergental, N. Heaton, D. Mirza, M.T.P.R. Perera, A. Quaglia, D. Holroyd, T. Vogel, C.C. Coussios, P.J. Friend, Liver transplantation after ex vivo normothermic machine preservation: A phase 1 (first-in-man) clinical trial, American Journal of Transplantation 16 (2016) 1779–1787. https://doi.org/10.1111/ajt.13708.

[420] D. Nasralla, C.C. Coussios, H. Mergental, M.Z. Akhtar, A.J. Butler, C.D.L. Ceresa, V. Chiocchia, S.J. Dutton, J.C. García-Valdecasas, N. Heaton, C. Imber, W. Jassem, I. Jochmans, J. Karani, S.R. Knight, P. Kocabayoglu, M. Malagò, D. Mirza, P.J. Morris, A. Pallan, A. Paul, M. Pavel, M.T.P.R. Perera, J. Pirenne, R. Ravikumar, L. Russell, S. Upponi, C.J.E. Watson, A. Weissenbacher, R.J. Ploeg, P.J. Friend, A randomized trial of normothermic preservation in liver transplantation, Nature 557 (2018) 50–56. https://doi.org/10.1038/s41586-018-0047-9.

[421] A. Schlegel, M. Mueller, X. Muller, J. Eden, R. Panconesi, S. von Felten, K. Steigmiller, R.X. Sousa Da Silva, O. de Rougemont, J.-Y. Mabrut, M. Lesurtel, M.C. Cerisuelo, N.D. Heaton, M.A. Allard, R. Adam, D. Monbaliu, I. Jochmans, M.P.D. Haring, R.J. Porte, A. Parente, P. Muiesan, P. Kron, M. Attia, D. Kollmann, G. Berlakovich, X. Rogiers, K. Petterson, A.L. Kranich, S. Amberg, B. Müllhaupt, P.-A. Clavien, P. Dutkowski, A multicenter randomized-controlled trial of hypothermic oxygenated perfusion (HOPE) for human liver grafts before transplantation, J Hepatol 78 (2023) 783–793. https://doi.org/10.1016/j.jhep.2022.12.030.

[422] W.R. Kim, J.R. Lake, J.M. Smith, D.P. Schladt, M.A. Skeans, S.M. Noreen, A.M. Robinson, E. Miller, J.J. Snyder, A.K. Israni, B.L. Kasiske, OPTN/SRTR 2017 Annual data report: Liver, American Journal of Transplantation 19 (2019) 184–283. https://doi.org/10.1111/ajt.15276.

[423] S.K. Niazi, E. Brennan, A. Spaulding, J. Crook, S. Borkar, A. Keaveny, A. Vasquez, M.T. Gentry, T. Schneekloth, C.B. Taner, Impact of recipient age at liver transplant on long-term outcomes, Transplantation 107 (2023) 654–663. https://doi.org/10.1097/TP.0000000000004426.

[424] J.B. Henson, M. Cabezas, L.M. McElroy, A.J. Muir, Rates of employment after liver transplant: A nationwide cohort study, Hepatol Commun 7 (2023) e0061–e0061. https://doi.org/10.1097/HC9.0000000000000061.

[425] C. Wu, C. Lu, C. Xu, Short-term and long-term outcomes of liver transplantation using moderately and severely steatotic donor livers, Medicine 97 (2018) e12026. https://doi.org/10.1097/MD.0000000000012026.

[426] L.R. Wingfield, C. Ceresa, S. Thorogood, J. Fleuriot, S. Knight, Using artificial intelligence for predicting survival of individual grafts in liver transplantation: A systematic review, Liver Transplantation 26 (2020) 922–934. https://doi.org/10.1002/lt.25772.

[427] J.P. Stevens, S. Gillespie, L. Hall, J. Tisheh, R. Ford, N.A. Gupta, Education and psychosocial factors predict odds of death after transfer to adult health care in pediatric liver transplant patients., J Pediatr Gastroenterol Nutr 75 (2022) 623–628. https://doi.org/10.1097/MPG.0000000000003549.

[428] T. Kitajima, S. Nagai, A. Segal, M. Magee, S. Blackburn, D. Ellithorpe, S. Yeddula, Y. Qadeer, A. Yoshida, D. Moonka, K. Brown, M.S. Abouljoud, Posttransplant complications predict alcohol relapse in liver transplant recipients, Liver Transplantation 26 (2020) 379–389. https://doi.org/10.1002/lt.25712.